Clinical Ultrasound

Angela Lindsay • Jordan Tozer
Michael J. Vitto • Michael Joyce
Lindsay Taylor
Editors

Clinical Ultrasound

A Pocket Manual

Second Edition

Springer

Editors
Angela Lindsay
Department of Emergency Medicine
Virginia Commonwealth University Health
Richmond, VA, USA

Michael J. Vitto
Department of Emergency Medicine
Virginia Commonwealth University Health
Richmond, VA, USA

Lindsay Taylor
Department of Emergency Medicine
Virginia Commonwealth University Health
Richmond, VA, USA

Jordan Tozer
Department of Emergency Medicine
Virginia Commonwealth University Health
Richmond, VA, USA

Michael Joyce
Department of Emergency Medicine
Virginia Commonwealth University Health
Richmond, VA, USA

ISBN 978-3-032-27642-1 ISBN 978-3-032-27643-8 (eBook)
https://doi.org/10.1007/978-3-032-27643-8

This Springer imprint is published by the registered company Springer Nature Switzerland AG
The registered company address is: Gewerbestrasse 11, 6330 Cham, Switzerland

If disposing of this product, please recycle the paper.

Preface

Ultrasound remains a powerful and rapidly evolving tool in the hands of clinicians at the bedside. As with any skill, mastering point-of-care ultrasound (POCUS) can initially feel overwhelming—especially for those new to image acquisition, interpretation, and the underlying technology. In this second edition, we build upon the foundation established in our first volume with expanded content that reflects the growing applications of POCUS in clinical practice.

New to this edition are dedicated chapters on advanced cardiac ultrasound, transesophageal echocardiography (TEE), and ultrasound-guided regional anesthesia—areas that continue to gain traction and importance across a wide range of clinical settings. These additions reflect both reader feedback and the evolving landscape of bedside imaging.

As the field continues to mature, so too does the expectation that clinicians integrate ultrasound seamlessly into real-time decision-making. Our goal with this edition is not only to provide updated techniques and expanded applications but also to offer a practical, confidence-building resource that supports learners at every stage—from novices taking their first steps with a probe to seasoned practitioners refining their craft. We remain committed to presenting information in a concise, accessible format that reflects the realities of clinical practice, where clarity and efficiency matter. Ultimately, we hope this manual continues to serve as a trusted companion at the bedside, empowering clinicians to deliver more informed, timely, and patient-centered care.

Richmond, VA, USA Angela Lindsay
Richmond, VA, USA Jordan Tozer
Richmond, VA, USA Michael J. Vitto
Richmond, VA, USA Michael Joyce
Richmond, VA, USA Lindsay Taylor

Contents

Contributors

Taylor Brittan Department of Emergency Medicine, University of Florida College of Medicine, UF Jacksonville, Jacksonville, FL, USA

Chelsea Bunce Department of Emergency Medicine, Virginia Commonwealth University Medical Center, Richmond, VA, USA

Melissa Edwards Department of Emergency Medicine, Virginia Commonwealth University Medical Center, Richmond, VA, USA

Holly Farkosh Department of Emergency Medicine, Virginia Commonwealth University Medical Center, Richmond, VA, USA

Zackary Funk Department of Emergency Medicine, Virginia Commonwealth University Medical Center, Richmond, VA, USA

Ashley Haggerty Department of Emergency Medicine, Division of Pediatric Emergency Medicine, Shady Grove Medical Center, Rockville, MD, USA

Noah Hillerbrand VCU Health, Department of Emergency Medicine, Richmond, VA, USA

Jason Jennings Department of Emergency Medicine, Virginia Commonwealth University Medical Center, Richmond, VA, USA

Michael R. Jones Department of Emergency Medicine, Virginia Commonwealth University Medical Center, Richmond, VA, USA

Michael Joyce Department of Emergency Medicine, Virginia Commonwealth University Health, Richmond, VA, USA

Angela Lindsay Department of Emergency Medicine, Virginia Commonwealth University Health, Richmond, VA, USA

Brian Makowski Department of Emergency Medicine, Cleveland Clinic, Akron, OH, USA

Corey Moore Department of Emergency Medicine, East Carolina University Medical Center, Greenville, NC, USA

Elizabeth Morrison Emergency Department, Bon Secours Mercy Health St. Rita's Medical Center, Lima, OH, USA

Ben Pastwik Department of Emergency Medicine, Virginia Commonwealth University Medical Center, Richmond, VA, USA

Robert Stenberg Department of Emergency Medicine, Cleveland Clinic, Akron, OH, USA

Lindsay Taylor Department of Emergency Medicine, Virginia Commonwealth University Health, Richmond, VA, USA

Jordan Tozer Department of Emergency Medicine, Virginia Commonwealth University Health, Richmond, VA, USA

Michael J. Vitto Department of Emergency Medicine, Virginia Commonwealth University Health, Richmond, VA, USA

Adam Weltler Department of Emergency Medicine, Virginia Commonwealth University, Richmond, VA, USA

Introduction: Basic Ultrasound Principles

1

Michael Joyce, Angela Lindsay, and Michael J. Vitto

This introductory chapter provides a concise overview of ultrasound fundamentals. We review the essential physics principles, terminology for image optimization, transducer types and their clinical applications, and key scanning modes including brightness (B) mode, motion (M) mode, and Doppler imaging. Common ultrasound artifacts, their mechanisms, and strategies for identification are also discussed. Whether you are new to ultrasound or returning to deepen your understanding, this chapter is designed to ground your learning in the key principles needed for confident image acquisition and interpretation.

Basic Terminology

- Brightness Mode (B-mode)
  - Standard ultrasound mode for all clinical imaging
  - Converts ultrasound waves into a grayscale image [1]
  - Figure 1.1—B-Mode imaging
  - Video 1.1—B-Mode imaging
- Motion Mode (M-mode)
  - Evaluates the movement of structures within the body [2].
  - Records movement of a structure over time

Supplementary Information The online version contains supplementary material available at https://doi.org/10.1007/978-3-032-27643-8_1.

M. Joyce (✉) · A. Lindsay · M. J. Vitto
Department of Emergency Medicine, Virginia Commonwealth University Health, Richmond, VA, USA
e-mail: john.joyce@vcuhealth.org; angela.creditt@vcuhealth.org; michael.vitto@vcuhealth.org

A. Lindsay et al. (eds.), *Clinical Ultrasound*,
https://doi.org/10.1007/978-3-032-27643-8_1

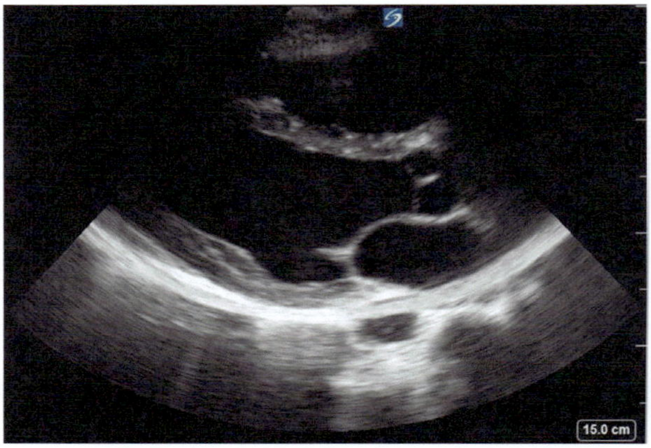

Fig. 1.1 B-Mode imaging. Brightness mode imaging of the heart. Brightness mode or B-mode is the standard ultrasound mode for all clinical imaging

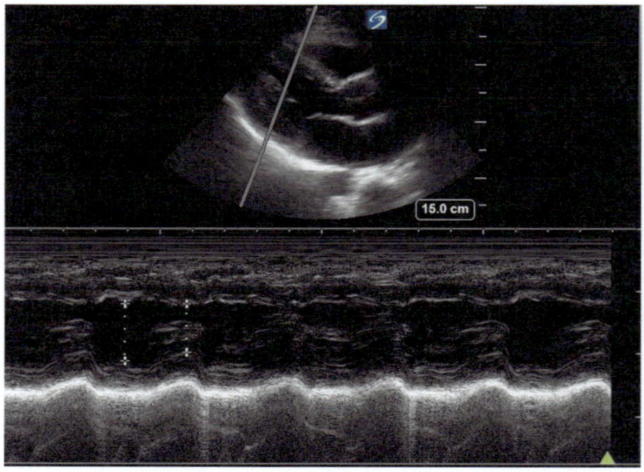

Fig. 1.2 M-mode imaging. Motion mode imaging of the heart. Motion mode or M-mode cardiac evaluates the movement of structures within the body. This image demonstrates the utilization of M-mode to evaluate movement of the left ventricle over time

    - A vertical line is placed through the structure of interest.
    - The machine then converts ultrasound echoes measured at this line onto the vertical axis of a graph with time on the horizontal axis [2].
  - Figure 1.2—M-mode imaging
- Frequency
  - The number of sound waves per unit time.
  - For clinical imaging, this typically ranges from 2 megahertz (MHz) to 15 MHz [1].
  - Higher frequency transducers have less tissue penetration, but provide more detailed image resolution.
  - Lower frequency transducers have greater tissue penetration, but sacrifice image resolution.
- Gain
  - Controls amplification of returning ultrasound waves [2].
  - This translates to brightness of the ultrasound image [2].

- Gain can be manually controlled by the sonographer and should be optimized for image clarity.
  - If the gain is too high, th e image will be bright.
    - Figure 1.3—High gain
  - If the gain is too low, the image will be dark.
    - Figure 1.4—Low gain
- Depth
  - Refers to how far sound travels prior to returning to the transducer, typically reported in centimeters.
    - If depth is increased, the ultrasound machine listens for returning echoes for a longer period of time to collect data [2] necessary to create an image.
    - If depth is decreased, the machine will listen for a shorter period of time.
  - This can be manually controlled by the sonographer.

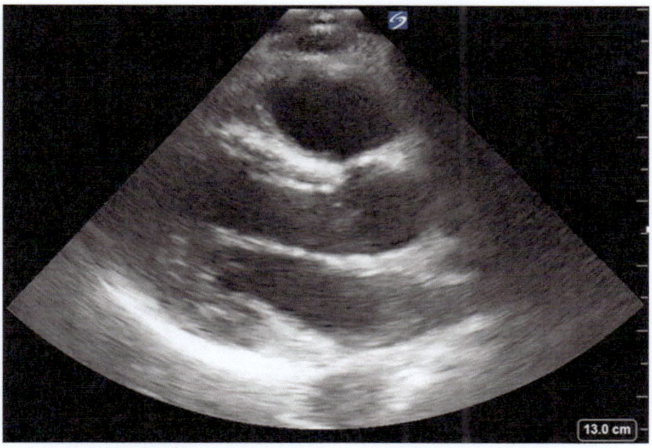

Fig. 1.3 High gain. This image demonstrates the parasternal long view of a heart with high gain. Gain is related to brightness of the image. When the gain is too high, the image will be bright, and details are lost

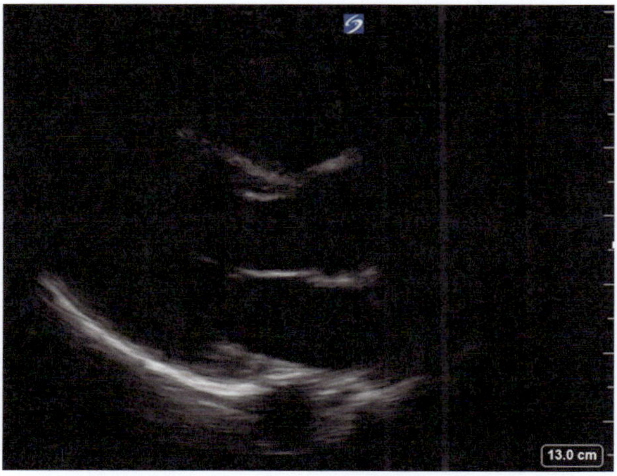

Fig. 1.4 Low gain. This image demonstrates the parasternal long view of a heart with low gain. Gain is related to brightness of the image. When the gain is too low, the image will be dark, and details are lost

  - Depth should be optimized so that the structure of interest is imaged within the center of the screen.
    - Figure 1.5—High depth
    - Figure 1.6—Shallow depth
    - Figure 1.7—Ideal depth
- Doppler
  - Measures frequency shift.
    - Doppler shift is defined as a change in frequency that occurs when sound reflects off a moving structure [2].
  - Calculates blood velocity
    - An increase in velocity causes an increase in Doppler shift.
  - Color Doppler
    - Shifts in velocity are color coded according to direction of flow in relationship to the transducer.

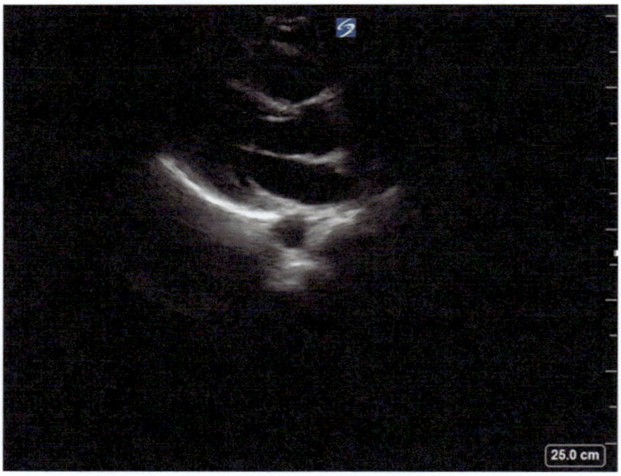

Fig. 1.5 High depth. This image demonstrates the parasternal long view of a heart with the depth set too deep. The structure of interest should be centered in the screen

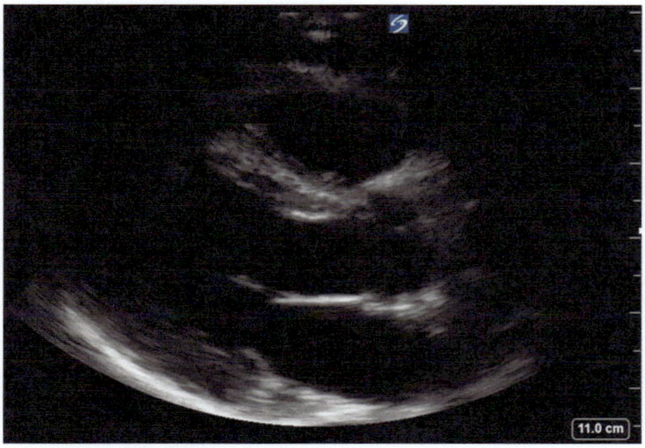

Fig. 1.6 Shallow depth. This image demonstrates the parasternal long view of a heart with the depth set too low. The structure of interest should be centered in the screen

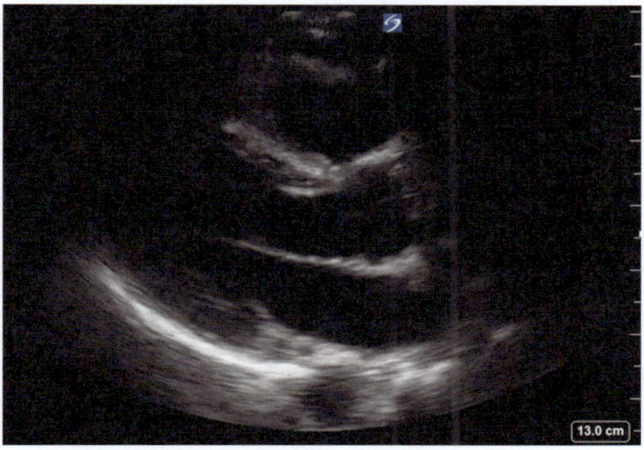

Fig. 1.7 Ideal depth. This image demonstrates the parasternal long view of a heart with ideal depth and gain settings to properly visions the entire structure of interest as well as the appropriate level of detail

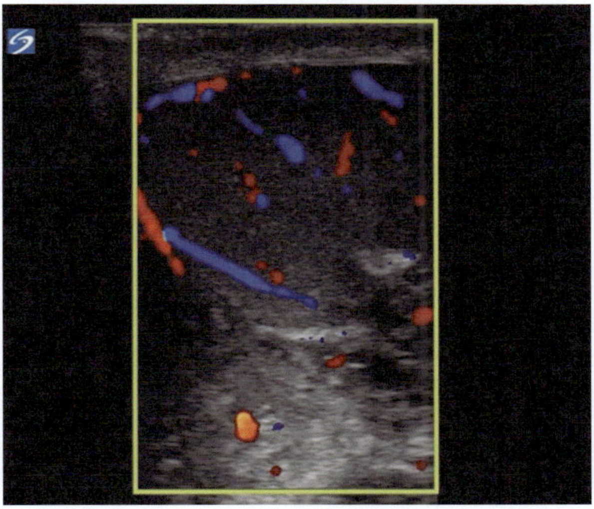

Fig. 1.8 Color Doppler. Color Doppler measures shifts in velocity, which are color coded according to direction of flow in relationship to the transducer; flow away from the transducer will appear blue, flow toward the transducer will appear red. Note that it does not relate to venous and arterial flow. In this image, the testicles are being assessed for vascular flow with color Doppler

    - Flow away from the transducer will appear blue.
    - Flow toward the transducer will appear red.
    - This can be remembered as "BART", *B*lue *A*way *R*ed *T*owards.
  - Figure 1.8—Color Doppler
  - Video 1.2—Color Doppler
- Power Doppler
  - Displays a signal in color if there is any motion detected at all.
    - Does not indicate velocity or direction.
  - Higher sensitivity than color Doppler allowing for imaging slower flow [2].
  - Good for low-flow applications such as testicular or ovarian exams.
  - Figure 1.9—Power Doppler
  - Video 1.3—Power Doppler

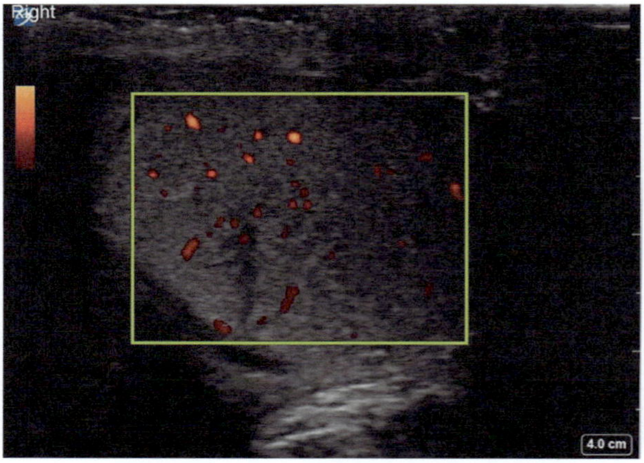

Fig. 1.9 Power Doppler. Power Doppler will display a signal in color if there is any motion at all. It does not indicate velocity or direction. In this image, the testicles are being assessed for vascular flow with power Doppler

- Transducer
  - Contains piezoelectric crystals that have the unique ability to translate electrical signal into sound waves.
    - Sound waves are sent to tissues, then reflected back to the transducer.
    - Reflected sound waves are translated into electric signals by the same piezoelectric crystals.
  - Computer software processes these signals into an ultrasound image.
- ALARA
  - "As low as reasonably achievable" [1, 2].
  - Ultrasound principle is to use the least amount of ultrasound possible on each patient.

Transducer Selection

- Curvilinear transducer
  - Low frequency with a wide field of view.
  - Greater tissue penetration allows for imaging of deeper structures.
  - Ideal for abdominal imaging.
  - Typical frequency range is 2–5 MHz [3].
    - Figure 1.10—Curvilinear transducer
- Phased array transducer
  - Smaller flat footprint
  - Uses electronic beam steering to produce a pie-shaped field of view.
  - Allows for imaging through small areas such as between ribs.
  - Most commonly used for cardiac imaging.
  - Typical frequency range is 2–7 MHz [4].
    - Figure 1.11—Phased array transducer

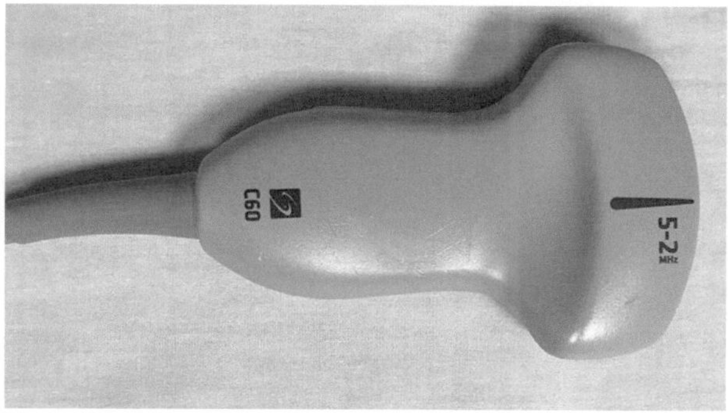

Fig. 1.10 Curvilinear transducer. Curvilinear transducers exhibit low frequency and a wide field of view

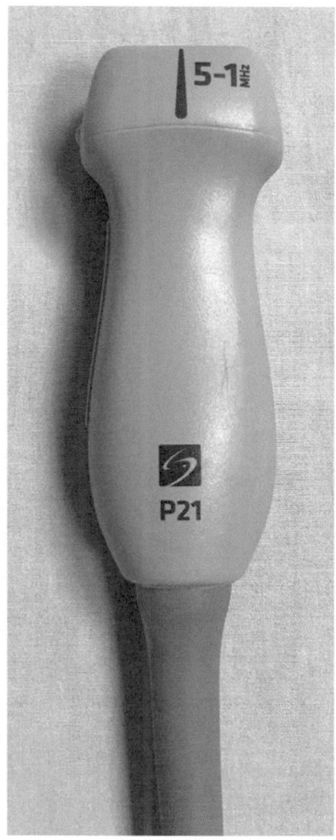

Fig. 1.11 Phased array transducer. Phased array transducers have smaller flat footprints and exhibit a pie-shaped field of view

- Linear array transducer
  - Produces a rectangular image.
  - High frequency makes this transducer ideal for imaging superficial structures including soft tissue, muscles, nerves, arteries, and veins.
  - Often used for procedural guidance.
  - Typical frequency range is 5–10 MHz [2]
    - Figure 1.12—Linear transducer

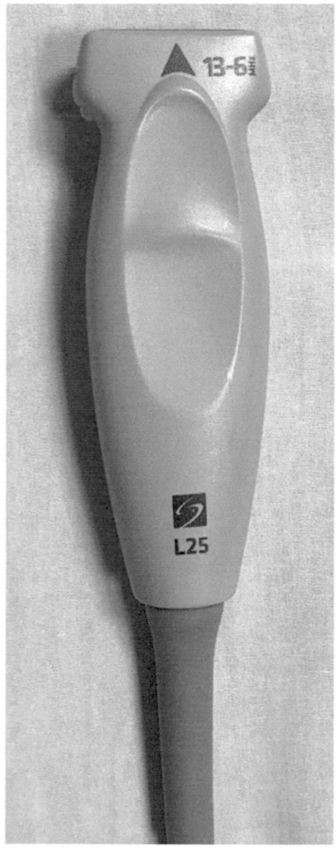

Fig. 1.12 Linear transducer. Linear Transducers produce rectangular images using high frequency

- Endocavitary transducer
  - Produces an image with a wide field of view, up to 180 degrees [2].
  - Specialized high-frequency curvilinear transducer that is commonly used for Obstetric, Gynecologic, or Ear, Nose, and Throat (ENT) applications.
  - Typical frequency range is 8–13 MHz [2].
    - Figure 1.13—Endocavitary transducer

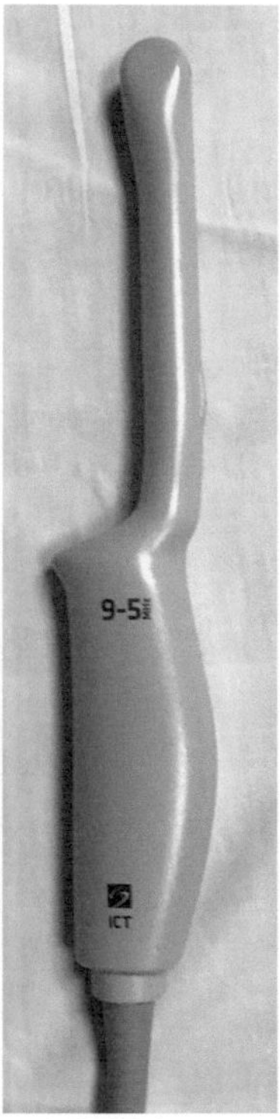

Fig. 1.13 Endocavitary transducer. Endocavitary Transducers exhibit high frequency and a wide field of view

Transducer Position

- Each transducer has a "marker" or position indicator.
  - The marker on the transducer corresponds to the marker indicator on the image screen, which will be identified as a blue dot.
  - This helps the sonographer with image orientation and facilitates an understanding of what is being seen on the screen.
    - Figure 1.14—Marker correlation
- Standard ultrasound imaging planes include: transverse, sagittal, and coronal.
  - Transverse
    - Also called cross-sectional or axial.
    - Transducer marker will be pointed toward patient's right.
    - Figure 1.15—Transverse plane

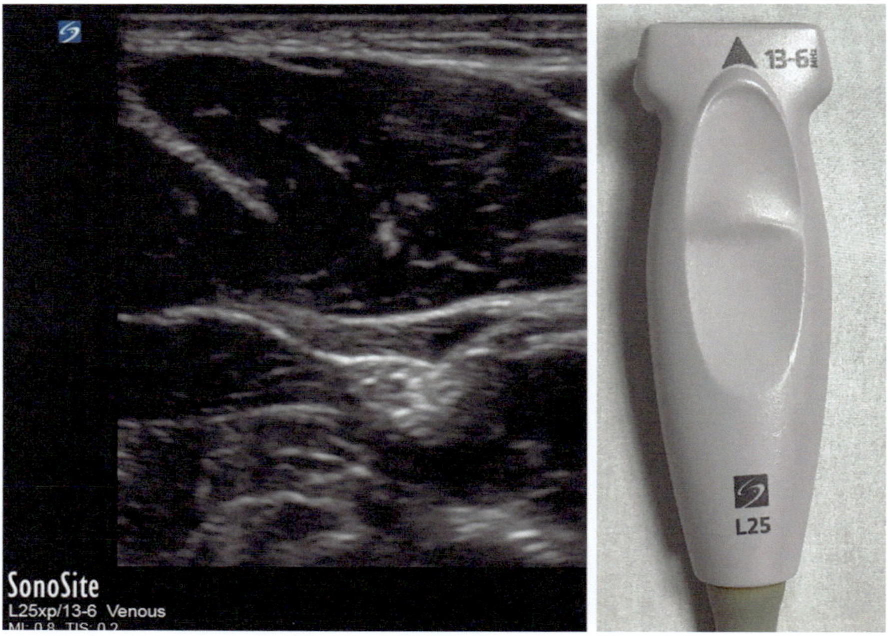

Fig. 1.14 Marker correlation. Transducer bump on the left side of the transducer corresponds to the blue box (or dot on some machines) on the left side of the image screen

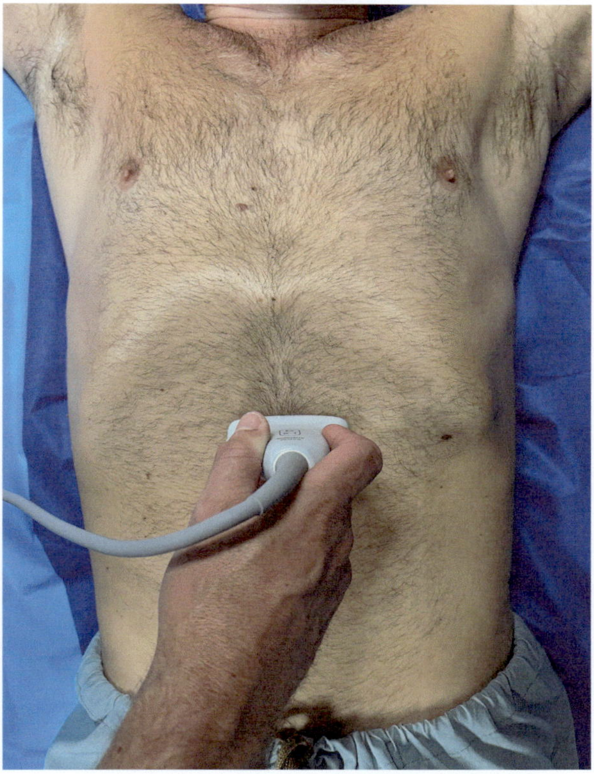

Fig. 1.15 Transverse plane. Transducer placement for imaging in a transverse plane. Transducer marker is directed toward the patient's right side

- Sagittal
  - With the transducer in an anterior or posterior position relative to the patient's body, the marker should point toward the patient's head or cephalad.
  - Figure 1.16—Sagittal plane
- Coronal
  - With the transducer in a lateral position relative to the patient's body, the marker should point toward the patient's head or cephalad.
  - Figure 1.17—Coronal plane
- Cardiac Imaging
  - With cardiac ultrasound, conventional transducer positioning does not apply.
  - For this technique, the marker position during cardiac imaging is variable depending on what image is being obtained.
  - See Chap. 3 (Transthoracic Echocardiography) for detailed information.

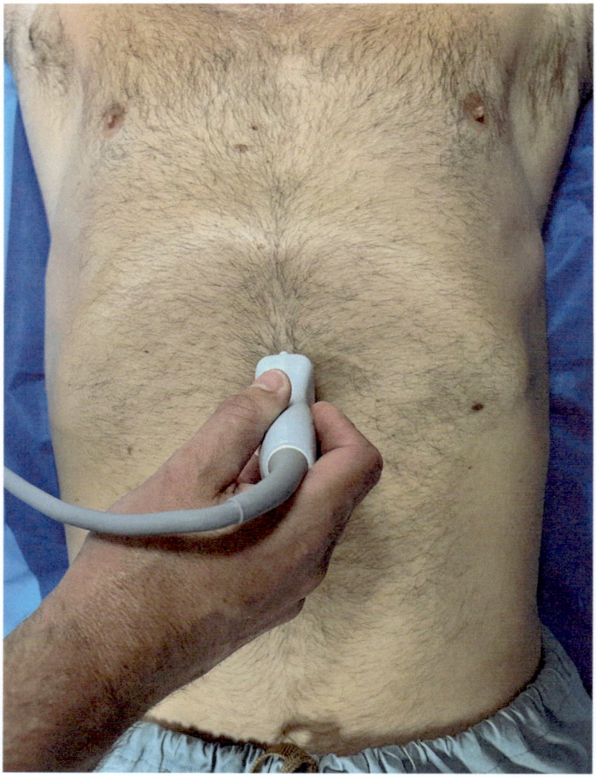

Fig. 1.16 Sagittal plane. Transducer placement for imaging in a sagittal plane. Transducer marker is directed toward the patient's head, and the transducer is positioned in the patient's midline

Fig. 1.17 Coronal plane. Transducer placement for imaging in a coronal plane. Transducer marker is directed toward the patient's head, and the transducer is positioned on the patient's lateral side

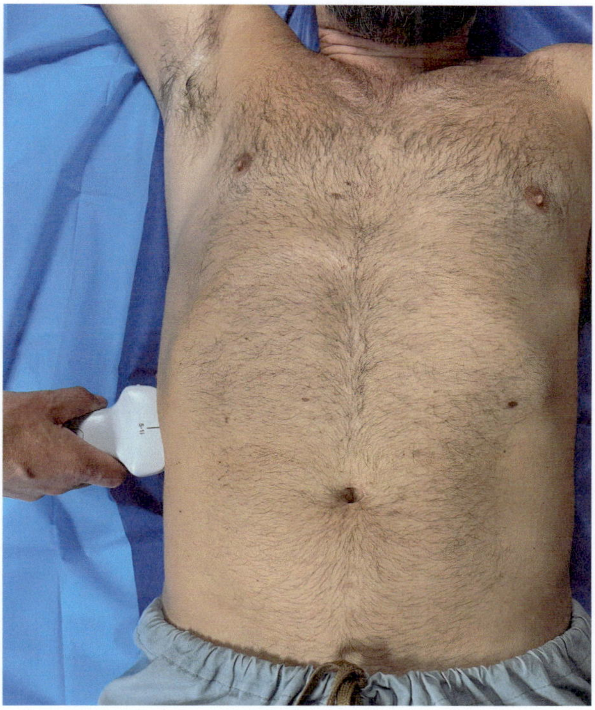

Ultrasound Artifact

- Artifacts in ultrasound imaging arise due to errors by the machine in interpreting the returning sound waves.
- A basic understanding of artifacts is necessary to identify normal and pathological findings.
- The most common artifacts are due to sound absorption or redirection, defined as falsely placing signals on the image screen that are not truly there.
- Types of artifacts
  - Posterior Acoustic Shadowing
    - Occurs when sound cannot pass through an impermeable or almost impermeable tissue such as bone or a calcified structure.
    - Figure 1.18—Bone shadowing
    - Video 1.4—Bone shadowing
    - Figure 1.19 Gallstone shadowing
    - Video 1.5—Gallstone shadowing
  - Posterior Acoustic Enhancement
    - Occurs when a sound passes through a fluid-filled structure, without significant attenuation causing in an increase in acoustic energy [1].

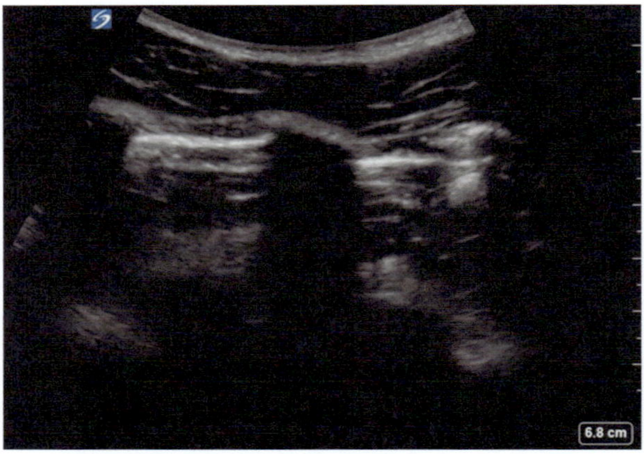

Fig. 1.18 Bone shadowing. Ribs exhibit posterior acoustic shadowing. Ultrasound waves cannot penetrate bone and calcified structures causing posterior acoustic shadowing

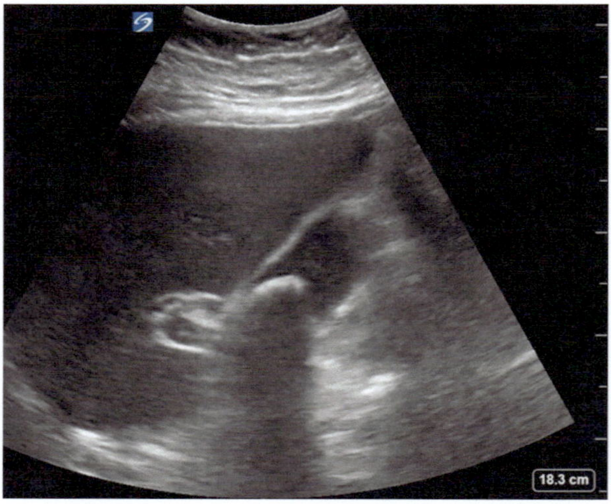

Fig. 1.19 Gallstone shadowing. Posterior acoustic shadowing helps properly identify gallstones within the gallbladder and can help distinguish stones from other structures such as polyps

  - This results in structures posterior to the fluid-filled structure appearing brighter or more echogenic.
  - Common examples include simple cysts, gallbladder, bladder, or large vessels.
  - Figure 1.20—Gallbladder with PAE
  - Video 1.6—Gallbladder with PAE
- Reverberation Artifact
  - Occurs when sound bounces between two greatly reflective structures [1] causing sound to reverberate over and over, creating a line of sound down the image screen.
  - Figure 1.21—Lung with reverberation artifact
  - Video 1.7—Lung with reverberation artifact

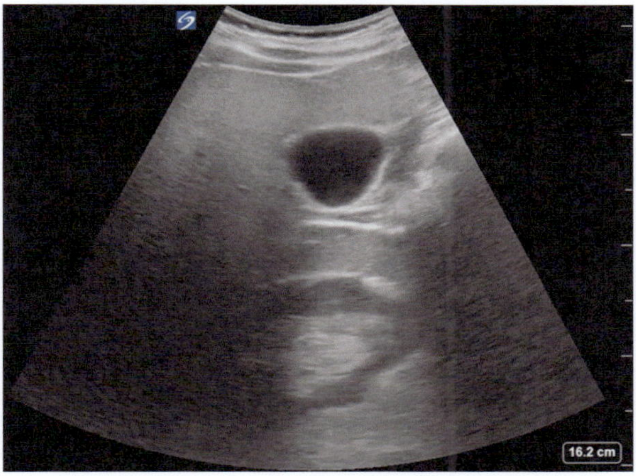

Fig. 1.20 Gallbladder with PAE. As sound passes through fluid-filled structures, such as the gallbladder seen here, acoustic energy is increased resulting in posterior acoustic enhancement in which the structures posterior to the structure appear brighter

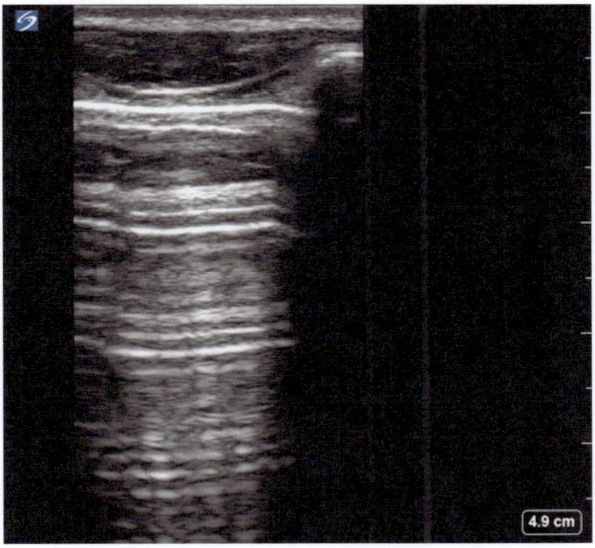

Fig. 1.21 Lung with reverberation artifact. When sound bounces between two greatly reflective structures, it will reverberate over and over creating a line of sound down the image screen known as reverberation artifact, as seen here with the pleural line of the lungs

- Mirror Artifact
  - When ultrasound waves hit a highly reflective structure, such as the diaphragm, the machine can interpret the images as coming back twice.
  - Figure 1.22—Liver with mirror artifact
  - Video 1.8—Liver with mirror artifact
- Edge Artifact
  - Caused by refraction of the ultrasound beam as it hits a highly reflective rounded structure, directing the beam away from the structure and not back to the transducer.
  - Can be mistaken for posterior acoustic shadowing

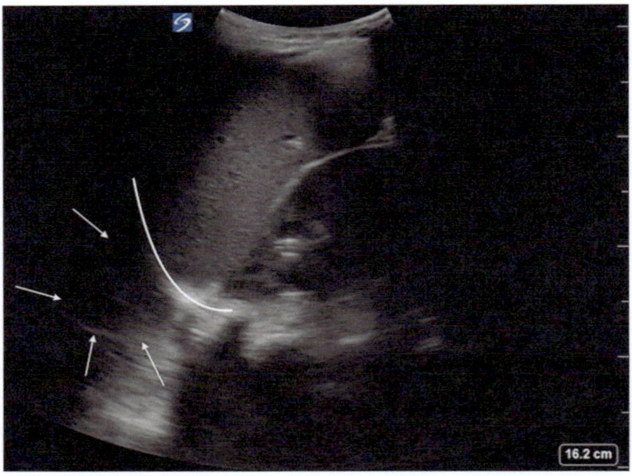

Fig. 1.22 Liver with mirror artifact. When ultrasound waves hit a highly reflective structure, such as the diaphragm, the machine can interpret the images as coming back twice. Here, there appears to be two livers, one above and one below the diaphragm

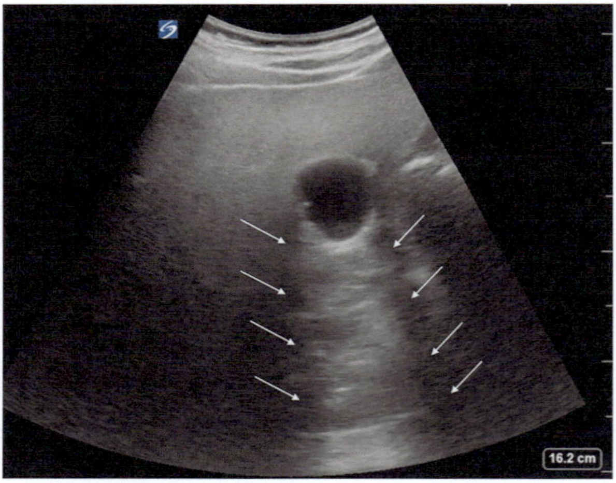

Fig. 1.23 Gallbladder with edge artifact. Edge artifact occurs when sound waves hit a highly reflective rounded structure, such as the walls of a gallbladder, the ultrasound beam is directed away from the structure creating a shadow effect similar to posterior acoustic shadowing

- Figure 1.23—Gallbladder with edge artifact
- Video 1.9—Gallbladder with edge artifact

Key Points

- Dim ambient lights to improve image on screen.
- Always adjust depth and gain first to optimize your image before trying to interpret.
- Increase contact with patient's body by applying pressure with the face of the transducer or increasing the amount of gel.

References

1. Hecht C, Manson W. Chapter 3: Physics and image artifacts. In: Ma OJ, Mateer JR, Reardon RF, Joing SA, editors. Emergency ultrasound. 3rd ed. China: McGraw-Hill Education; 2014. p. 33–46.
2. Scruggs W, Fox JC. Chapter 2: Equipment. In: Ma OJ, Mateer JR, Reardon RF, Joing SA, editors. Emergency ultrasound. 3rd ed. China: McGraw-Hill Education; 2014. p. 15–32.
3. Saul T, Del Rios Rivera M, Lewiss R. Focus on: ultrasound image quality. ACEP News website. 2011. https://www.acep.org/Content.aspx?id=79787. Accessed 17 Apr 2017.
4. Rasalingham R, Makan M, Perez JE. The Washington manual of echocardiography. Saint Louis: Department of Medicine, Washington University School of Medicine, Lippincott Williams & Wilkins; 2013.

2 Extended Focused Assessment with Sonography for Trauma

Melissa Edwards, Jordan Tozer, Angela Lindsay, and Michael J. Vitto

Ultrasound has revolutionized our ability to rapidly and noninvasively assess life-threatening injuries requiring operative intervention in patients who have sustained blunt or penetrating trauma. The Extended Focused Assessment with Sonography for Trauma, or the EFAST exam, allows physicians to look inside the abdomen to assess for hemorrhage, the heart for pericardial effusion or tamponade, and the lungs for pneumothorax or hemothorax. In an unstable trauma patient, the EFAST exam will help determine proper disposition including immediate operative intervention versus additional workup such as with computed tomography imaging. This chapter will review indications for performing an EFAST exam, basic anatomy, image acquisition, normal ultrasound anatomy, interpretation of EFAST pathology, and common pitfalls to imaging.

Clinical Application and Indications

- Blunt trauma
- Penetrating trauma
- Unexplained hypotension or altered mental status

Supplementary Information The online version contains supplementary material available at https://doi.org/10.1007/978-3-032-27643-8_2.

M. Edwards (✉)
Department of Emergency Medicine, Virginia Commonwealth University Medical Center, Richmond, VA, USA
e-mail: melissa.edwards@vcuhealth.org

J. Tozer · A. Lindsay · M. J. Vitto
Department of Emergency Medicine, Virginia Commonwealth University Health, Richmond, VA, USA
e-mail: jordan.tozer@vcuhealth.org; Angela.creditt@vcuhealth.org; michael.vitto@vcuhealth.org

A. Lindsay et al. (eds.), *Clinical Ultrasound*, https://doi.org/10.1007/978-3-032-27643-8_2

Normal EFAST Anatomy

- The basic EFAST exam evaluates the abdomen for free intraperitoneal fluid, the heart for pericardial fluid, and the lungs for pneumothorax or hemothorax.
- Right Upper Quadrant (RUQ)
  - Visualize the liver and kidney looking for the potential space between the two called the hepatorenal recess.
  - The diaphragm is seen at the superior edge of the liver as a hyperechoic curved stripe.
  - Lower right lung base will be located above the diaphragm.
- Left Upper Quadrant (LUQ)
  - Visualize the spleen and left kidney with the potential space between the two organs called the splenorenal recess.
  - The diaphragm can be seen at the superior edge of the spleen as a hyperechoic curved stripe.
  - Lower left lung base will be located above the diaphragm.
- Pelvis
  - Visualize the bladder, which will appear as a hypoechoic collection of fluid surrounded by a well-defined echogenic border.
  - To the right and left of the bladder will be a paracolic gutter.
  - Uterus or prostate can be seen posterior to the bladder.
- Subxiphoid
  - Visualize the heart, pericardial sac, and potential space between the heart and pericardium.
  - The liver will be seen anterior to the heart.
  - Posterior to the liver will be the right ventricle and right atrium.
  - The most posterior structures will be the left ventricle and left atrium.
  - Please see the cardiac chapter for more detailed cardiac anatomy.
- Lung Apices
  - The lungs sit within the thorax encaged by the ribs and muscular chest wall.
  - Each lung is surrounded by a visceral pleura and parietal pleura with a potential space between the two.
  - The pleural line will appear as a hyperechoic horizontal line between two rib spaces.
  - Please see the thoracic chapter for more detailed lung anatomy.
- Inferior Vena Cava
  - The inferior vena cava (IVC) is the largest vein in the human body.
  - The IVC will be seen posterior to the liver entering the right atrium.
  - The IVC normally collapses with inspiration and dilates with expiration.
- Free intraperitoneal fluid or blood accumulates within dependent areas of the abdomen including:
  - Hepatorenal recess between the liver and kidney within the RUQ, also known as Morrison's pouch.
  - Splenorenal recess between the spleen and kidney within the LUQ.
  - Left subphrenic space between the diaphragm and spleen.

  - Paracolic gutters within the pelvis.
  - Rectovesicular pouch, the most dependent area in the supine male.
  - Rectouterine pouch, also known as the pouch of Douglas, the most dependent area in the supine female.
- Fluid can accumulate around the heart, within the pericardium.
- Fluid can accumulate within the pleural cavity.

Image Acquisition

1. Transducer Selection
   (a) Curvilinear
   (b) Phased array
2. Patient Position
   (a) The patient should be lying supine
   (b) Can also place patient in Trendelenburg or reverse Trendelenburg to increase the dependency of the fluid
3. Standard Exam Views
   (a) Right upper quadrant
      - Place the transducer over the patient's right flank between mid-axillary and anterior axillary line with the transducer marker directed toward the patient's head.
        - Morrison's pouch is usually best imaged between rib 8 and 9
        - Figure 2.1—Transducer placement RUQ
        - Figure 2.2—RUQ normal EFAST
        - Video 2.1—RUQ normal EFAST
      - When scanning through the liver-renal interface, be sure to image the tip of the left side of the liver, as this is where blood or fluid will accumulate first in a supine patient [1].
        - Figure 2.3—Liver tip
        - Video 2.2—EFAST liver tip
      - Scan through the area including the inferior right hemithorax located above the diaphragm.
        - Figure 2.4—RUQ EFAST view with hemithorax
   (b) Left upper quadrant
      - Place the transducer over the patient's left flank between the mid and posterior axillary line near the 10th rib space with the marker pointed toward the patient's head.
        - Figure 2.5—Transducer placement LUQ
        - Figure 2.6—LUQ standard view
        - Video 2.3—LUQ standard view
      - There is also a potential space located between the spleen and diaphragm; therefore, it is important to image above the spleen
        - Figure 2.7—LUQ above spleen view

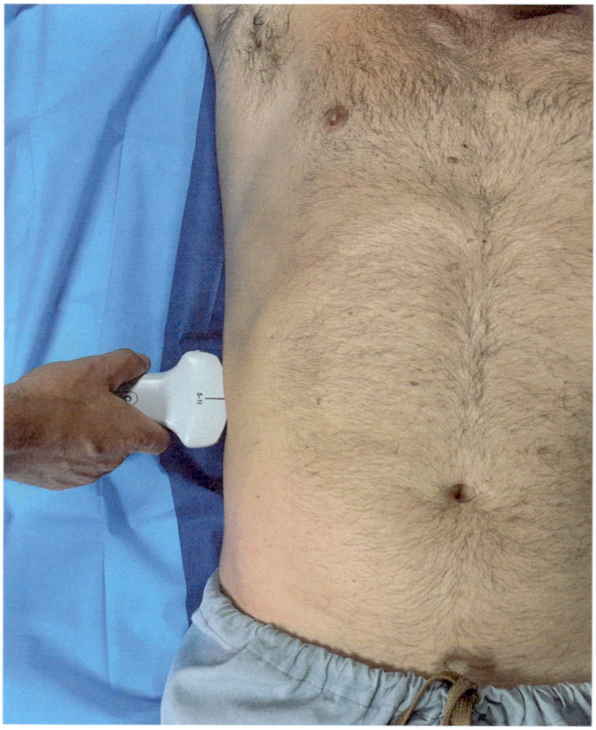

Fig. 2.1 Transducer placement RUQ: Place the transducer over the patient's right flank between the mid-axillary and anterior axillary line with the transducer marker directed toward the patient's head

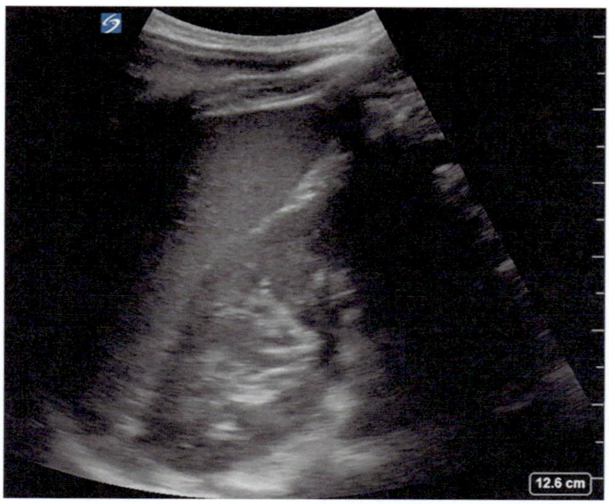

Fig. 2.2 RUQ normal EFAST: Normal RUQ EFAST showing no free fluid. Imaging should include the tip of the liver, area between the liver and right kidney, and the diaphragm above the liver

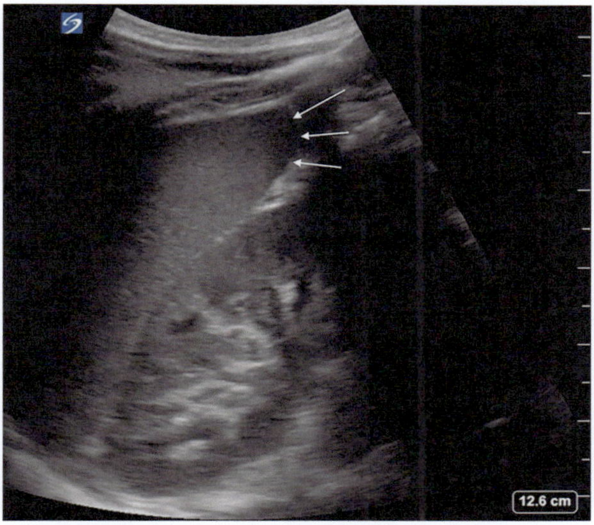

Fig. 2.3 EFAST liver tip: RUQ view demonstrating the liver tip above the right kidney. Hemoperitoneum can be detected first around the liver tip; therefore, it is important to image this specific area of the RUQ

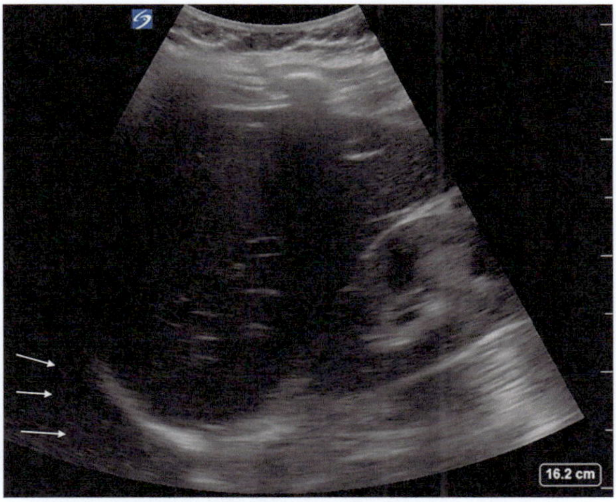

Fig. 2.4 RUQ EFAST view with hemithorax: Evaluation of the RUQ should include the right hemithorax, visualized above the liver and hyperechoic diaphragm

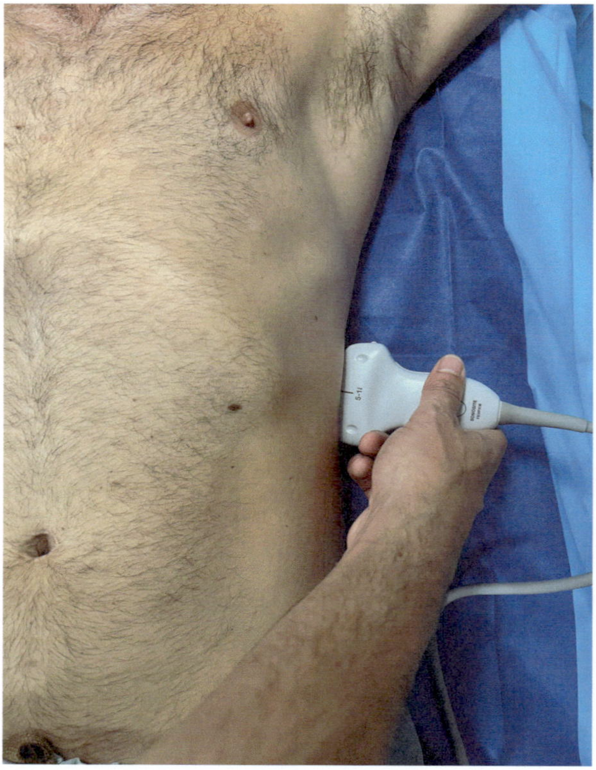

Fig. 2.5 Transducer placement LUQ: Place the transducer over the patient's left flank between the mid-axillary and posterior axillary line near the 10th rib space with the marker pointed toward the patient's head

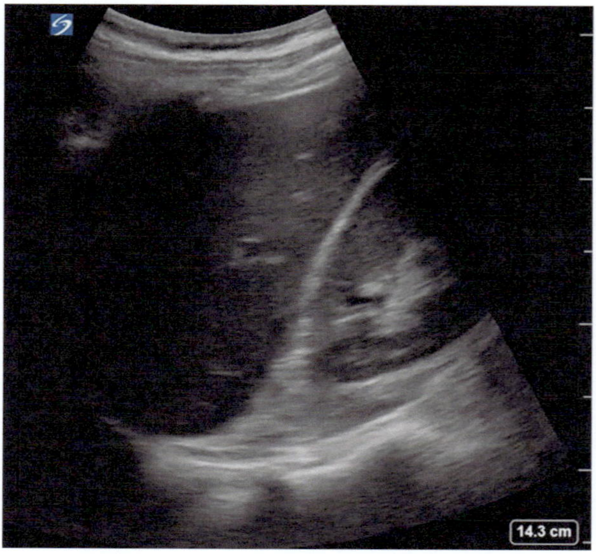

Fig. 2.6 LUQ standard view: LUQ EFAST view showing no free fluid. Imaging should include the spleen, area between the spleen and left kidney, and views of the diaphragm above the spleen

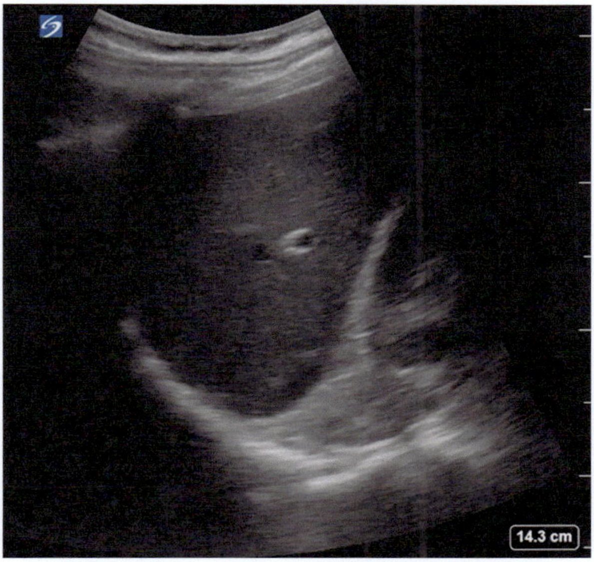

Fig. 2.7 LUQ EFAST imaging above the spleen: Free fluid will typically accumulate above the spleen first in the LUQ, making it important to always image this area

- Scan through the area including the left hemithorax located above the diaphragm.
  - Figure 2.8—Left hemithorax

(c) Pelvis

- Place the transducer superior to the pubic bone angled inferiorly with the transducer marker pointed toward the patient's right in the transverse plane.
  - Figure 2.9—Transducer placement pelvis, transverse
- Scan through from superior to inferior to visualize the paracolic gutters and area posterior to the bladder.
  - Figure 2.10—Paracolic gutters in transverse
  - Video 2.4—Paracolic gutters in transverse
- Rotate the transducer 90° clockwise to image the pelvis in sagittal plane with the transducer marker pointed to patient's head
  - Figure 2.11—Transducer placement bladder in sagittal
  - Figure 2.12—Sagittal view of the pelvis
  - Video 2.5—Sagittal view of the pelvis
- Scan through by fanning from right to left

(d) Subxiphoid

- Place the transducer inferior to the xiphoid process with the marker oriented toward the patient's right.
  - EFAST should be completed in abdominal mode on the ultrasound machine; however, if in cardiac mode, to image the heart, be sure to hold the transducer with the marker pointed toward the patient's left.

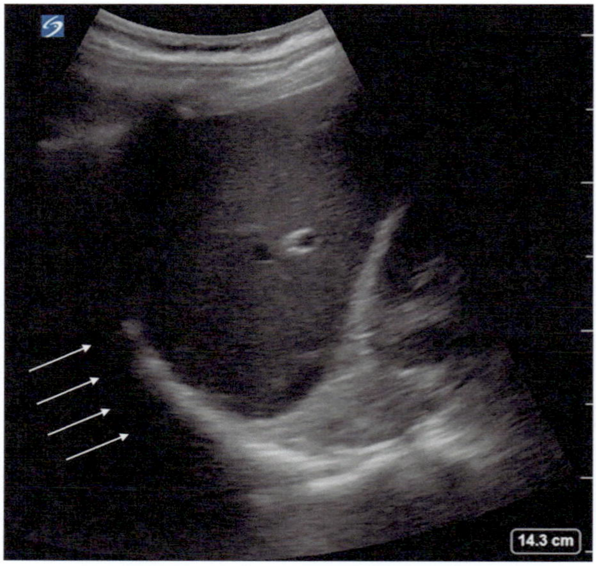

Fig. 2.8 LUQ EFAST view with left hemithorax: Evaluation of the LUQ should include the left hemithorax, visualized above the spleen and hyperechoic diaphragm

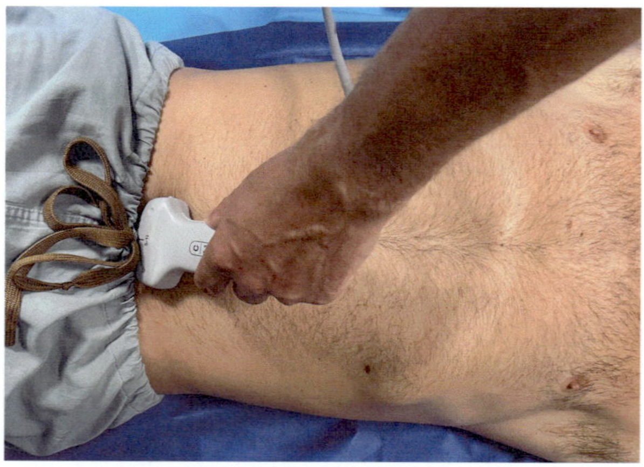

Fig. 2.9 Transducer placement pelvis, transverse: Place the transducer superior to the pubic bone angled inferiorly with the transducer marker pointed toward the patient's right in the transverse plane

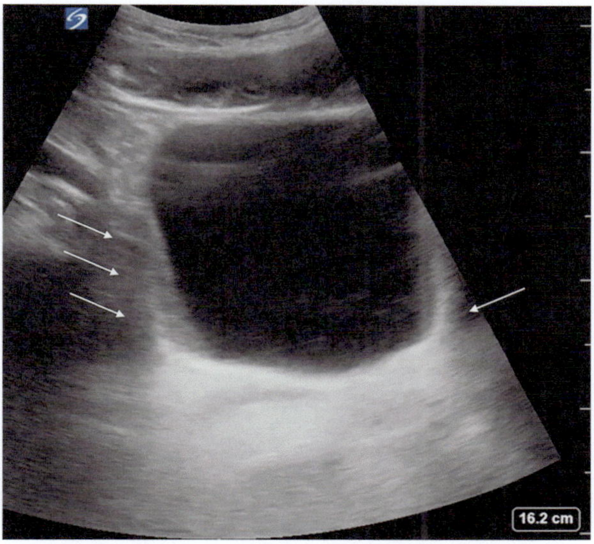

Fig. 2.10 Paracolic gutters in transverse: Normal pelvis and bladder EFAST view in a transverse plane. Arrows point to bilateral paracolic gutters on each side of the bladder

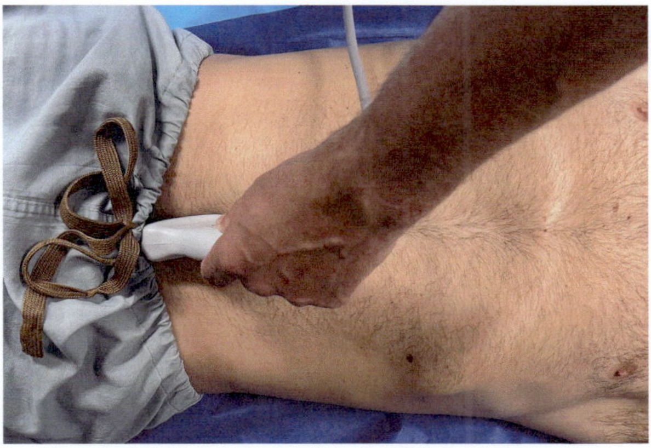

Fig. 2.11 Transducer placement bladder in sagittal: From a transverse position, rotate the transducer 90° clockwise to image the pelvis in sagittal plane with the transducer marker pointed to patient's head

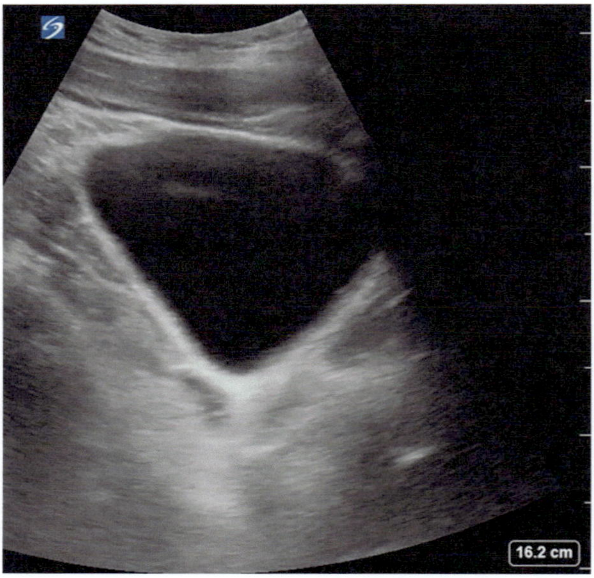

Fig. 2.12 Sagittal view of bladder: Normal pelvis and bladder EFAST view in a sagittal plane

- Operator should use an overhand grip on the transducer and use a moderate amount of force to press the transducer into the patient's abdomen, with the angle of the transducer superior and leftward toward the left shoulder.
  - Figure 2.13—Subxiphoid EFAST transducer placement
- Adjust depth to adequately visualize the entire heart
- Figure 2.14—Subxiphoid EFAST view
- Video 2.6—Subxiphoid EFAST view

(e) Bilateral lung apices

- Can use curvilinear, linear, or phased array transducer.
- Place the transducer on the anterior chest in a sagittal orientation with the marker pointed toward the patient's head over the 2nd intercostal space.
  - Figure 2.15—Transducer placement lungs
  - Figure 2.16—Lung view EFAST
  - Video 2.7—Lung sliding
- Evaluate for lung sliding using a shallow depth.
- Lung sliding appears as horizontal movement of two thin hyperechoic lines in a to-and-fro movement.
- Decrease the gain to help visualize the pleura.
- Use M-mode to confirm findings or if unable to determine the presence of lung sliding.
  - Place the M-mode line between two ribs, so it crosses perpendicularly over the pleura.
  - Identify "seashore sign" with normal lung sliding.

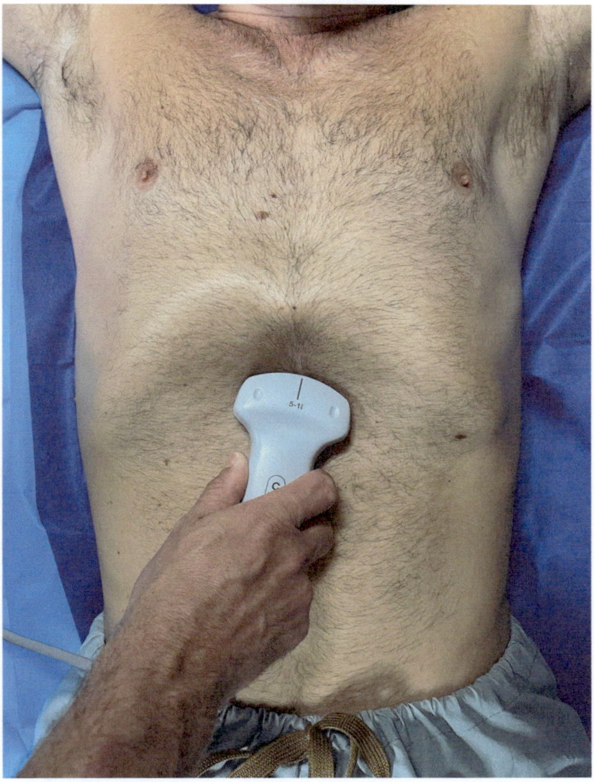

Fig. 2.13 Subxiphoid EFAST transducer placement: Place the transducer inferior to the xiphoid process with the marker oriented toward the patient's right. Place operator's hand on top of the transducer, use a moderate amount of force to press the transducer into the patient's abdomen, and angle the transducer superior and leftward toward the left shoulder

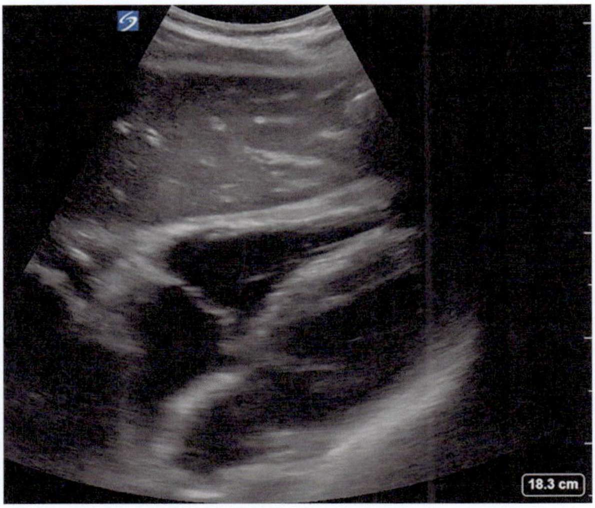

Fig. 2.14 Subxiphoid EFAST view: Normal EFAST demonstrating a subxiphoid view of the heart. The liver is used as the acoustic window to view cardiac structures and pericardium. The right heart sits closest to the liver

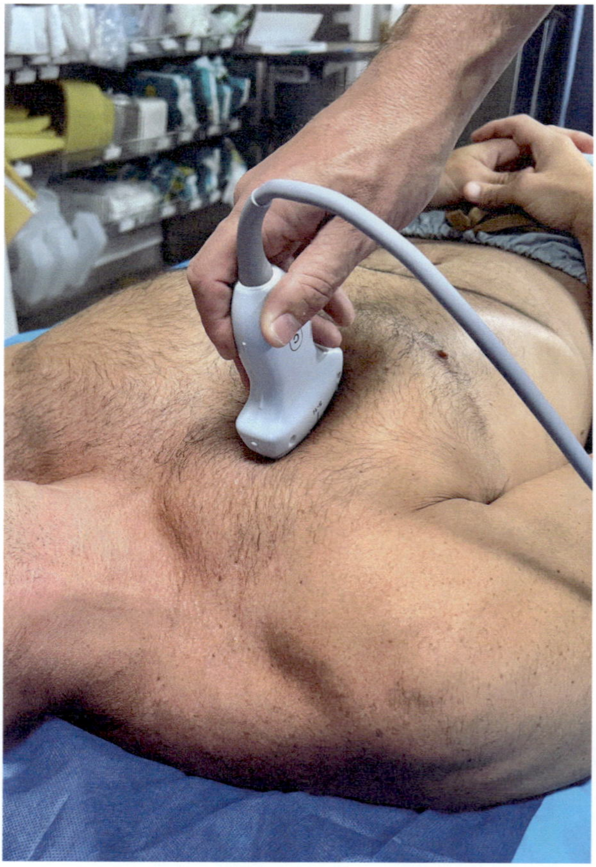

Fig. 2.15 Transducer placement lungs: Place the transducer on the anterior chest in a sagittal orientation with the marker pointed toward the patient's head over the 2nd intercostal space

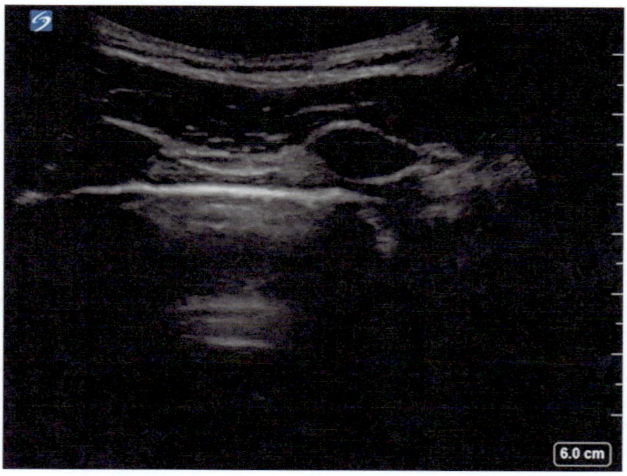

Fig. 2.16 Lung view EFAST: Normal EFAST demonstrating lung sliding. Note two anechoic ribs with posterior acoustic shadowing and the hyperechoic pleural line between them

  - Horizontal lines represent the static chest wall [2].
  - Granular pattern represents movement of the lung beyond the pleural line [2].
  - Figure 2.17—M-mode spike position
  - Figure 2.18—Normal sliding lung M-mode

(f) Inferior vena cava

  - Place the transducer inferior to the xiphoid process, slightly to the right of midline, with the marker oriented toward the patient's head.
  - Figure 2.19—Transducer placement IVC
  - Figure 2.20—IVC view
  - Video 2.8—IVC view

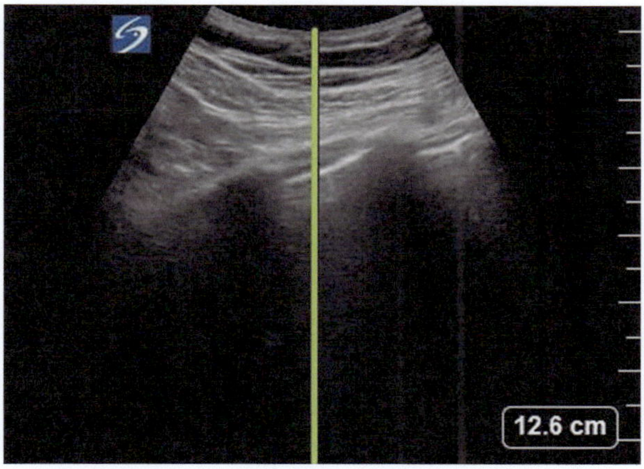

Fig. 2.17 M-mode spike position: The M-mode spike should be placed between the two rib shadows overlying the hyperechoic pleural line

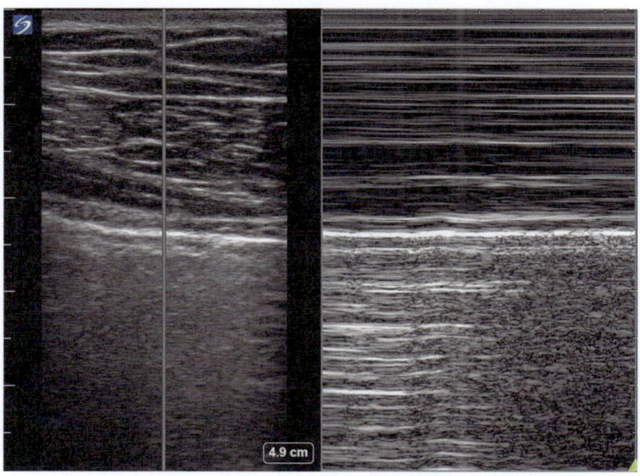

Fig. 2.18 Normal sliding lung M-mode: M-mode ultrasonography of a normal lung demonstrates the static chest wall in the top half of image and movement of the lungs in the bottom half consistent with normal respiration. Sometimes referred to as "seashore" sign

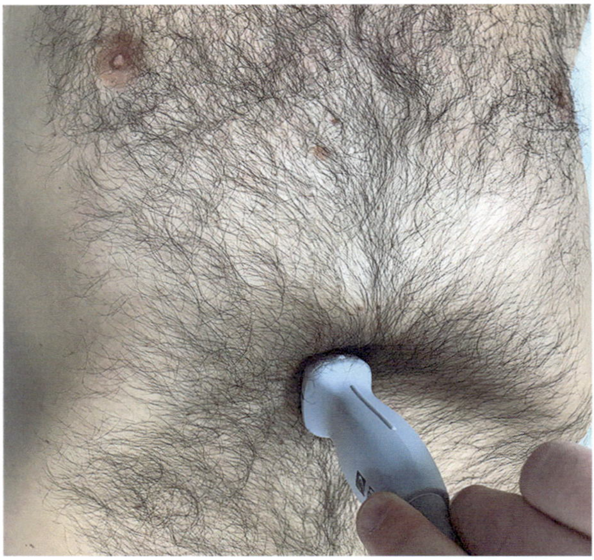

Fig. 2.19 Transducer placement IVC: Place the transducer inferior to the xiphoid process, slightly to the right of midline, with the marker oriented toward the patient's head

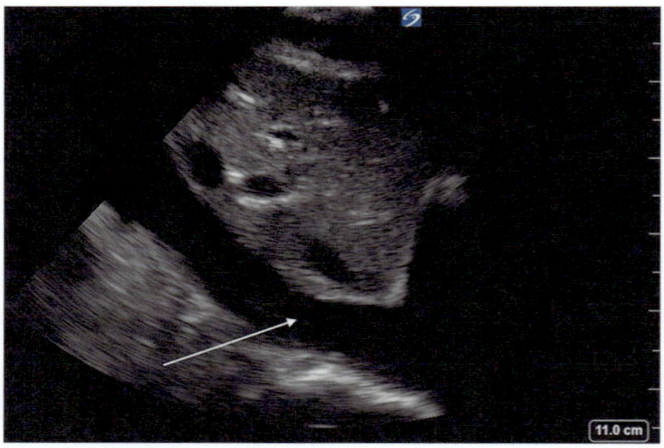

Fig. 2.20 IVC view: Normal EFAST view of the IVC as it passes by the liver and drains into the right atrium of the heart

EFAST Pathology

(a) Hemoperitoneum

- Accumulation of blood within the peritoneum
- Blood will be seen as an anechoic, hypoechoic, or echogenic fluid collection:
  - Between the liver and kidney
    - Figure 2.21—Positive EFAST Morrison's pouch
    - Video 2.9—Positive EFAST Morrison's pouch
  - Around the liver tip
    - Figure 2.22—Positive EFAST liver tip
    - Video 2.10—Positive EFAST liver tip

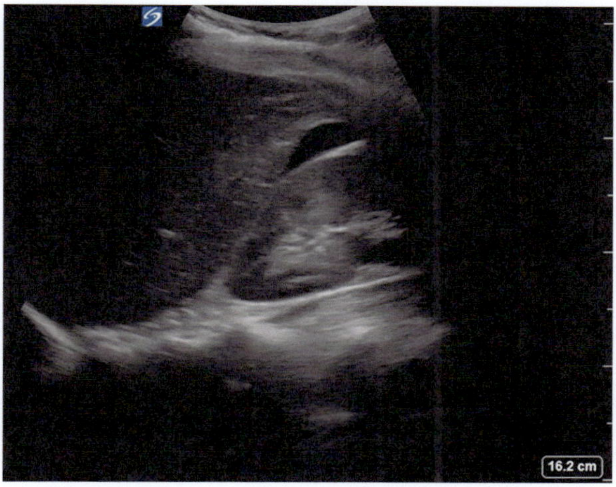

Fig. 2.21 Positive EFAST Morrison's pouch: Free fluid is located within Morrison's pouch between the liver and right kidney

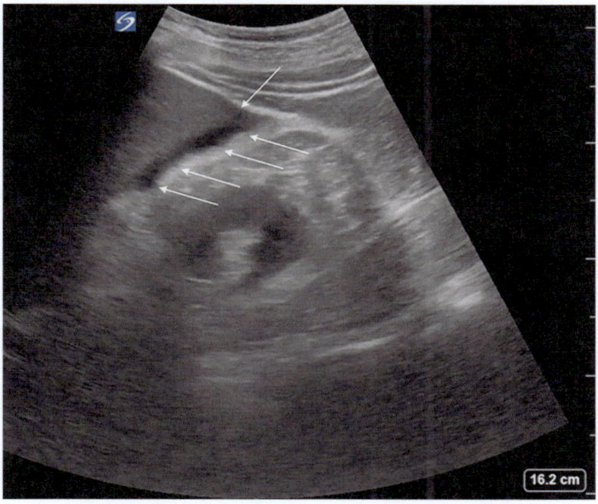

Fig. 2.22 Positive EFAST liver tip: Free fluid is seen here surrounding the liver tip (*arrows*)

  - Between the spleen and kidney
    - Figure 2.23—Positive EFAST LUQ
    - Video 2.11—Positive EFAST LUQ
  - Between the spleen and diaphragm
    - Figure 2.24—Positive EFAST LUQ above the spleen
    - Video 2.12—Positive EFAST LUQ above the spleen
  - Posterior to or on either side of the bladder
    - Figure 2.25—Positive EFAST bladder transverse
    - Video 2.13—Positive EFAST bladder transverse
    - Figure 2.26—Positive EFAST bladder sagittal
    - Video 2.14—Positive EFAST bladder sagittal
- Depending on the amount, free fluid can be a large pocket or a small anechoic stripe

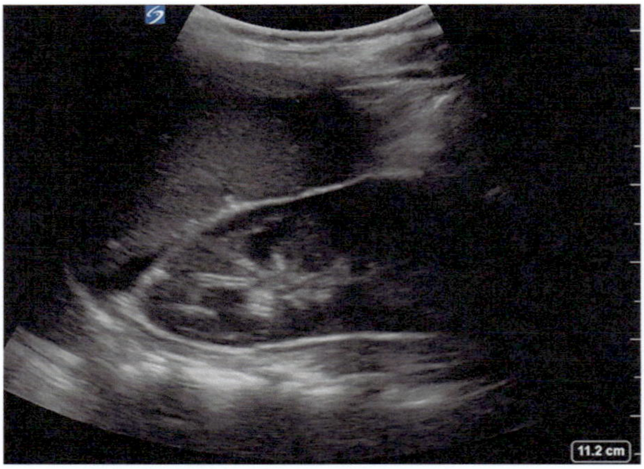

Fig. 2.23 Positive EFAST LUQ: Free fluid is seen here between the spleen and left kidney

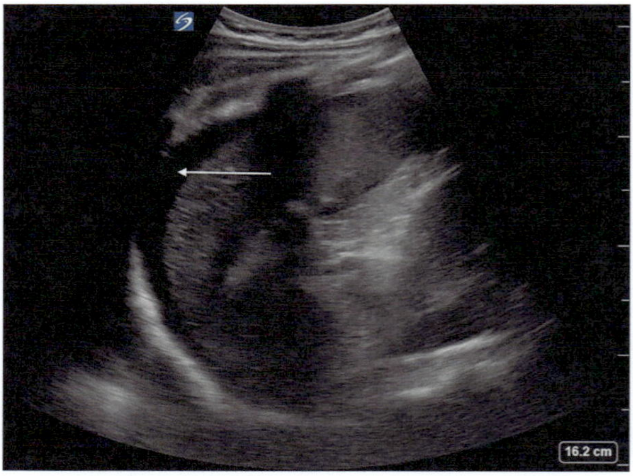

Fig. 2.24 Positive EFAST LUQ above spleen: Free fluid is located superior to the spleen and inferior to the diaphragm (*arrow*). Fluid will typically accumulate above the spleen first in the LUQ making it important to always image this area

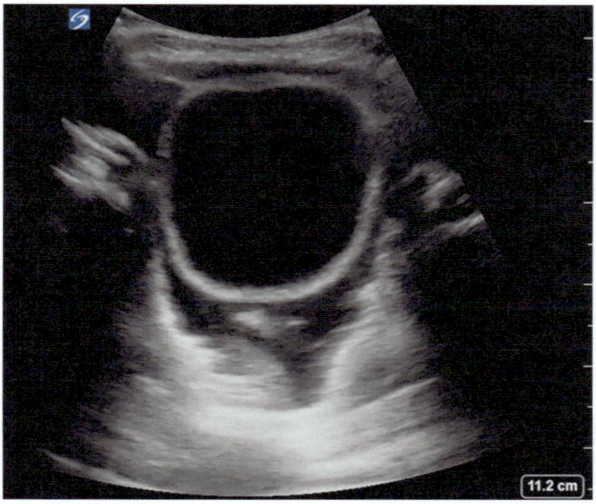

Fig. 2.25 Positive EFAST bladder transverse: Free fluid is surrounding the bladder in a transverse plane. Note the anechoic fluid posterior to the bladder and in both paracolic gutters

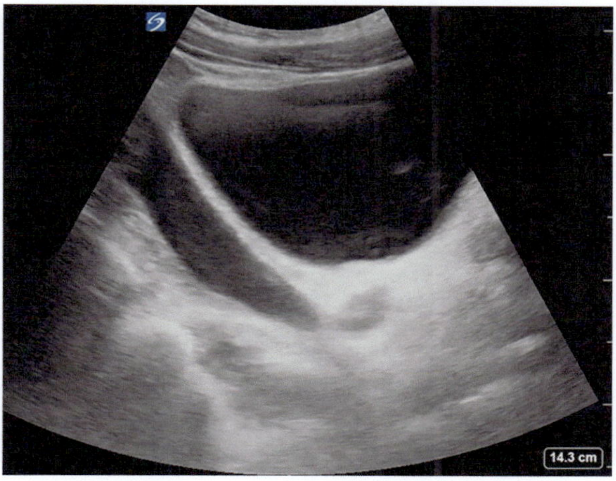

Fig. 2.26 Positive EFAST bladder sagittal: Free fluid is found around the bladder in the sagittal plane

(b) Hemothorax or Pleural Effusion
- Abnormal accumulation of blood or fluid between the two pleural layers.
- Anechoic or hypoechoic fluid collected above the diaphragm within the thoracic cavity between the visceral and parietal pleura.
  - Can be seen when imaging the right or left upper quadrants.
  - Will accumulate posteriorly if the patient is supine and inferiorly between the diaphragm and lung if the patient is upright.
  - Figure 2.27—Pleural effusion
  - Video 2.15—Pleural effusion
- May see "curtain" or "flag" sign which occurs with the lung slides into the effusion during respirations.
  - Figure 2.28—Large pleural effusion with flag sign
  - Video 2.16—Large pleural effusion with flag sign

(c) Pneumothorax
- Caused by separation of the lung pleura away from the chest wall, resulting in a collapsed lung.
- Absent lung sliding due to the separation of the visceral pleura from the parietal pleura [2].
  - Video 2.17—Absent lung sliding
- If lung sliding is absent, move the transducer superior or inferior to locate the lung point sign.
  - Lung point sign is the transition point between normal lung sliding and a pneumothorax with the absence of lung sliding.
  - This is not always present, especially with a large pneumothorax [2].
  - Lung point sign is 100% specific for pneumothorax [2].
  - Video 2.18—Lung point
- Use M-mode to confirm the absence of sliding as described above

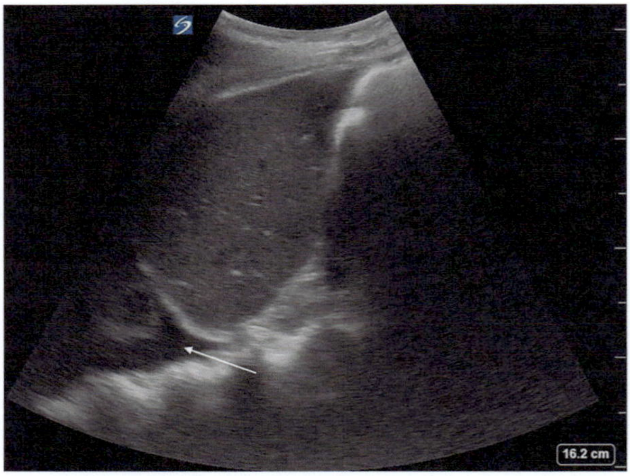

Fig. 2.27 Positive pleural fluid above the diaphragm: A small pleural effusion (*arrow*) is noted above the diaphragm

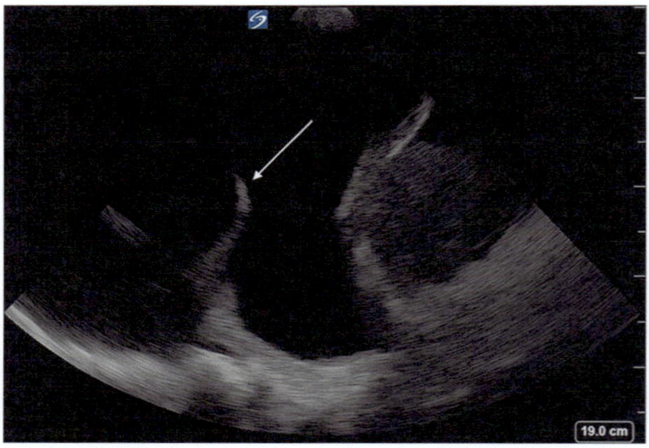

Fig. 2.28 Large pleural effusion with flag sign: With large pleural effusions, the lung will appear to be floating in the fluid (*arrow*), creating what looks like a flag flapping in the wind (flag sign)

  - M-mode will demonstrate no movement of the lungs, which is sometimes referred to as barcode sign due to the horizontal lines seen throughout the entire image [2].
  - Figure 2.29—Barcode sign

(d) Hemopericardium or Pericardial Effusion

- Accumulation of blood or fluid between the visceral and parietal pericardium surrounding the heart.
- Appears as a hypoechoic stripe between the heart and brightly echogenic pericardium at the inferior border of the heart, which can be seen next to the liver.
  - Figure 2.30—Pericardial effusion
  - Video 2.19—Pericardial effusion
- The sonographer can distinguish a left pleural effusion from a pericardial effusion by the pattern of fluid.

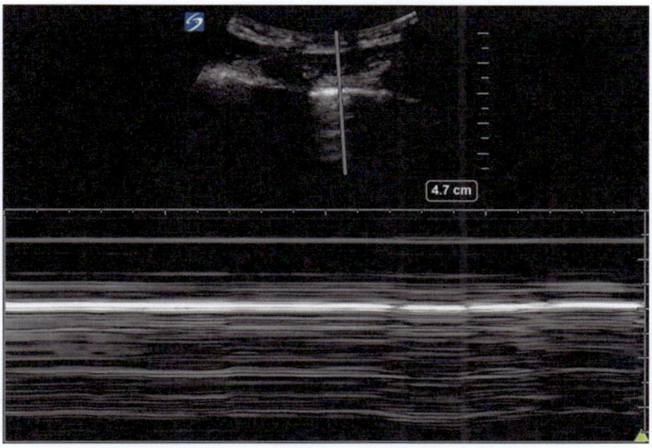

Fig. 2.29 Barcode sign: M-mode through the pleural line demonstrates no movement as evidenced by the horizontal lines in the bottom half of the image. This is sometimes referred to as "barcode sign" given the similar appearance to retail barcodes

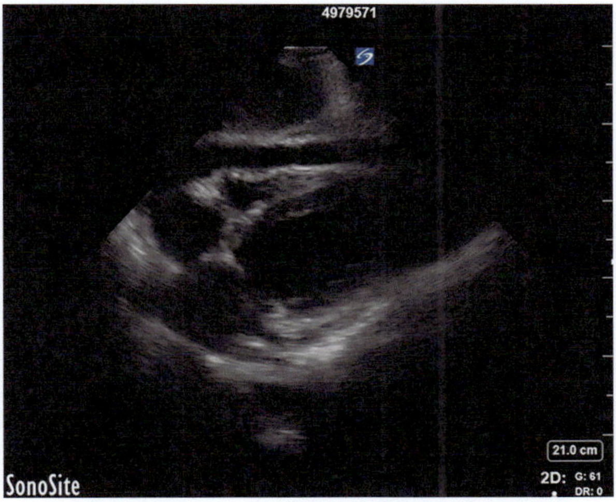

Fig. 2.30 Pericardial effusion: Anechoic fluid surrounds the right heart indicating a pericardial effusion

- Pericardial fluid will be present posterior to the left ventricular wall and anterior to the descending aorta [3].
- Left-sided pleural effusion will occur posterior to the left ventricular wall and will not be present anterior to the descending aorta [3].
- Figure 2.31—Comparing pleural fluid vs. pericardial fluid.

(e) Cardiac Tamponade

- Occurs when fluid within the pericardium generates excessive external pressure, which then impairs the ability for the heart chambers to fill eventually causing hypotension and shock
  - Affects the thin-walled right atrium and right ventricle first.
  - Right atrial systolic collapse [3, 4] is the most sensitive sign of tamponade.
    - Usually, the first echocardiographic sign.
    - Figure 2.32—Right atrial systolic collapse in tamponade
    - Video 2.20—Right atrial systolic collapse in tamponade

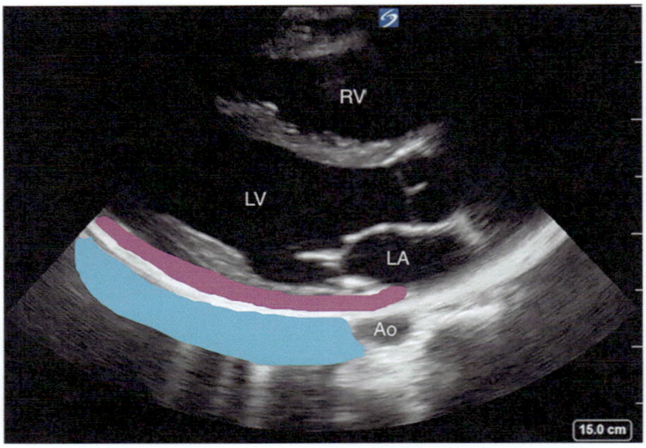

Fig. 2.31 Comparing pleural fluid and pericardial fluid: In a parasternal long view, pericardial fluid will be present posterior to the left ventricular wall and anterior to the descending aorta (*pink stripe*). A left-sided pleural effusion will occur posterior to the left ventricular wall and will not be present anterior to the descending aorta (*blue stripe*)

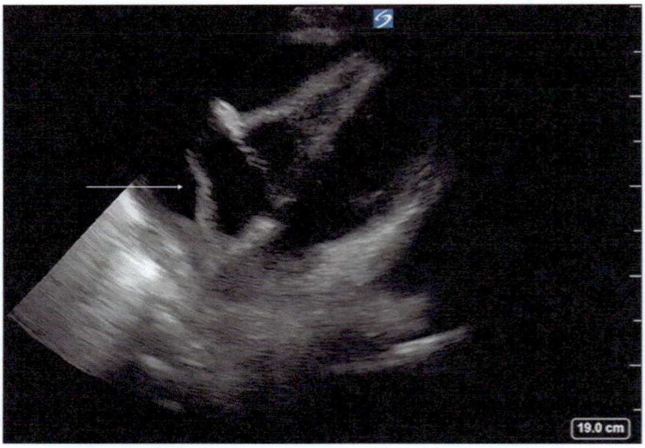

Fig. 2.32 Right atrial systolic collapse in tamponade (*arrow*): In cardiac tamponade, the pressure within the pericardium exceeds the pressure within the right atrium causing it to collapse during systole

- Right ventricular diastolic collapse [4] is the most specific sign of tamponade [3]
  - Figure 2.33—Right ventricle collapse
  - Video 2.21—Right ventricle collapse
- Will also see a dilated IVC with minimal collapse [4]
  - Figure 2.34—Plethoric IVC
  - Video 2.22—Plethoric IVC

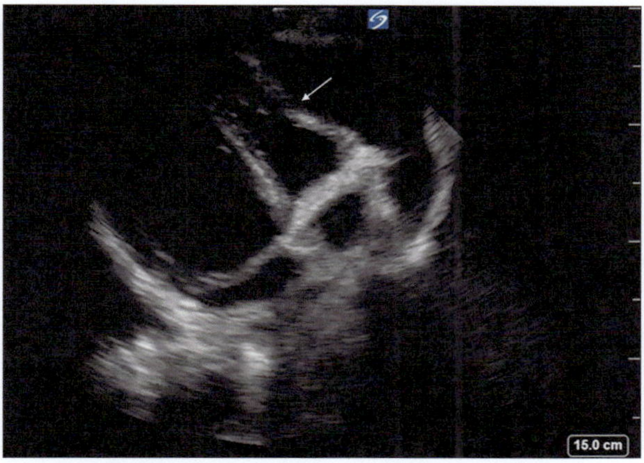

Fig. 2.33 Right ventricle collapse (*arrow*): In cardiac tamponade, the pressure within the pericardium exceeds the pressure within the right ventricle causing it to collapse during diastole

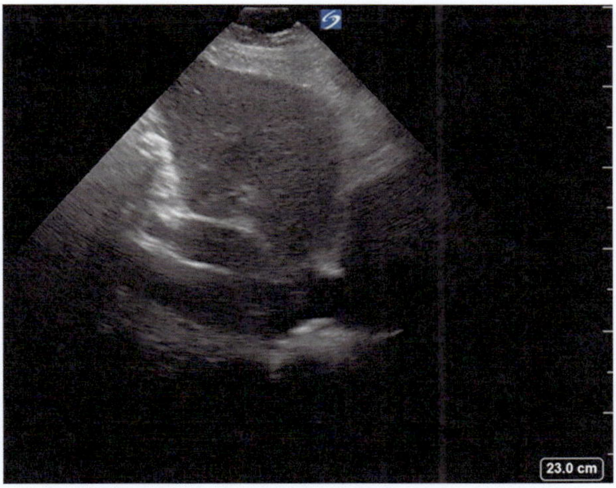

Fig. 2.34 Plethoric IVC: Here, the IVC is visualized passing the liver and draining into the right atrium. Note that the IVC is quite large indicating the IVC is plethoric

EFAST Pitfalls

- False Positives
  - Right Upper Quadrant (RUQ)
    - Use caution and perform a complete fan-through of hepatorenal space as the well-circumscribed gallbladder can often be erroneously identified as free fluid, but is more often found anteriorly.
      - Figure 2.35—Gallbladder
      - Video 2.23—Gallbladder
    - Beware of the "double line sign"—a wedge-shaped hypoechoic area bordered by echogenic lines on both sides representing perinephric fat [5].
      - Figure 2.36—"Double line sign"
      - Video 2.24—"Double line sign"

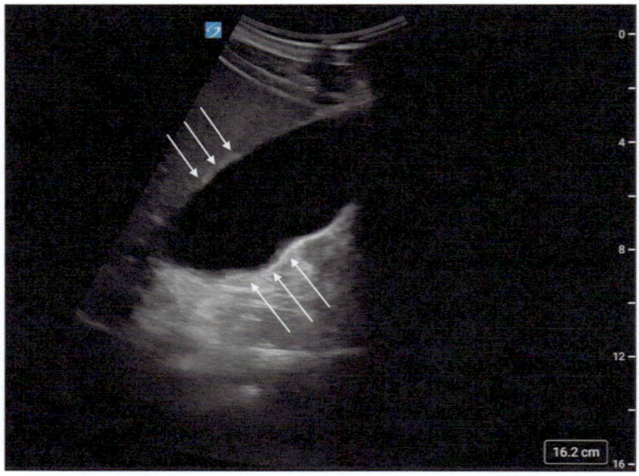

Fig. 2.35 Gallbladder: This can be mistaken for free fluid within the hepatorenal space. Note that the gallbladder (*arrows*) is well-defined with hyperechoic borders as opposed to sharp, irregular free fluid tracking in this space

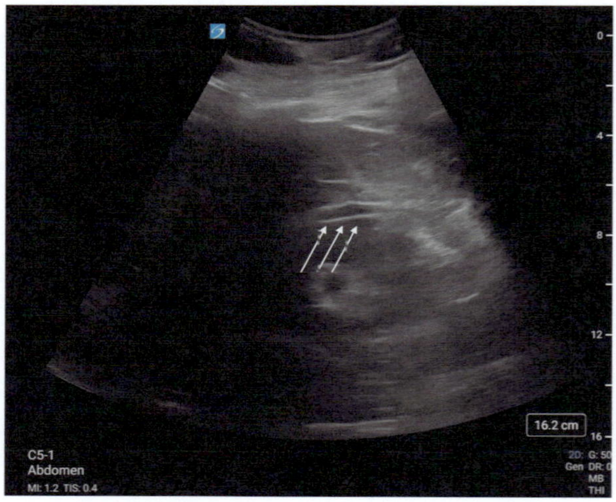

Fig. 2.36 "Double Line Sign": Here, there is a wedge-shaped hypoechoic space bordered by two hyperechoic lines representing perinephric fat rather than free fluid

  - Ultrasound may reveal a thin anechoic line adjacent to the inferior border of the liver or spleen near the caudal tip, known as "lipliner sign", which is thought to be artifactual due to advanced signal processing [6]
    - Figure 2.37 (a) RUQ Lipliner sign, (b) LUQ Lipliner sign
    - Video 2.25—RUQ Lipliner sign
- Left Upper Quadrant (LUQ)
  - In a patient who has recently eaten, the stomach can be mistaken for pathology.
  - The stomach will often be located posterior and have a well-defined border.

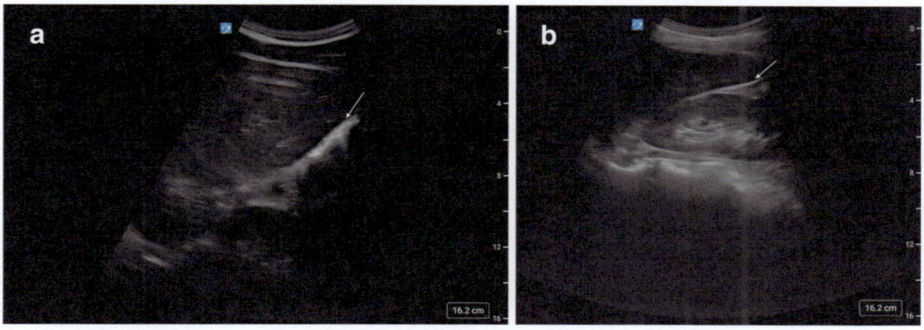

Fig. 2.37 "Lipliner Sign": (**a**) Thin anechoic stripe (arrow) that abuts the inferior border near the liver tip within the RUQ; (**b**) Thin anechoic strip (arrow) along the inferior border near the splenic tip within the LUQ

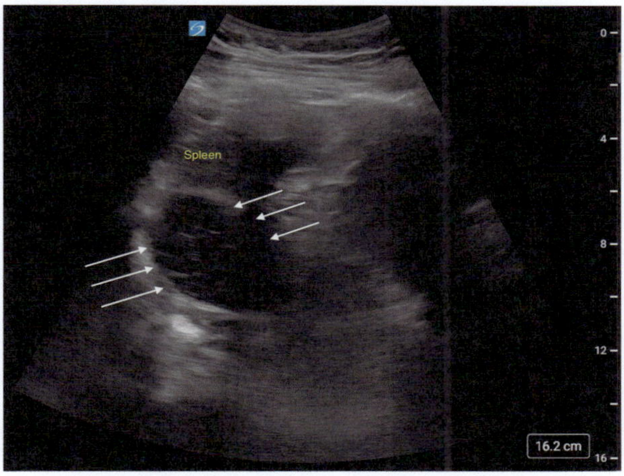

Fig. 2.38 Stomach: This can often be erroneously identified in the LUQ EFAST view (*arrows*), but typically is well-circumscried and filled with mixed densities and bubbling representing digested food particles. It is also typically identified more posteriorly

- Mixed hypoechoic/hyperechoic densities and bubbling may be seen representing digested food particles.
  - Figure 2.38—Stomach
  - Video 2.26—Stomach
- Pelvis
  - In a male patient, seminal vesicles can often be mistaken for free fluid in the transverse orientation. This can be discovered by rotating the probe into a sagittal position to see the seminal vesicles as a contiguous structure with the prostate.
    - Figure 2.39—Seminal vesicles in transverse.
    - Video 2.27—Seminal vesicles in transverse.
  - In a female patient, ovarian cysts, fibroids, and even physiological free fluid can be mistaken for hemoperitoneum.
    - Figure 2.40—Ovarian cysts
    - Video 2.28—Ovarian cysts

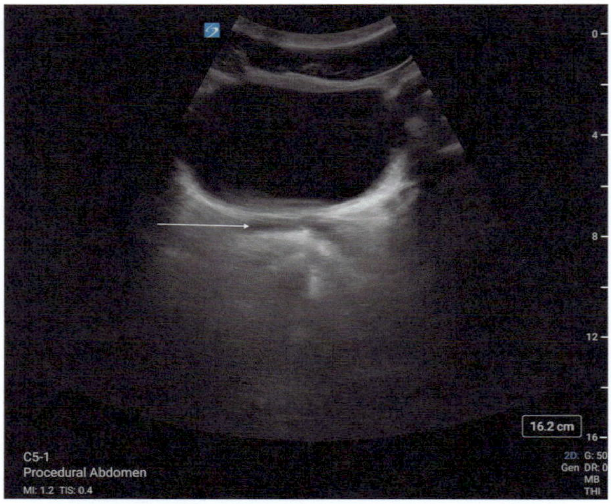

Fig. 2.39 Seminal vesicles in transverse (arrow); located between the bladder and prostate in males, can be mistaken for free fluid

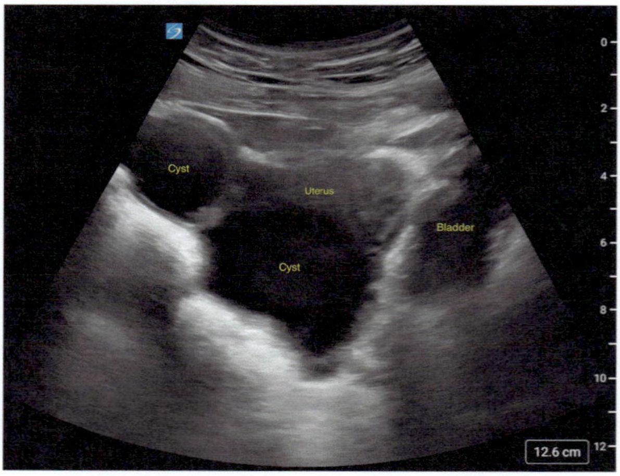

Fig. 2.40 Ovarian cysts: Here, in this sagittal view of the pelvis, there are well-circumscribed anechoic densities that can range from simple to complex depending on pathology. Notice, however, that there does not appear to be free fluid between the uterus and the bladder

- Pericardial
  - When evaluating for a pericardial effusion, an epicardial fat pad can be confused with a small pericardial effusion.
  - An epicardial fat pad will be anterior to the right ventricle in the parasternal long view.
  - Can sometimes be distinguished from blood or fluid by a speckled appearance [3].
  - More common in diabetics, obese, elderly, and females [3].
    - Figure 2.41—Epicardial fat pad in parasternal long
    - Video 2.29—Epicardial fat pad in parasternal long

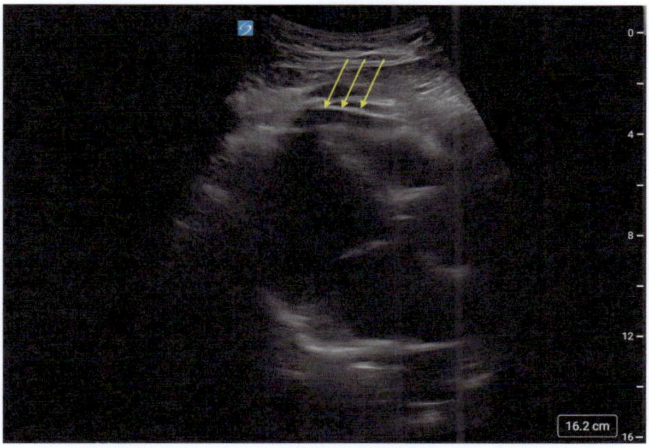

Fig. 2.41 Epicardial fat pad in parasternal long: Note the small anechoic space between the heart and pericardium representing the epicardial fat pad (*arrows*). The anechoic fluid that you would expect in a pericardial effusion is not circumferentially surrounding the heart in this example

- Pleura
  - If near enough to the pericardium on the left lung, pulsation from the heart can mimic a lung point sign.
  - Try evaluating a more superior rib space and utilizing M-mode when necessary as described previously.
    - Video 2.30—Pulsation of pericardium

Key Points

- To have a positive EFAST, as little as 100 cc of fluid can be detected with ultrasound [1, 7].
- Use EFAST as a serial screening exam; rapidly repeat with any change in patient status.
- Hemoperitoneum can be anechoic or echogenic depending on if clot formation has begun.
  - If presentation following trauma is delayed, blood within the peritoneum will often be clotted and can be missed [8].
- Morrison's pouch is the most sensitive location of identifying hemoperitoneum.
  - In children, fluid will accumulate in the pelvis before the RUQ.
- Fluid will most often accumulate between the diaphragm and spleen first, before splenorenal recess, when there is blood in the LUQ [1].
  - However, blood from a splenic injury will usually accumulate in the RUQ before demonstrating evidence of hemoperitoneum in the LUQ.
- Placing the patient in Trendelenberg and reverse Trendelenberg and waiting about 5 min for fluid to accumulate by gravity will increase the sensitivity of the EFAST exam.
- Ultrasound cannot determine the etiology of the fluid within the abdomen. Fluid that is seen on ultrasound may or may not be blood and may or may not be the result of trauma.

- The sonographer cannot visualize the retroperitoneum using the EFAST exam. Therefore, bleeding from retroperitoneal structures such as the kidneys or aorta will be difficult to assess.
- Use both transverse and sagittal views to examine for intraperitoneal fluid in the pelvis.
- Care must be taken to differentiate between intra-abdominal organs and fluid, such as bowel.
- If unable to visualize the heart adequately in a subxiphoid window, obtain an image using a parasternal long technique (see Chap. 3 for more details).
  - Can also try having the patient take a deep breath in and hold it, which may push the cardiac structures into view.
- EFAST exam will be limited by morbid obesity and subcutaneous emphysema.
- EFAST has been shown to have a higher sensitivity than chest X-ray when evaluating for pneumothorax [9].

References

1. Ma OJ, Mateer JR, Kirkpatrick AW. Chapter 5: Trauma. In: Ma OJ, Mateer JR, Reardon RF, Joing SA, editors. Emergency ultrasound. 3rd ed. China: McGraw-Hill Education; 2014. p. 61–92.
2. Husain LF, Hagopian L, Wayman D, Baker WE, Carmody KA. Sonographic diagnosis of pneumothorax. J Emerg Trauma Shock. 2012;5(1):76–81. https://www.ncbi.nlm.nih.gov/pmc/articles/PMC3299161/. Accessed 26 Apr 2017
3. Rasalingam R, Makan M, Perez JE. The Washington manual of echocardiography. Philadelphia: Wolters Kluwer Health/Lippincott Williams & Wilkins; 2013.
4. Mallin M, Dawson M. Introduction to bedside ultrasound: volume 2. United States of America: Emergency Ultrasound Solutions; 2013. iBook. https://itun.es/us/ueELM.l.
5. Sierzenski PR, Schofer JM, Bauman MJ, Nomura JT. The double-line sign: a false positive finding on the focused assessment with sonography for trauma (FAST) examination. J Emerg Med. 2011;40(2):188–9. https://doi.org/10.1016/j.jemermed.2009.07.029.
6. Parker MA, Hicks BG, Kaili M, Silver A, Zhu M, Feuerherdt M, et al. The lipliner sign: potential cause of a false positive focused assessment with sonography in trauma (FAST) examination. J Emerg Med. 2024;67(6):e553–9. https://doi.org/10.1016/j.jemermed.2024.06.013. Epub 2024 Jun 28. PMID: 39366788.
7. Fleming S, Bird R, Ratnasingham K, Sarker SJ, Walsh M, Patel B. Accuray of FAST scan in blunt abdominal trauma in a major London trauma centre. Int J Surg. 2012;10(9):470–4. http://www.sciencedirect.com/science/article/pii/S1743919112001082. Accessed 20 Apr 2017.
8. Lewiss RE, Saul T, Del Rios M. Focus on: EFAST—extended focused assessment with sonography for trauma. ACEP News Website. 2009. https://www.acep.org/Clinical%2D%2D-Practice-Management/Focus-On%2D%2DEFAST%2D%2D-Extended-Focused-Assessment-With-Sonography-for-Trauma/. Accessed 20 Apr 2017.
9. Abdulrahman Y, Musthafa S, Hakim SY, Nabir S, Qanbar A, Mahmood I, Siddiqui T, Hussein W, Ali HH, Afifi I, El-Menyar A, Al-Thani H. Utility of extended FAST in blunt chest trauma: is it the time to be used in the ATLS algorithm? World J Surg. 2015;39(1):172–8. https://link.springer.com/article/10.1007%2Fs00268-014-2781-y. Accessed 20 Apr 2017.

Transthoracic Echocardiography

3

Corey Moore, Jordan Tozer, Michael J. Vitto,
Angela Lindsay, and Michael Joyce

Cardiac ultrasound, often referred to as echocardiography, is a very broad and technical field. It can take years to master the intricacies; however, with simple training and education of basic heart function and image acquisition, echocardiography can be performed well and accurately by a novice sonographer. Patients, young and old, can benefit from point-of-care echocardiography to diagnose and guide treatment, disposition, and further care for their condition. This chapter will introduce the basic skills needed for obtaining standard echocardiographic views that can be used in all fields of medicine. It will review cardiac ultrasound indications, basic anatomy, image acquisition, normal ultrasound anatomy, and interpretation of pathology.

Clinical Application and Indications

- Visualize overall cardiac activity and gross estimation of ejection fraction
- Guide resuscitation during cardiac arrest
- Evaluate for cardiac cause of undifferentiated hypotension

Supplementary Information The online version contains supplementary material available at https://doi.org/10.1007/978-3-032-27643-8_3.

C. Moore (✉)
Department of Emergency Medicine, East Carolina University Medical Center, Greenville, NC, USA
e-mail: Corey.moore@ecuhealth.org

J. Tozer · M. J. Vitto · A. Lindsay · M. Joyce
Department of Emergency Medicine, Virginia Commonwealth University Health, Richmond, VA, USA
e-mail: jordan.tozer@vcuhealth.org; angela.creditt@vcuhealth.org; john.joyce@vcuhealth.org

A. Lindsay et al. (eds.), *Clinical Ultrasound*,
https://doi.org/10.1007/978-3-032-27643-8_3

- Evaluate for wall motion abnormalities in patients with suspected myocardial infarction
- Evaluate for pericardial effusion or cardiac tamponade
- Evaluate for signs of right ventricular strain
- Evaluate inferior vena cava

Normal Cardiac Anatomy

- The heart is a four-chambered structure that is surrounded by a pericardium and lies within the mediastinum.
- Atria are fluid-filled thin-walled structures.
- The most anterior chamber is the right ventricle, which has thicker walls than the atria but thinner than the left ventricle.
- The left ventricle has the thickest wall and lies posterior to the right ventricle, separated by the interventricular septum.
- Central Circulation
  - Blood enters the heart through the inferior and superior vena cava, draining directly into the right atrium.
  - It then passes through the tricuspid valve and enters the right ventricle.
  - During systole, blood is ejected from the right ventricle through the pulmonary valve and into the pulmonary arteries.
  - Blood returns from the pulmonary circulation through the four pulmonary veins and drains directly into the left atrium.
- Blood passes through the mitral valve and enters the left ventricle.
  - During systole, blood is ejected from the left ventricle through the aortic valve and into the proximal aorta.
- Valves
  - Mitral valve has two leaflets—anterior and posterior [1].
  - Aortic valve has three leaflets—left, right, and noncoronary [1].
    - Congenital bicuspid valve occurs in 1–2% of the population [1].
  - Tricuspid valve has three cusps—anterior, posterior, and septal [1].
  - The pulmonary valve has three cusps—anterior, right, and left [1].

Image Acquisition

- Transducer Selection
  - Phased array
    - Be sure to select cardiac mode on the ultrasound machine
- Standard Exam Views
  - Parasternal long axis
  - Parasternal short axis
  - Apical four-chamber
  - Apical two-chamber

- Subxiphoid
- Inferior vena cava (IVC)
- Patient Position and Procedure
  - Place the patient in a supine position.
  - For subxiphoid views, the patient should have their knees bent to relax abdominal muscles for easier visualization.
  - A left lateral decubitus position can bring the heart closer to the chest wall and improve cardiac windows, especially for apical views.

Parasternal Long Axis

- Transducer Placement
  - Place the transducer on the anterior chest at the second or third intercostal space to the left of the sternum with the transducer marker toward the patient's right shoulder.
  - Slide the transducer inferior or superior, one rib space at a time, to find the optimal cardiac window.
  - Figure 3.1—Parasternal long transducer placement
- Ultrasound Anatomy
  - Figure 3.2—Parasternal long
  - Apex points toward the left of the screen with the base of the heart and great vessels on the right of the screen.
  - Right ventricle is the most anterior chamber of the heart and will be visualized at the top of the screen.
  - Left ventricle at the bottom of the screen with the left atrium to the lower right.
  - Systole will be visualized when the mitral valve is closed and the left ventricular walls are shortened.

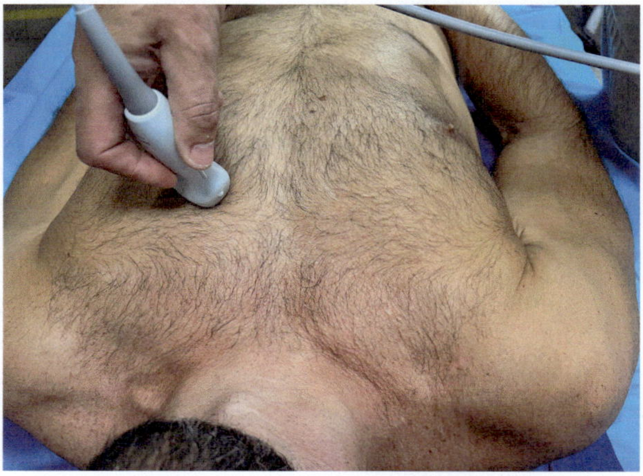

Fig. 3.1 Parasternal long transducer placement: Place the transducer on the anterior chest at the second or third intercostal space to the left of the sternum with the transducer marker toward the patient's right shoulder

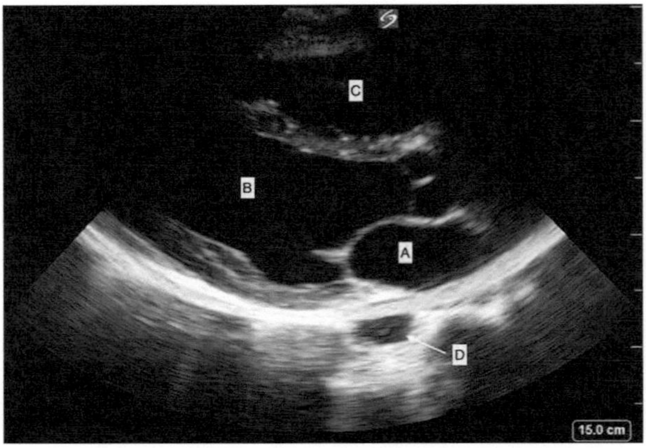

Fig. 3.2 Parasternal long: Parasternal long cardiac view in between cardiac cycles with both mitral and aortic valves closed. Blood flows from the left atrium (**a**) through the mitral valve, into the left ventricle (**b**), and out to the body through the aortic valve. The right ventricle can be seen at the top of the screen (**c**). The descending thoracic aorta is posterior to the heart (**d**)

  - During systole, the aortic valve will be open as blood flows from within the left ventricle to the ascending aortic arch.
- Diastole will be visualized when the mitral valve is open, and the left ventricle fills with blood.
  - During diastole, blood flows from the left atrium through the mitral valve into the left ventricle.
- The descending aorta is visualized immediately posterior to the bright, echogenic pericardial sac.
- Video 3.1—Parasternal long

Parasternal Short Axis

- Transducer Placement
  - From the long axis position, rotate the transducer approximately 90° clockwise so the marker points toward the left shoulder.
  - This will give you a cross-sectional view of the left ventricle.
  - Figure 3.3—Parasternal short transducer placement
- Ultrasound Anatomy
  - Figure 3.4—Parasternal short
  - Left ventricle appears as a muscular circle that, in the absence of pathology, contracts concentrically.
  - The bicuspid mitral valve is located centrally within the left ventricle that has the appearance of a “fish mouth” opening and closing.
    - Figure 3.5—Mitral valve fish mouth in parasternal short
    - Video 3.2—Parasternal short at the mitral valve
  - Sliding or fanning the transducer toward the apex will allow visualization of the two papillary muscles in short axis.
    - Each papillary muscle is usually located at 4 and 8 o’clock within the circular left ventricle.
    - Video 3.3—Parasternal short at the apex

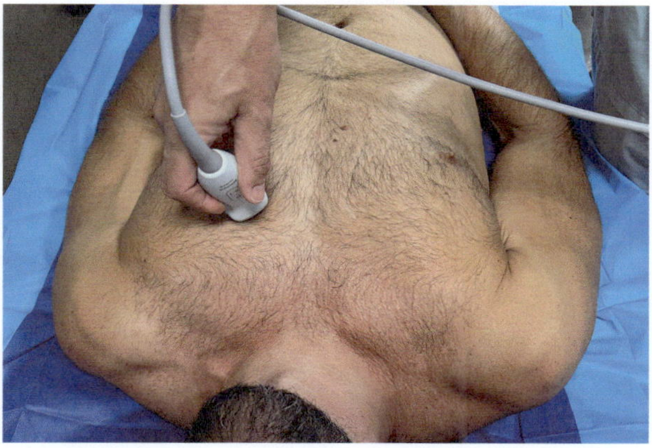

Fig. 3.3 Parasternal short transducer placement: From the long axis position, rotate the transducer approximately 90° clockwise so the marker points toward the left shoulder

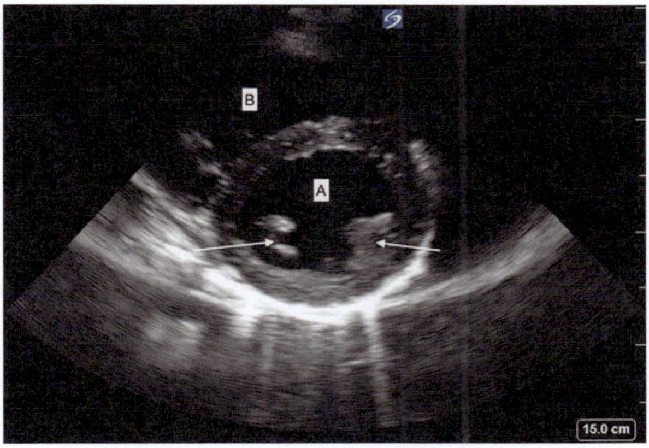

Fig. 3.4 Parasternal short labeled: Parasternal short cardiac view at the level of the papillary muscles (arrows). LV cavity (**a**) is circular, not elongated or ovoid. The RV cavity (**b**) can be seen in upper left

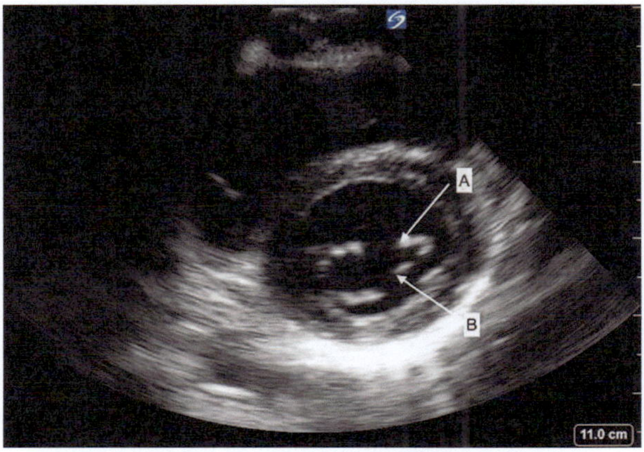

Fig. 3.5 Mitral valve fish mouth in parasternal short: Mitral valve parasternal short view displaying the "fish mouth" of the mitral valve in short axis. The anterior leaflet (**a**) can be seen above the posterior leaflet (**b**)

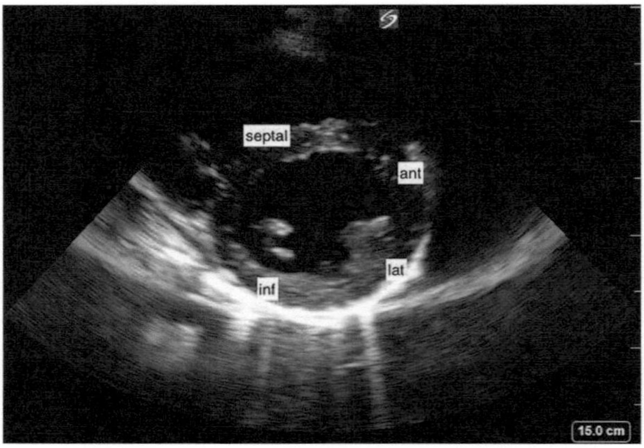

Fig. 3.6 Walls of LV labeled in parasternal short: Parasternal short cardiac view at the level of the papillary muscles showing the relative wall sections

- Right ventricle will appear as a "C"-shaped structure on the left side of the screen, separated from the left ventricle by the septal wall.
- Myocardial infarction or ischemia can be identified by wall motion abnormalities and a loss of concentric contraction of the left ventricle.
  - Anterior wall is closest to the transducer
  - Septal wall is to the left of the screen
  - Lateral wall is to the right of the screen
  - Interior wall is in the far field
  - Figure 3.6—Walls of LV labeled in parasternal short

Apical Four- and Two-Chamber

(a) Transducer Placement
- Place the transducer on the point of maximal impulse (PMI) with the marker pointed toward the patient's left elbow.
  - Figure 3.7—Apical four-chamber transducer placement
  - This will allow visualization of the four chambers of the heart, viewed from apex to base.
- Rotate the transducer counterclockwise, positioning the probe indicator toward the head, to obtain a two-chamber view of the left atrium and left ventricle.

(b) Ultrasound Anatomy
- Four-chamber
  - Figure 3.8—Apical four-chamber ultrasound image
  - Left ventricle and atrium will be seen on the right side of the screen.
    - The left ventricle wall on the far right is the lateral wall.
  - The septal wall separates the two ventricles and is in the middle of the screen in a vertical orientation.
  - Right ventricle and atrium will be seen on the left side of the screen.
  - Video 3.4—Apical four-chamber

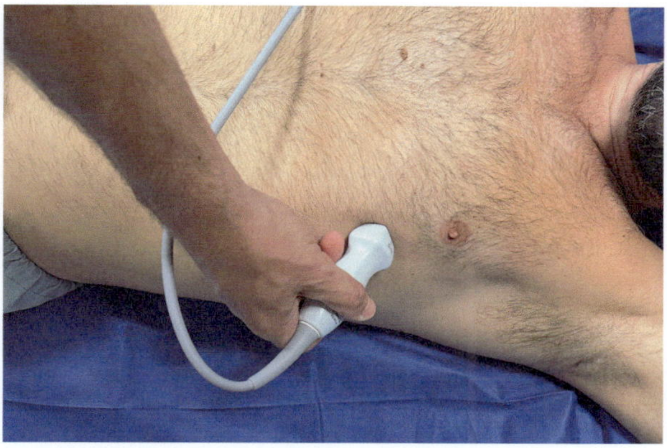

Fig. 3.7 Apical four-chamber transducer placement: Place the transducer on the point of maximal impulse (PMI) with the marker pointed toward the patient's left elbow

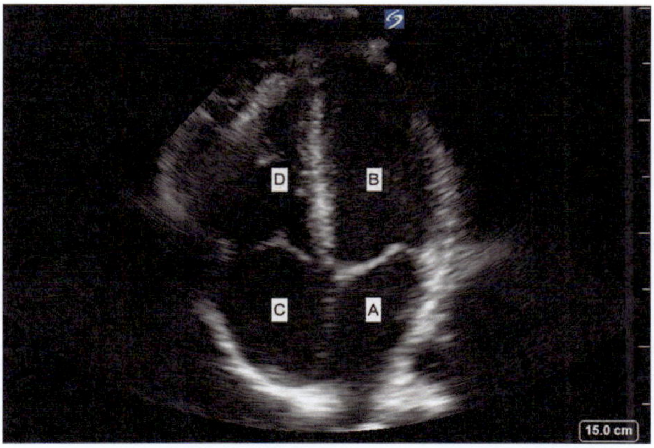

Fig. 3.8 Apical four-chamber: Apical four-chamber view in systole, with apex of the heart located at the *top* of the screen, base located at the *bottom*. Ideal orientation is with septal wall (between **d** and **b**) located in vertical orientation, perpendicular to the face of the cardiac transducer. Cardiac chambers are as follows: left atrium (**a**), left ventricle (**b**), right atrium (**c**), and right ventricle (**d**)

- Two-chamber
  - Figure 3.9—Apical two-chamber
  - Only the left ventricle and left atrium will be seen in this view.
  - This view allows visualization of the anterior and inferior walls of the left ventricle.
  - Video 3.5—Apical two-chamber

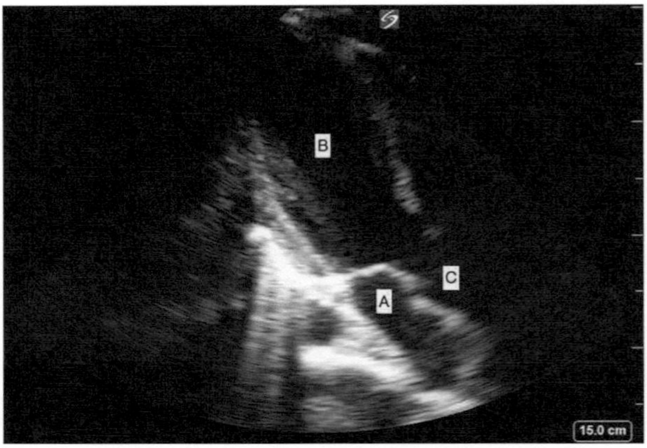

Fig. 3.9 Apical two-chamber: Apical two-chamber cardiac view demonstrating vertical orientation of the heart. Inferior wall of the left ventricle (**b**) is to the left of the image, anterior wall to the right. Left atrium (**a**) and aortic outflow (**c**) are also demonstrated

Subxiphoid

- Transducer Placement
  - Place the transducer just below the xiphoid process with the marker pointed toward the patient's left.
  - Place the operator's hand on top of the transducer, use a moderate amount of force to press the transducer into the patient's abdomen, and angle the transducer superior and toward the left shoulder, nearly flattened against the abdomen.
  - Adjust depth to adequately visualize the entire heart.
  - Figure 3.10—Subxiphoid transducer placement
- Ultrasound Anatomy
  - Figure 3.11—Subxiphoid ultrasound image
  - The liver is anterior to the heart.
  - Posterior to the liver is the right ventricle and right atrium.
  - Posterior to the right heart is the left ventricle and left atrium.
  - Video 3.6—Subxiphoid

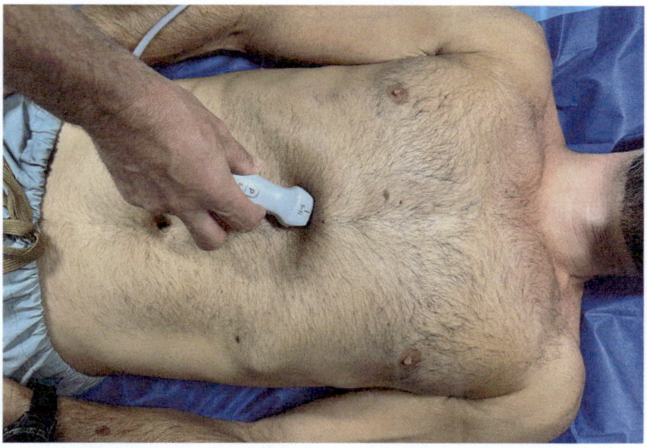

Fig. 3.10 Subxiphoid transducer placement: Place the transducer just below the xiphoid process with the marker pointed toward the patient's left

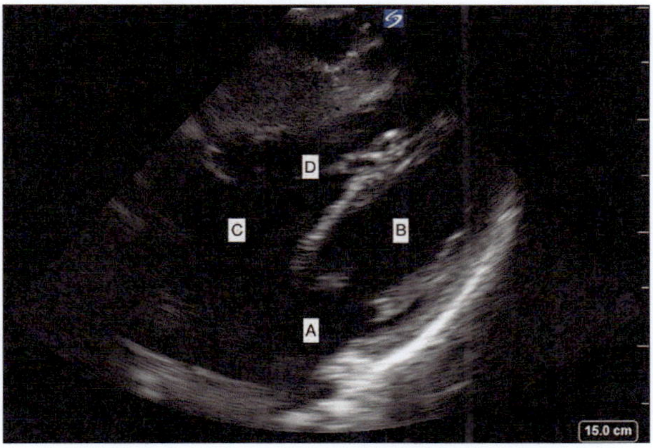

Fig. 3.11 Subxiphoid: Subxiphoid cardiac view demonstrating the heart viewed through the liver window. Cardiac chambers are identified as follows: left atrium (**a**), left ventricle (**b**), right atrium (**c**), right ventricle (**d**)

Inferior Vena Cava

(a) Transducer Placement
- Place the transducer just below the xiphoid process, slightly to the right of midline, with the marker pointed toward the patient's head.
- The transducer should be perpendicular to the spine.
- Figure 3.12—IVC transducer placement

(b) Ultrasound Anatomy
- Figure 3.13—IVC ultrasound image
- IVC will be seen posterior to the liver entering the right atrium.
  - Video 3.7—IVC
- IVC normally collapses with inspiration and dilates with expiration.
  - Dilated IVC with minimal collapse indicates volume overload; impaired cardiac filling, such as with tamponade; outflow obstruction, such as with PE; or cardiogenic shock.

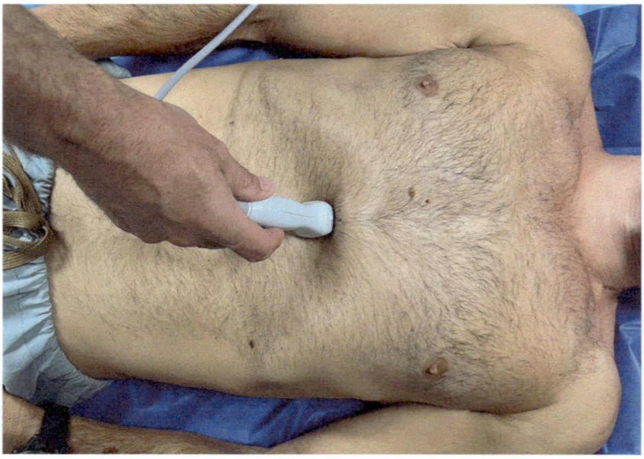

Fig. 3.12 IVC transducer placement: Place the transducer just below the xiphoid process, slightly to the right of midline, with the marker pointed toward the patient's head

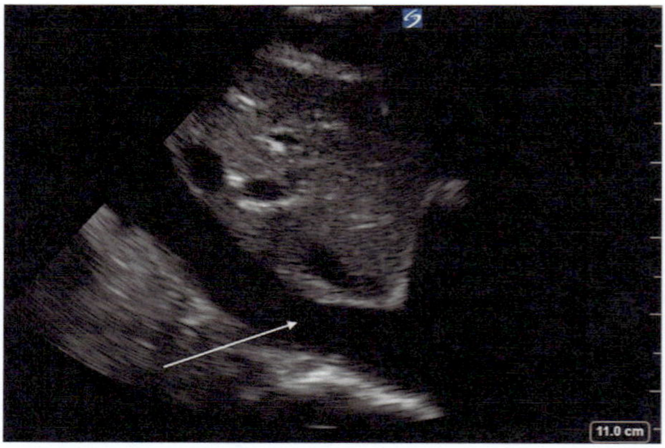

Fig. 3.13 IVC: Inferior vena cava demonstrated in long axis passing by the liver and emptying into the right atrium

    - Figure 3.14—Dilated IVC
    - Video 3.8—Dilated IVC
  - Increased IVC collapse may indicate hypovolemia.
    - Figure 3.15—Collapsed IVC
    - Video 3.9—Collapsed IVC
  - Aorta may be visualized in this view and will be toward patients right with the vertebral body ridges directly posterior to it.
  - In contrast, the IVC traverses the liver so when viewed in sagittal should have liver tissue both anterior and posterior to it.

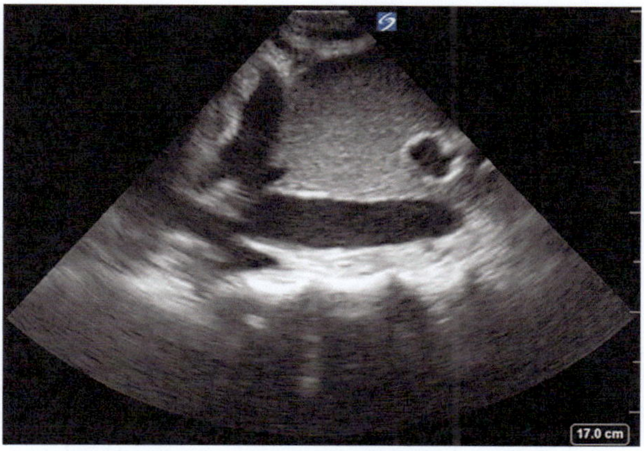

Fig. 3.14 Dilated IVC: Dilated IVC passing by the liver and emptying into the right atrium

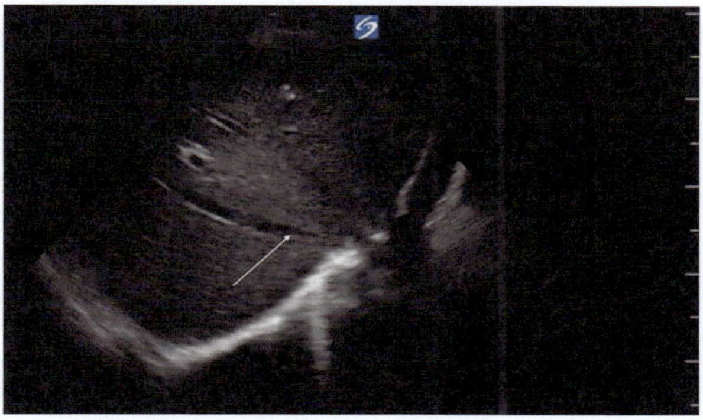

Fig. 3.15 Collapsed IVC: Collapsed IVC (arrow) passing the liver on its course to the right atrium. At times, a collapsed IVC can be so small that it can be difficult to find and image

Measuring Global Left Ventricular Systolic Function

(a) Qualitative scale includes normal, mildly reduced, moderately reduced, or severely reduced:
- Video 3.10—Normal LV systolic function
- Video 3.11—Mildly reduced LV systolic function
- Video 3.12—Moderately reduced LV systolic function
- Video 3.13—Severely reduced LV systolic function

(b) This corresponds to the following quantitative scale:
- Normal ejection fraction (EF) = greater than 50% [2]
- Mildly reduced = 40–49%
- Moderately reduced = 30–39%
- Severely reduced = less than 25% [2]
- Ejection fracture is the percent of blood ejected from the left ventricle into systemic circulation via the aorta

(c) If possible, obtain all cardiac views to evaluate:
- Endocardial wall motion and left ventricular wall thickening during systole.
  - Degree of contractility correlates with left ventricular wall thickening during contraction.
  - Normally the entire left ventricular wall should thicken during systole as the left ventricular cavity decreases in size.
- Left ventricular cavity size during cardiac cycle
  - Left ventricular cavity size should decrease by slightly more than half, indicating a normal ejection fraction.
  - Abnormal cavity size can be seen with dilated and hypertrophic cardiomyopathy.
- Mitral valve movement during diastole and mitral annulus movement during cardiac cycle.
  - Visualize movement of the anterior leaflet of the mitral valve.
    - Anterior leaflet will be closest to transducer.
  - With normal left ventricular function, the anterior leaflet of the mitral valve should touch or come very close to the septum during diastole.
  - Figure 3.16—Mitral valve leaflet touching septum
  - Video 3.14—Normal EF with mitral valve touching the septum

(d) To summarize, with overall reduced function:
- Endocardial walls have less contractility.
- Walls may be hypertrophied or the chamber dilated.
- Anterior leaflet of the mitral valve will not touch the septum.

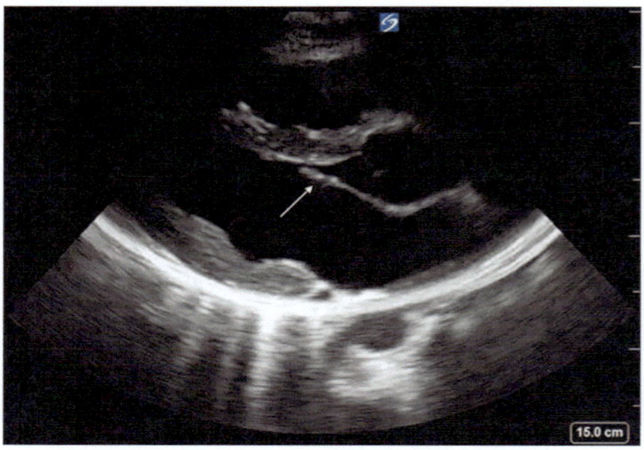

Fig. 3.16 Mitral valve leaflet touching septum: Parasternal long axis image with anterior leaflet of mitral valve (arrow) touching septum during diastole, which is the common state associated with normal ejection fraction

Cardiomyopathies

- Dilated Cardiomyopathy
  - Dilation and decreased left ventricular function [3].
  - Left ventricle will appear like a "water balloon".
  - Characterized by decreased wall thickness and enlarged cavity size.
  - Little change in cavity size during the cardiac cycle.
  - Figure 3.17—Dilated cardiomyopathy
  - Video 3.15—Dilated cardiomyopathy
- Hypertrophic Cardiomyopathy
  - Left ventricular walls appear uniformly thickened with increased overall mass [1].
  - EF can be normal, increased, or decreased.
  - Figure 3.18—Hypertrophic cardiomyopathy
  - Video 3.16—Hypertrophic cardiomyopathy

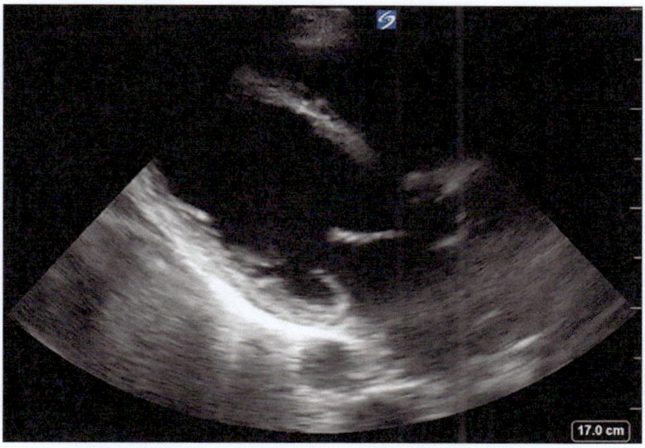

Fig. 3.17 Dilated CM: Parasternal long axis image demonstrating ballooning of LV typical of dilated cardiomyopathy

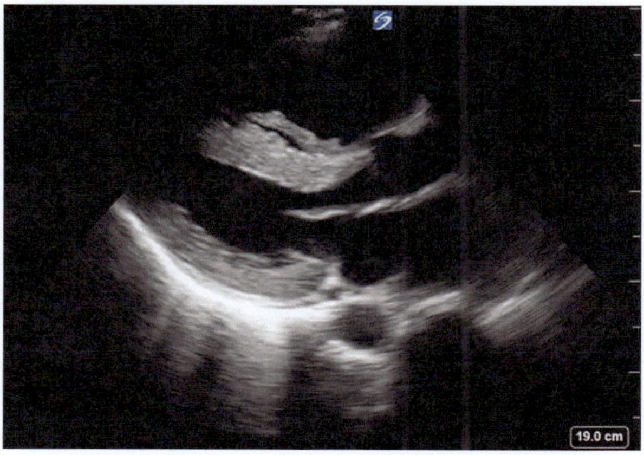

Fig. 3.18 Hypertrophic CM: Parasternal long axis image demonstrating thickened left ventricular walls indicating hypertrophic cardiomyopathy

- Takotsubo Cardiomyopathy
  - Also known as Stress-induced cardiomyopathy.
  - Left ventricle will have apical ballooning and dyskinesis [3].
  - Base of the left ventricle maintains its normal structure.
  - Figure 3.19—Takotsubo cardiomyopathy
  - Video 3.17—Takotsubo cardiomyopathy
- Hypertrophic Obstructive Cardiomyopathy
  - Septal hypertrophy that leads to impaired outflow due to obstruction [1].
  - Can cause sudden cardiac death in young adults with exercise.
  - Figure 3.20—Hypertrophic obstructive cardiomyopathy
  - Video 3.18—Hypertrophic obstructive cardiomyopathy

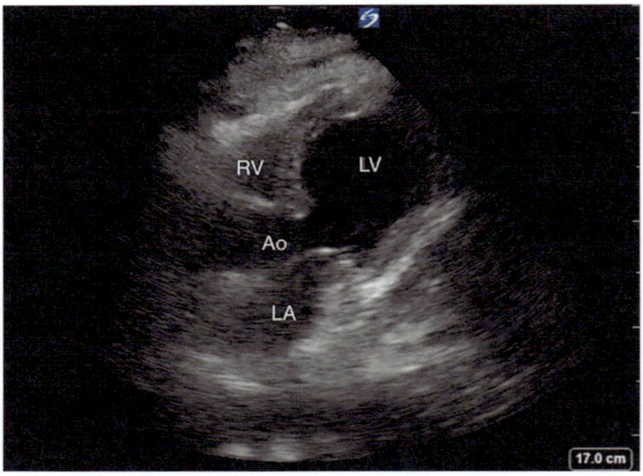

Fig. 3.19 Takotsubo cardiomyopathy: Note the isolated apical dilation of the left ventricle (LV) in this subxiphoid view of takotsubo cardiomyopathy, named after the Japanese word for octopus trap

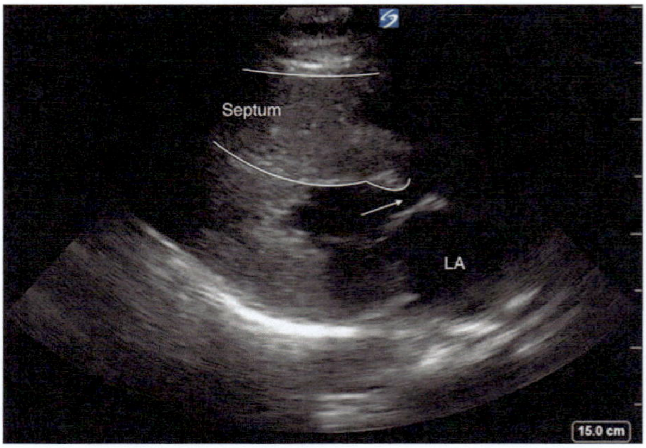

Fig. 3.20 Hypertrophic obstructive cardiomyopathy: This is a parasternal long view of HOCM. Note the enlarged septum denoted by white lines and the subsequent small outflow tract (arrow)

Right Ventricular Dilation

(a) Right ventricular imaging is used to evaluate for enlargement or strain, particularly in the setting of acute pulmonary embolism (PE).
(b) In a nonacute setting, it can be used to evaluate for other causes of elevated right heart pressures such as pulmonary hypertension.
(c) Evaluate the heart using all cardiac views if possible.
- Parasternal long
  - May see right ventricle enlargement or flattening of the septal wall into the left ventricle cavity [2].
  - Figure 3.21—Parasternal long dilated RV
  - Video 3.19—PSL dilated RV
- Parasternal short
  - Allows size comparison of the right ventricle to the left ventricle.
  - Enlarged right ventricle may cause the left ventricle to appear "D"-shaped indicating septal flattening or bowing into the left ventricular cavity [2].
    - Highly suggestive of acute PE in the appropriate clinical setting.
    - Figure 3.22—Parasternal short with dilated RV
    - Video 3.20—PSS with dilated RV
- Apical four-chamber
  - Optimal view to directly compare the right and left ventricle cavity size.
  - Normal RV/LV cavity ratio is 0.6:1 in diastole [4]
    - Ratio of 0.7–1:1 suggests mild to moderate enlargement [4].
    - Ratio of greater than 1:1 represents severe dilation [4] and is highly suggestive of acute pulmonary embolism in the in appropriate clinical setting.
  - Figure 3.23—Apical four-chamber RV dilation
  - Video 3.21—Apical four-chamber with RV dilation
- Inferior vena cava (IVC)
  - With an acutely enlarged right ventricle, evaluating the IVC will provide adjunctive information.
  - Dilated, plethoric IVC further supports the diagnosis of elevated right heart pressures.

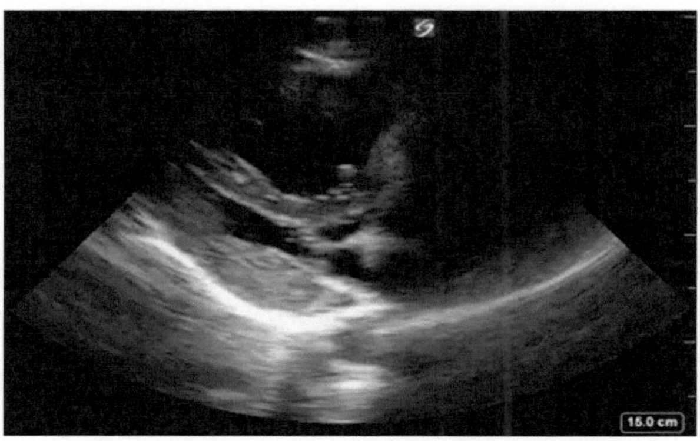

Fig. 3.21 Parasternal long dilated right ventricle: Parasternal long axis image showing severely dilated right ventricle and associated collapsed left ventricle

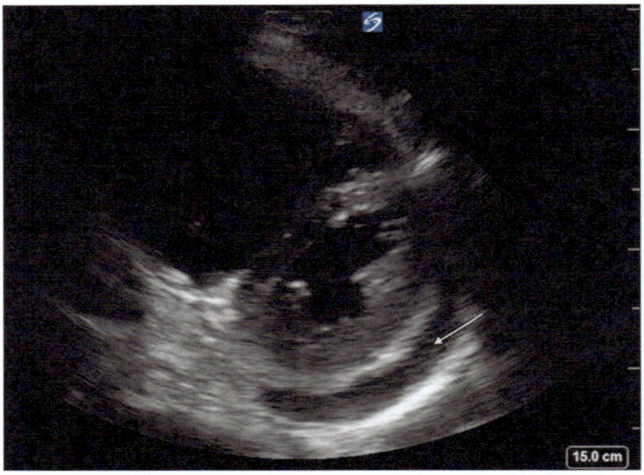

Fig. 3.22 Parasternal short dilated right ventricle: Parasternal short axis image showing enlarged RV when compared to the LV. This results in septal bowing toward the LV that causes it to appear "D-shaped." Small effusion denoted by arrow

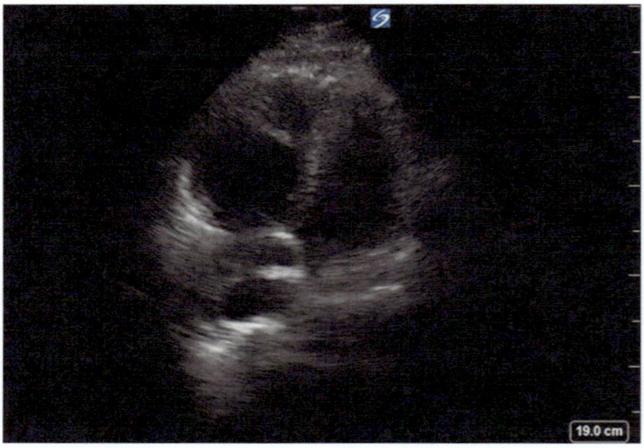

Fig. 3.23 Apical four-chamber right ventricle dilation: Apical four-chamber image showing RV/LV ratio of greater than 1:1, indicating severe RV dilation

Pericardial Effusion and Tamponade

(a) Pericardial effusion occurs when fluid accumulates between the visceral and parietal pericardium.
- There can be approximately 10–50 mL of fluid within the pericardial space, which is considered physiologic and often not visualized on echocardiography [5].
- Appears as a hypoechoic stripe between the heart and brightly echogenic pericardium.
  - Figure 3.24—Pericardial effusion
  - Video 3.22—Pericardial effusion parasternal long
  - Video 3.23—Pericardial effusion parasternal short

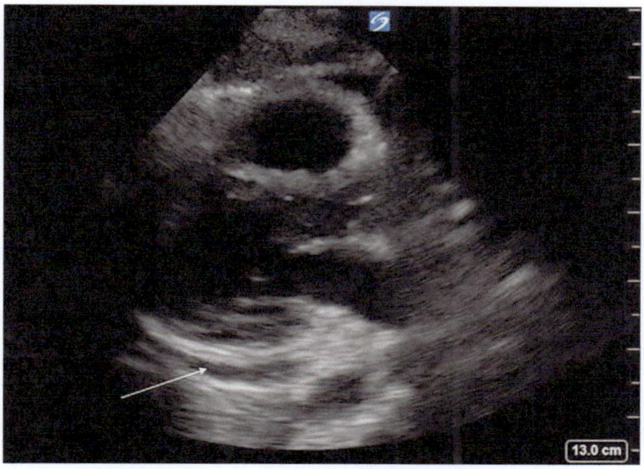

Fig. 3.24 Pericardial effusion: Small pericardial effusion (arrow) seen in parasternal long view, seen during diastole. Note the fluid extending anterior to the descending thoracic aorta, differentiating it from pleural effusion

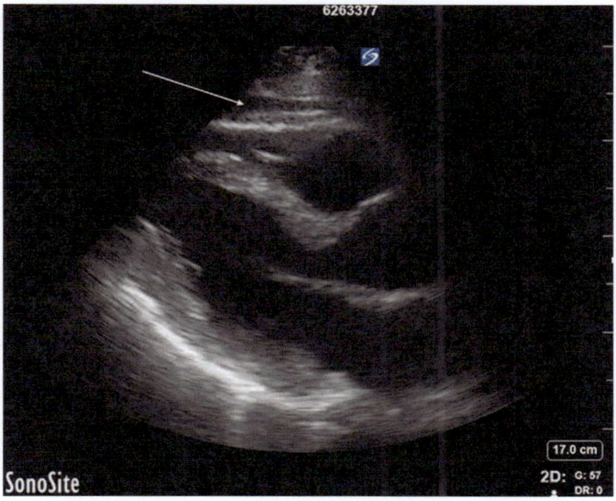

Fig. 3.25 Epicardial fat pad: An epicardial fat pad may be present anterior to the right ventricle and can be very similar in appearance to a small pericardial effusion in a parasternal long view; often they can be indistinguishable. However, small pericardial effusions will typically be seen posterior to the left ventricle, and an epicardial fat pad will be seen anterior to the right ventricle

- An epicardial fat pad may be present anterior to the right ventricle and can be confused with small pericardial effusion in the parasternal long view.
  - An epicardial fat pad will be anterior to the right ventricle in the parasternal long view.
  - Can sometimes be distinguished from blood or fluid by a speckled appearance [1].
  - More common in diabetics, obese, elderly, and females [1].
  - Figure 3.25—Epicardial fat pad
- You can distinguish a left pleural effusion from a pericardial effusion by the pattern of fluid.
  - Pericardial fluid will be present posterior to the left ventricular wall and anterior to the descending aorta [1].

   - Left-sided pleural effusion will occur posterior to the left ventricular wall and will not be present anterior to the descending aorta [1].
   - Figure 3.26—Pericardial effusion vs. left-sided pleural effusion

(b) Pericardial Effusion Grading
   - Trace pericardial effusions appear as a thin stripe of dependent hypoechoic fluid between the two pericardial layers.
   - For circumferential effusions:
     - Small effusions have a hypoechoic stripe measuring less than 5 mm [1, 3].
       - Figure 3.27—Small pericardial effusion (<0.5 cm)
     - Moderate effusions have approximately 5–20 mm of separation between pericardial layers [1, 3].
       - Figure 3.28—Moderate pericardial effusion (0.5–2 cm)

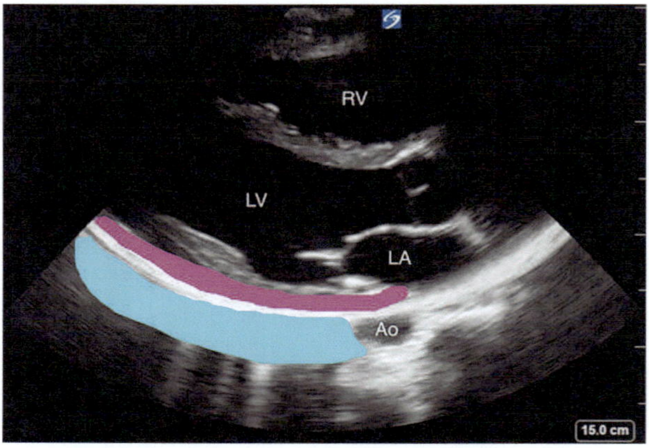

Fig. 3.26 Pericardial effusion vs. left-sided pleural effusion: This parasternal long view demonstrates the distinguishing features of the relative locations for where pericardial effusions (pink) and pleural effusions (blue) would appear. Notice the pericardial effusion will travel anterior to the descending aorta, whereas the pleural effusion will not

Fig. 3.27 Small pericardial effusion (<0.5 cm): Small-sized pericardial effusion seen posterior to the left ventricle (arrow) in this parasternal long view

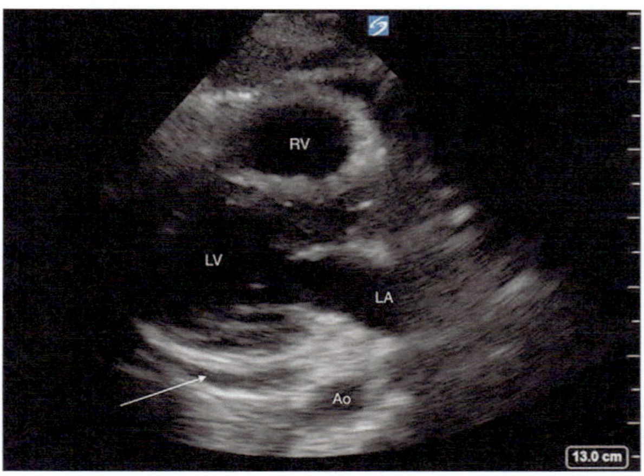

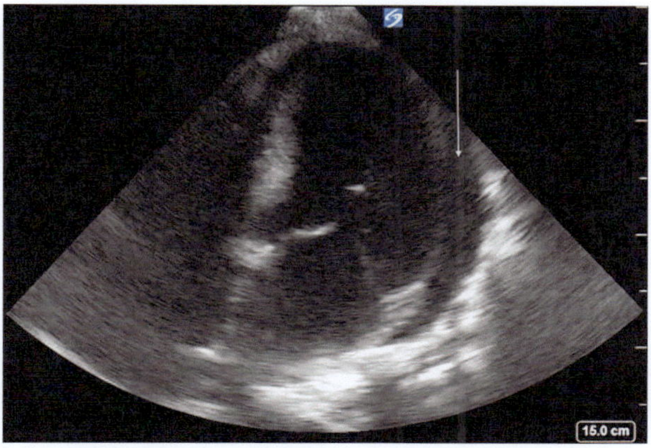

Fig. 3.28 Moderate pericardial effusion (0.5–2 cm): Moderate-sized pericardial effusion (arrow) seen in an apical four-chamber view

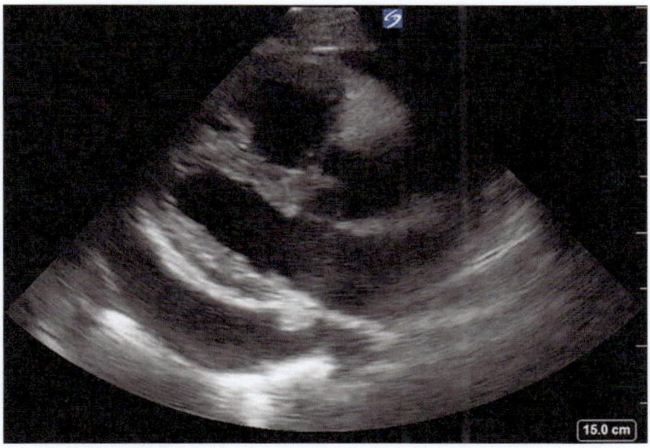

Fig. 3.29 Large pericardial effusion (>2 cm): Large-sized pericardial effusion is noted here in this parasternal long view

- Large effusions have greater than 20 mm of separation from the left ventricular wall [1, 3].
  - Corresponds to greater than 500 mL of fluid [5]
  - Figure 3.29—Large pericardial effusion (>2 cm)

(c) Tamponade

- Occurs when fluid within the pericardium generates excessive external pressure, which then impairs the ability for the heart chambers to fill eventually causing hypotension and shock.
  - Affects the thin-walled right atrium and right ventricle first
    - Video 3.24—Tamponade parasternal long
    - Video 3.25—Tamponade subxiphoid
  - Right atrial systolic collapse [3, 4] is the most sensitive sign of tamponade
    - Usually the first echocardiographic sign
    - Figure 3.30—RA collapse in tamponade

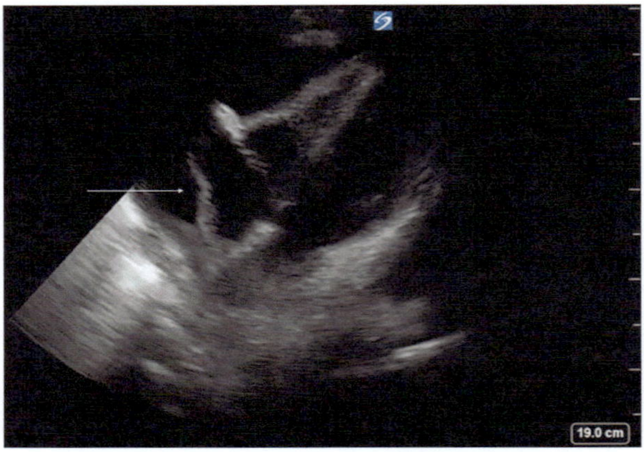

Fig. 3.30 RA collapse in tamponade: RA collapse in pericardial tamponade (arrow). This is the most sensitive sign for pericardial tamponade

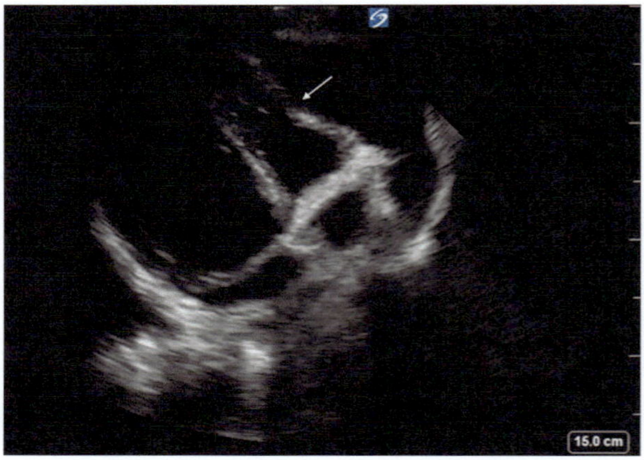

Fig. 3.31 RV collapse in tamponade: RV collapse during diastole is seen here (arrow) in this subxiphoid view of pericardial tamponade. This is the most specific sign for pericardial tamponade

- Right ventricular diastolic collapse [3, 4] is the most specific sign of tamponade
  - Figure 3.31—RV collapse in tamponade
- These findings may be subtle, M-mode can be used to help better visualize the amount of collapsibility.
  - Using M-Mode, place the cursor through the RV free wall, tracking through the mitral valve.
  - This will give you an image traced over time, which shows how these chambers change throughout the cardiac cycle.
  - In tamponade, the RV free wall will collapse during diastole, or when the mitral valve opens.
  - Figure 3.32—M-mode showing RV collapse during tamponade
- Plethoric IVC with minimal collapse will also be evident [4]

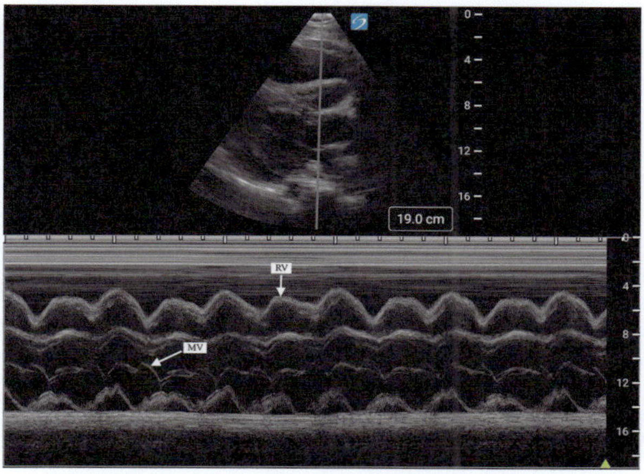

Fig. 3.32 RV collapse in tamponade: RV (arrow) diastolic collapse, while MV open (arrow)

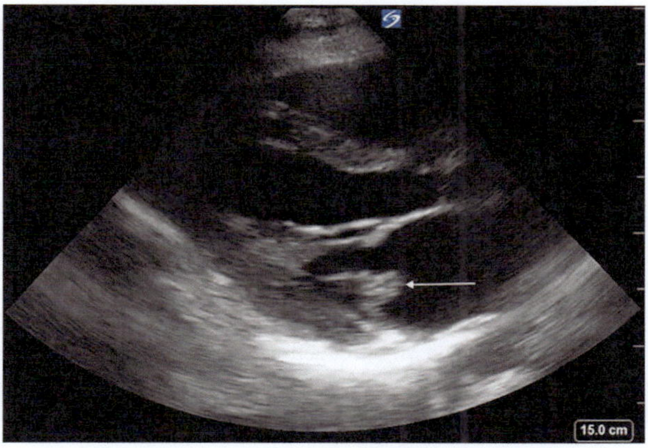

Fig. 3.33 Endocarditis: Parasternal long image showing posterior mitral valve leaflet vegetation (arrow) on upstream atrial side of leaflet

Endocarditis

(a) Endocarditis occurs when bacteria in the blood stream coagulate on the downstream side of valve leaflets. It can be possible to diagnose endocarditis by transthoracic echocardiography, but this modality is less sensitive than transesophageal echocardiography, which is the gold standard.
- Endocarditis can be diagnosed by visualizing an echogenic, mobile lucency attached to one or more valves.
  - Figure 3.33—Endocarditis
  - Video 3.26—Endocarditis

Key Points

- Echocardiography is a difficult skill and requires repeated practice to become competent.
- Depending on the patient, you may have to adjust your transducer or move up or down a rib space to find the optimal window.
- Placing the patient in a left lateral decubitus position, with the left arm above the head, can improve image quality by moving the heart closer to the chest wall and opening rib spaces.
- Each TTE involves systemic evaluation for key functions of the heart and evaluation for the presence of key pathology: reduced ejection fraction, enlarged RV, and pericardial effusion.
- Limitations to adequate transthoracic echocardiography include:
  - Morbidly obese patients
  - COPD
  - Positive pressure ventilation
  - Subcutaneous emphysema
  - Patients' status post-midline sternotomy

References

1. Rasalingam R, Makan M, Perez JE, editors. The Washington manual of echocardiography. Philadelphia: Wolters Kluwer Health/Lippincott Williams & Wilkins; 2013.
2. Reardon RF, Laudenbach A, Joing SA. Chapter 6: Cardiac. In: Ma OJ, Mateer JR, Reardon RF, Joing SA, editors. Emergency ultrasound. 3rd ed. New York: McGraw-Hill Education; 2014. p. 93–168.
3. Otto CM. Textbook of clinical echocardiography. 5th ed. Philadelphia: Elsevier Saunders; 2013.
4. Mallin M, Dawson M. Introduction to bedside ultrasound: volume 2. United States of America: emergency ultrasound solutions; 2013. iBook. https://itun.es/us/ueELM.l.
5. Jung HO. Pericardial effusion and pericardiocentesis: role of echocardiography. Korean Circ J. 2012;42(11):725–34. https://www.ncbi.nlm.nih.gov/pmc/articles/PMC3518705/. Accessed 30 Apr 2017.

4 Advanced Transthoracic Echocardiography

Michael R. Jones, Jordan Tozer, and Michael J. Vitto

Advanced cardiac echocardiography builds upon foundational transthoracic imaging to offer a more detailed, dynamic, and clinically nuanced evaluation of cardiovascular function. As cardiac pathology becomes increasingly complex and management more time-sensitive, advanced echocardiographic techniques—such as quantitative cardiac output measurements, dynamic valve evaluations, and right heart imaging—have emerged as essential tools in both diagnostic precision and therapeutic decision-making. This chapter explores these advanced modalities, emphasizing their clinical applications, technical considerations, and interpretive challenges organized by various pathologies. By integrating evolving technology with bedside clinical acumen, advanced echocardiography continues to redefine the role of noninvasive imaging in modern medical care.

Supplementary Information The online version contains supplementary material available at https://doi.org/10.1007/978-3-032-27643-8_4.

M. R. Jones (✉)
Department of Emergency Medicine, Virginia Commonwealth University Medical Center, Richmond, VA, USA
e-mail: michael.jones6@vcuhealth.org

J. Tozer · M. J. Vitto
Department of Emergency Medicine, Virginia Commonwealth University Health, Richmond, VA, USA
e-mail: jordan.tozer@vcuhealth.org; michael.vitto@vcuhealth.org

A. Lindsay et al. (eds.), *Clinical Ultrasound*,
https://doi.org/10.1007/978-3-032-27643-8_4

Reduced Ejection Fraction

- E-point Septal Separation (EPSS)
  - As indicated in the basic cardiac ultrasound chapter, ejection fraction (EF) can be estimated by visualizing how closely the anterior leaflet of the mitral valve comes to the septum during diastole.
  - This distance can be measured to provide an estimate of ejection fraction.
  - To obtain this measurement:
    - Obtain the parasternal long-axis view.
    - Place your M-mode cursor through the septum and the anterior mitral valve leaflet.
    - Obtain your M-mode tracing and freeze the image produced.
    - You will see a tracing of the anterior mitral valve leaflet with two distinct peaks.
      - The first is called the E wave for "early diastolic" filling.
      - The second is called the A wave for the "atrial kick."
    - Measure the distance between the peak of the E wave and the septum.
  - A measurement of less than 7 mm supports a normal ejection fraction [1].
  - A measurement of greater than 10 suggests a reduced ejection fraction [1].
    - Figure 4.1
- Mitral Annular Plane Systolic Excursion (MAPSE)
  - When the heart suffers from ischemia, it is often the endocardial fibers that are the first to be affected. This is because these fibers are furthest from the blood supply.
  - The endocardial fibers are primarily arrayed in the longitudinal plane, contributing to longitudinal contraction of the myocardium.
  - MAPSE is a surrogate measurement of myocardial contraction in the longitudinal plane and can be used to evaluate myocardial contraction and ejection fraction.
  - To obtain this measurement:
    - Obtain the apical four-chamber view.
    - Place your M-mode cursor through the lateral mitral annulus.
    - Obtain your M-mode tracing and freeze the image produced.

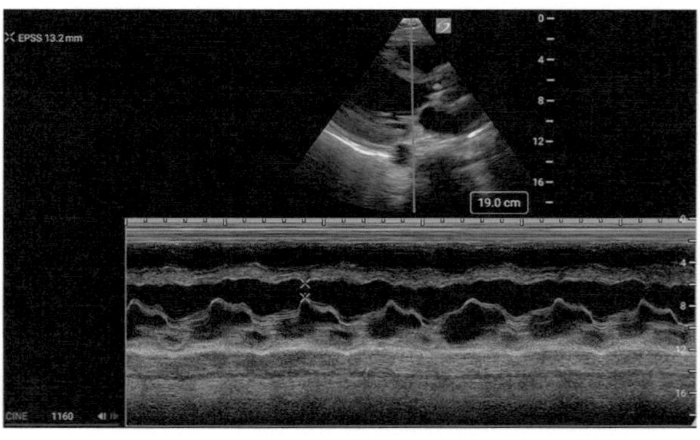

Fig. 4.1 E-point septal separation (EPSS) measurement obtained using M-mode and measuring the distance from the E-point to the septum. An EPSS measurement of 13.2 as demonstrated here indicates reduced ejection fraction

- You will see a tracing with a sine wave appearance, having peaks and troughs.
  - The peak indicates when the mitral annulus is closest to the cardiac apex, indicating contraction of the myocardial fibers (systole).
  - The trough indicates when the mitral annulus is furthest away from the cardiac apex, indicating relaxation of the myocardial fibers (diastole).
- Measure the vertical distance between the peak and the trough.
- A measurement of greater than 12 mm supports a normal ejection fraction [2].
  - Figure 4.2
- A measurement of less than 7 mm suggests a reduced ejection fraction [3].

- Simpson's Method of Discs
  - Because ejection fraction is the volume of blood ejected with each contraction, the most accurate method of measuring this would be to measure the volume of the LV cavity during diastole and the volume of the LV during systole and obtain the percent difference.
  - These volumes can be estimated in a noninvasive manner with ultrasound by tracing the border of the LV endocardium in two orthogonal planes.
  - Advanced calculation packages of bedside ultrasound machines have the ability to estimate volume by adding a series of "discs" together that can be obtained by tracing the endocardial border of the LV in two orthogonal planes.
  - The addition of these volumetric "discs" generated by tracing the LV endocardial border in end diastole and end systole allow for calculation of the percent change.
  - This is called Simpson's Method of Discs or simply Simpson's Method for estimating ejection fraction.
  - To obtain this measurement:
    - You will first need to ensure your ultrasound machine has the calculation package that includes Simpson's Method

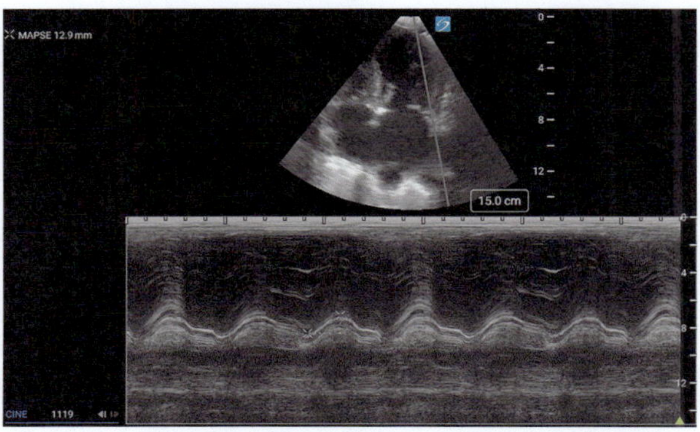

Fig. 4.2 Mitral annular plane systolic excursion (MAPSE) measurement calculated by obtaining an M-mode tracing of the lateral mitral annulus during multiple cardiac cycles. MAPSE is measured by obtaining the vertical distance between the peak and trough of the mitral annular movement. A MAPSE measurement of 12.9 as demonstrated here indicates normal ejection fraction

  - Obtain your apical four-chamber view
    - Freeze the view in end diastole
    - Trace the endocardial border
      - Begin at the medial mitral valve annulus and end at the lateral valve annulus.
      - Include the papillary muscles in the volumetric estimate.
      - Save your tracing
    - Cycle forward or backward to freeze the view in end systole.
    - Trace the endocardial border using the same technique as above and save your tracing
  - Obtain the apical two-chamber view by rotating the probe 90° counter-clockwise from the apical four-chamber view.
    - Freeze the view in end diastole.
    - Trace the endocardial border using the same technique as above and save your tracing.
    - Cycle forward or backward to freeze the view in end systole.
    - Trace the endocardial border using the same technique as above and save your tracing.
  - Your calculation package will display an ejection fraction.
    - Figure 4.3
- The percentage calculated for ejection fraction will correspond to ejection fraction percentage to diagnose normal, mildly reduced, moderately reduced, or severely reduced ejection fraction [4, 5].

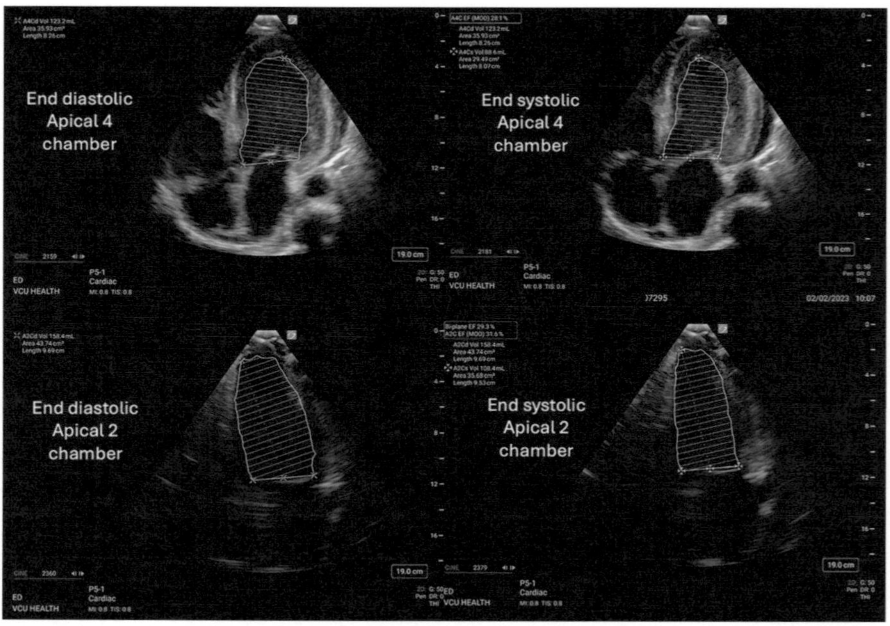

Fig. 4.3 Simpson's method of discs for measuring ejection fraction is demonstrated here. The myocardial border is traced in end diastole and end systole in both the apical four-chamber and apical two-chamber views. Using a calculation package, an ejection fraction can be obtained

Cardiac Output

- When evaluating for reduced ejection fraction, it can also be useful to estimate the patient's cardiac output. However, this can also be useful in determining fluid responsiveness in addition to other applications.
- This will estimate the patient's cardiac output in liters of blood per minute, which can then be converted to cardiac index by incorporating the patient's body surface area.
- Indications:
  - Reduced EF
  - Cardiogenic shock
  - Fluid responsiveness
- Concepts behind this method:
  - Cardiac output is defined as follows: CO = SV × HR
    - SV: Stroke volume
    - HR: Heart rate
  - We can calculate stroke volume with ultrasound and multiply by heart rate to obtain cardiac output.
  - Stroke volume can be obtained by measuring the volume of blood ejected with each contraction.
    - Volume is area multiplied by length or distance.
    - We can calculate the cylinder of blood ejected with each contraction as follows:
    - Obtain the area of your "cylinder" of blood ejected by measuring the diameter of the LVOT. Your machine will estimate the area based upon the diameter.
    - Obtain the length of your "cylinder" of blood by taking the velocity time integral (VTI) of the pulse wave Doppler tracing during ejection of blood through the LVOT.
- How to obtain this measurement:
  - Obtain the parasternal long-axis view.
    - Freeze the image in mid-systole
    - Measure the diameter of the LVOT at the proximal aortic valve leaflets.
      - Figure 4.4
    - Save the diameter measurement
  - Obtain the apical five-chamber view (similar to the apical four-chamber view, but fanned slightly more anteriorly to see the LVOT–see Video 4.1)
    - Place the pulse wave Doppler gate at the LVOT where you measured the diameter.
    - Begin your pulse wave Doppler tracing and freeze the image when you obtain multiple systolic tracings.
      - Ideally, your tracing should have a sharp upstroke and minimal spectral broadening.

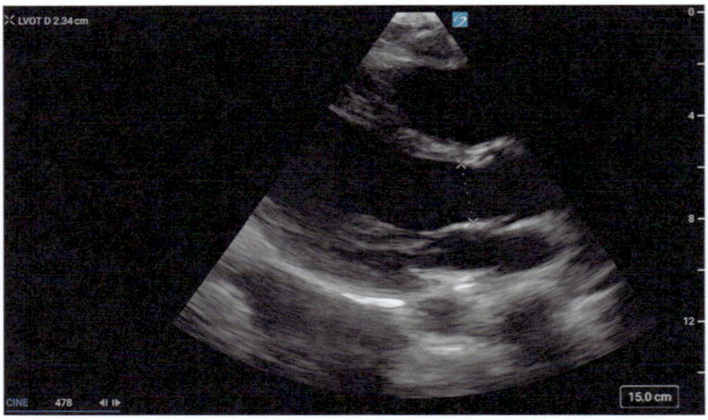

Fig. 4.4 Left ventricular outflow tract (LVOT) measurement in the parasternal long axis

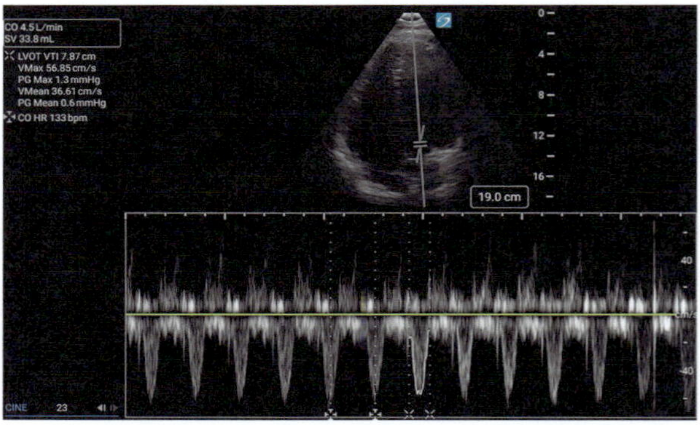

Fig. 4.5 Pulse wave Doppler tracing through the left ventricular outflow tract (LVOT) is demonstrated here. The Doppler tracing is then traced, and the velocity time integral (VTI) is calculated. This is multiplied by the heart rate to obtain the cardiac output

        - Obtain the velocity time integral by tracing the Doppler tracing from the beginning to the end of the cardiac cycle.
        - Save the measurement
            - Figure 4.5
    - The machine's calculation package should calculate a VTI and stroke volume.
    - Calculate the heart rate by placing calipers on each systolic peak.
    - The machine's calculation package will calculate cardiac output based on the stroke volume and heart rate [6].
- Expected measurements for cardiac output:
    - Normal at rest: 4–8 L/min [7]
    - Abnormal: Less than 4 L/m or greater than 8 L/min [7]
- Expected measurement for cardiac index:
    - Normal at rest: 2.5–4 L/min/m^2 [7]
    - Abnormal: Less than 2 L/min/m^2 [7]

Bedside Echo Assessment in Left Ventricular Assist Devices (LVAD)

- In some patients, ejection fraction and cardiac output will become so low that they may require a left ventricular assist device (LVAD) to support their cardiac output.
- LVADs change cardiac physiology and can have complications, which can be assessed by using ultrasound.
- When assessing a patient with an LVAD, the following views should be obtained:
  - Parasternal long axis
    - Figure 4.6, Video 4.2
    - Evaluate the left ventricular walls. If they are coming too close together, this could indicate a suction event.
    - Evaluate the aortic valve. If it appears to be opening significantly, this could indicate pump thrombosis.
    - Evaluate the mitral valve with a color flow box. This can indicate whether severe mitral regurgitation is present.
  - Parasternal short axis
    - Video 4.3
    - Evaluate the LV walls again for evidence of a suction event.
    - Evaluate the cannula to see if it appears to be in the correct place.
  - Apical four chamber
    - Video 4.4
    - Evaluate the LV and RV walls
    - Evaluate the MV and TV
    - Evaluate the cannula
  - Subxiphoid
    - Repeat above
  - IVC
    - Evaluate for evidence of hypovolemia, which could precipitate a suction event or hypervolemia, which could indicate fluid overload

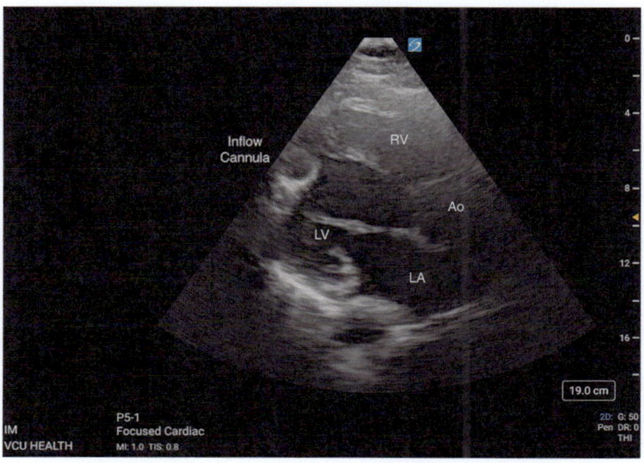

Fig. 4.6 Left ventricular assist device (LVAD) with inflow cannula visible at the apex of the left ventricle. LA left atrium, LV left ventricle, RV right ventricle, Ao Aortic outflow tract

Aortic Dissection

- Aortic dissection is a rare, but life-threatening diagnosis which ultrasound can be instrumental in evaluating.
  - Ultrasound may visualize a dissection flap, which would be diagnostic.
  - Ultrasound may also pick up secondary findings of a dissection, which can lead to the diagnosis.
  - The SPEED protocol [8] is an ultrasound protocol used for the evaluation of aortic dissection. Within this protocol, look for the following findings:
    - Intimal dissection flap
      - Figure 4.7a [9], b, Video 4.5
    - Dilated aortic outflow tract
      - Figure 4.8, Video 4.5
    - Pericardial effusion
      - Figure 4.9
    - If one of these findings is detected, it is considered a positive test.
- How to perform the SPEED protocol for aortic dissection:
  - Obtain the parasternal long-axis view and visualize the aortic outflow tract.
    - Look for an intimal dissection flap in the aortic outflow tract.
    - Look for aortic outflow track diameter measuring more than 35 mm.
    - Look for pericardial effusion posterior to the left ventricle, but anterior to descending aorta.
    - Look for an intimal dissection flap in the descending aorta in cross-section visualized in the far field of the parasternal long axis.
  - Obtain a subxiphoid view of the heart
    - Rotate 90° and visualize the aorta (left of the IVC) in the long axis.
    - Look for an intimal dissection flap in the abdominal aorta.
      - Video 4.6
    - If a dissection flap is identified, confirm this finding by obtaining an image of the dissection flap in the short axis.
      - Rotate 90° while keeping the aortic dissection flap in view.
      - Video 4.7

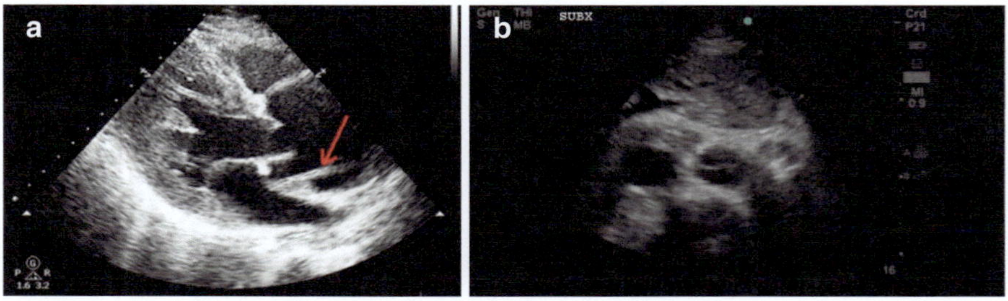

Fig. 4.7 (**a**) Dissection flap demonstrated in the parasternal long axis with evidence of dilated aortic root [9]. (**b**) Dissection flab demonstrated in the transverse subxiphoid view of the aorta

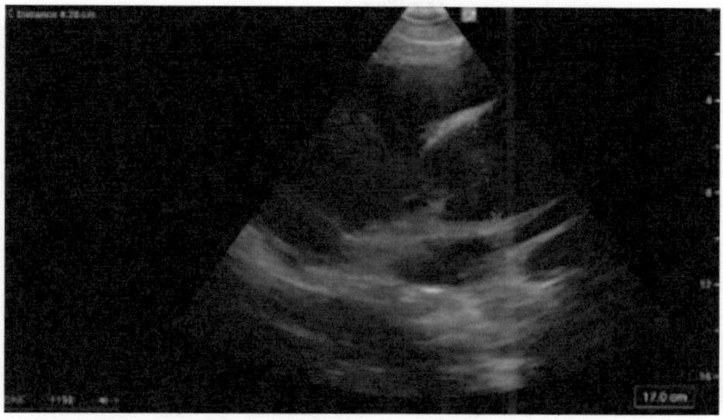

Fig. 4.8 Dilated aortic root is demonstrated as a secondary sign of dissection

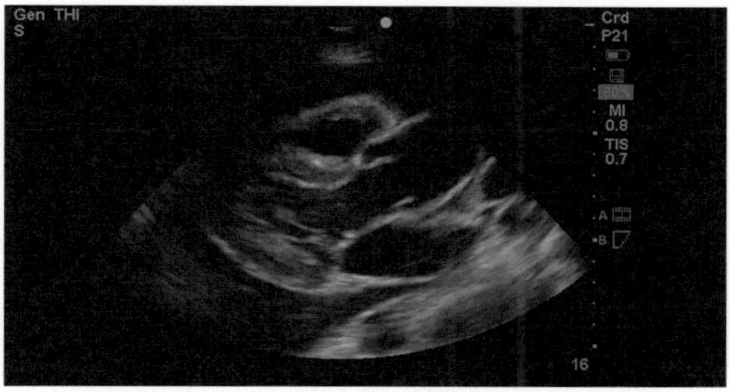

Fig. 4.9 Pericardial effusion demonstrated as a secondary sign of dissection

  - The SPEED protocol provided the following test characteristics:
    - Sensitivity of 93.2% and specificity of 90.9 [8]
    - Positive and negative predictive values of 26.3% and 99.7% [8]
- The suprasternal notch view, which is an additional view to evaluate the aortic arch
  - Obtain the suprasternal notch view by placing the probe with the indicator to the patient's left (in cardiac orientation).
  - Visualize the aortic arch and its branches (brachiocephalic, carotid, subclavian).
  - Look for an intimal dissection flap.
    - Figure 4.10
    - Video 4.8

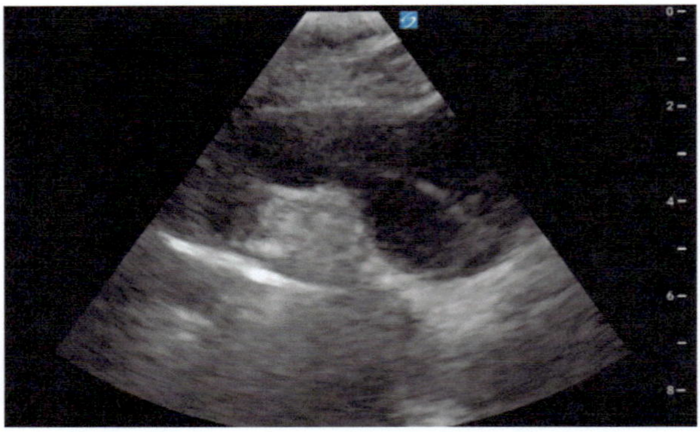

Fig. 4.10 Dissection flap demonstrated in the suprasternal notch view

Aortic Valve

- When evaluating the aortic valve, it is important to identify both aortic stenosis and aortic regurgitation. While there are many methods and measurements for these conditions, we will focus on the simplest and most accessible methods for ease of implementation.
- Aortic stenosis
  - Aortic stenosis can be evaluated qualitatively by viewing the aortic valve in the parasternal long axis, parasternal short axis, and apical five-chamber view.
    - Evaluate the valve to estimate whether the aortic valve appears to be opening completely.
    - Evaluate the valve to see if there are calcifications to suggest sclerosis.
      - This would appear as more prominently hyperechoic aortic valve leaflets.
      - There may be posterior acoustic shadowing due to calcifications.
  - AS can also be measured quantitatively by planimetry (measuring the aortic valve area opening during systole).
    - How to obtain this measurement:
      - Obtain a parasternal short-axis view.
      - Slide up the axis of the heart toward the base of the heart until you see the aortic valve orifice.
      - Visualize the "Mercedes-Benz" sign of the aortic valve.
        - Figure 4.11
        - Video 4.9
      - Measure the maximum area of the valve orifice opening during systole.
        - Figure 4.12 [10]

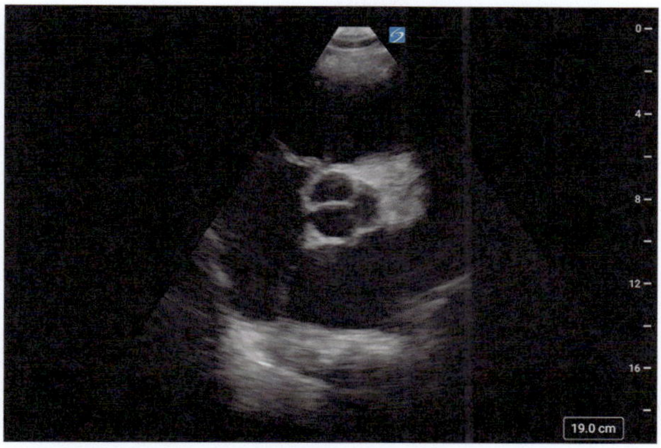

Fig. 4.11 "Mercedes Benz" sign of the aortic valve demonstrated in the parasternal short axis of the heart with slight adjustment of probe toward the base of the heart

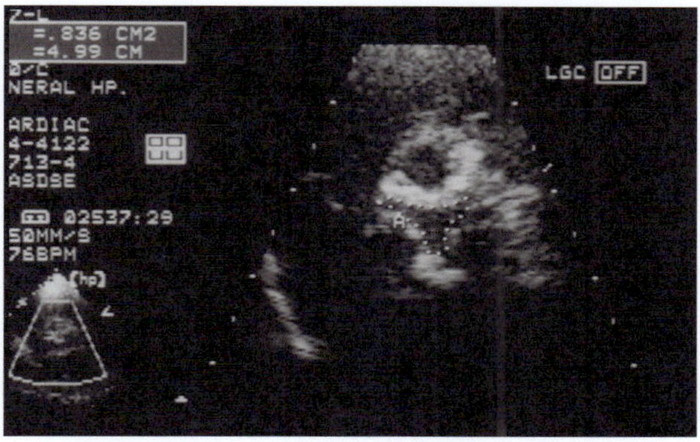

Fig. 4.12 Aortic stenosis demonstrated by measurement of 2D planimetry of the aortic valve during systole in the parenteral short axis of the heart [10]

    - AS grading using this method is as follows:
      - Mild: >1.5 cm^2
      - Moderate: 1.5–1 cm^2
      - Severe: <1 cm^2 [10]
  - AS can also be measured quantitatively by measuring the peak velocity across the aortic valve.
    - How to obtain this measurement:
      - Acquire the apical five-chamber view of the heart with the aortic outflow tract and aortic valve in view.
        - Video 4.1
      - Place continuous wave Doppler through the aortic outflow tract with the focus just distal to the aortic valve.
      - Begin the continuous wave Doppler tracing and freeze after multiple cardiac cycles.
      - Measure the peak velocity through the aortic outflow tract.
        - Figure 4.13

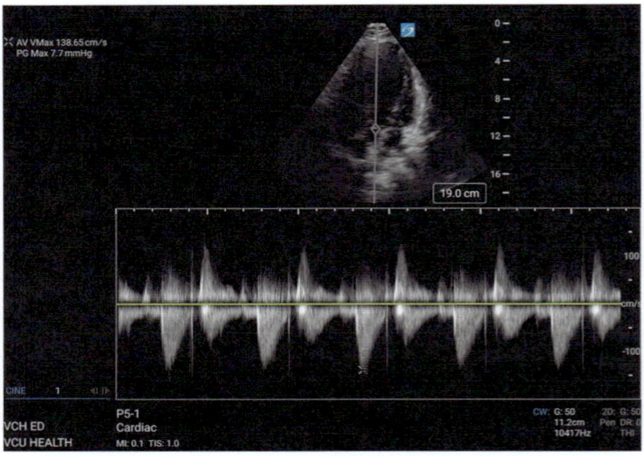

Fig. 4.13 Peak velocity measurement of flow through the aortic valve using continuous wave Doppler. This figure demonstrates normal peak velocity

    - Aortic stenosis severity grading is as follows
      - Mild: 250–300 cm/s
      - Moderate: 300–400 cm/s
      - Severe: >400 cm/s [11, 12]
    - While simple, this method of measurement has significant limitations:
      - Not reliable in patients with reduced cardiac output.
      - Patients with atrial fibrillation need an average of multiple measurements.
  - AS can be measured quantitatively by the continuity equation
    - This equation is based on the principle: $A_1 \times VTI_1 = A_2 \times VTI_2$.
      - We can easily measure the area of the LVOT and the VTI at the LVOT (A_1 and VTI_1, respectively).
      - We can measure the peak velocity distal to the aortic valve (VTI_2) and solve for the area of stenosis (A2).
    - How to obtain this measurement:
      - Obtain the apical five-chamber view of the heart.
        - Video 4.1
      - Measure the LVOT and save (A_1)
        - Figure 4.4
      - Measure the VTI at the LVOT using pulse wave Doppler and save (VTI_1)
        - Figure 4.14
      - Measure the VTI distal to the aortic valve using continuous wave Doppler and save (VTI_2)
      - Solve for A_2.
        - $A_2 = (A_1 \times VTI_1)/VTI_2$
    - AS grading using this method is as follows:
      - Mild: >1.5 cm^2
      - Moderate: 1.5–1 cm^2
      - Severe: <1 cm^2 [12]

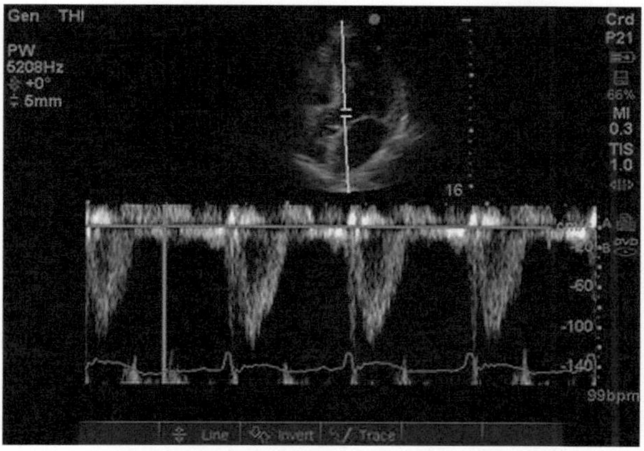

Fig. 4.14 Peak velocity of flow at the left ventricular outflow tract (LVOT) obtained by pulse wave Doppler at the LVOT. This can be used in the continuity equation or dimensionless index for evaluation of aortic stenosis. (Hlaing and Panzer [13]—Scientific Figure on ResearchGate

  - AS can be measured quantitatively by the dimensionless index
    - Using the principle of the continuity equation, a ratio of the velocity proximal and distal to the aortic valve can be calculated to give an index of aortic stenosis severity. This eliminates the need to measure the diameter of the LVOT and thus reduces potential error from inaccurate measurement of the LVOT.
    - How to perform this measurement:
      - Obtain the apical five-chamber view of the heart.
      - Measure the peak velocity at the LVOT using pulse wave Doppler and save (V_1).
      - Measure the peak velocity distal to the aortic valve using continuous wave Doppler and save (V_2)
      - Calculate V1/V2.
    - AS grading using this method is as follows:
      - Mild: >0.5
      - Moderate: 0.5–0.25
      - Severe: <0.25 [14]
    - The dimensionless index may also be calculated using VTI instead of peak velocity. However, this method has been shown to introduce more variability as compared to peak velocity [15].
- Aortic regurgitation
  - Aortic regurgitation (AR) can be identified by noticing subtle qualitative signs, but it is more accurate to perform quantitative measurements.
  - Qualitative signs of AR:

        - Increased E-point septal separation (EPSS) with an otherwise normal appearing ejection fraction
        - High-frequency fluttering of the anterior mitral leaflet
        - "Reverse doming" of the anterior mitral valve leaflet
    - A simple semi-quantitative method for evaluation AR is measurement of the vena contracta width. The vena contracta is the narrowest width of the regurgitant jet.
        - How to perform:
            - Obtain the parasternal long-axis view of the heart
            - Place the color flow box over the aortic valve
                - Video 4.10
                - Figure 4.15
            - Measure the narrowest portion of regurgitant flow that occurs at or immediately downstream of the regurgitant flow.
        - Grading of AR using this method is as follows:
            - Mild: <0.3 cm
            - Moderate: 0.3–0.6 cm
            - Severe: >0.6 cm [16]
    - Another similar semi-quantitative method is measuring the jet width to LVOT ratio.
        - How to perform:
            - Obtain the parasternal long-axis view of the heart.
            - Place the color flow box over the aortic valve.
            - Measure the width of the regurgitant jet just below the leaflets of the aortic valve at the vena contracta.
            - Measure the width of the LVOT.
            - Calculate the jet width to LVOT ratio.

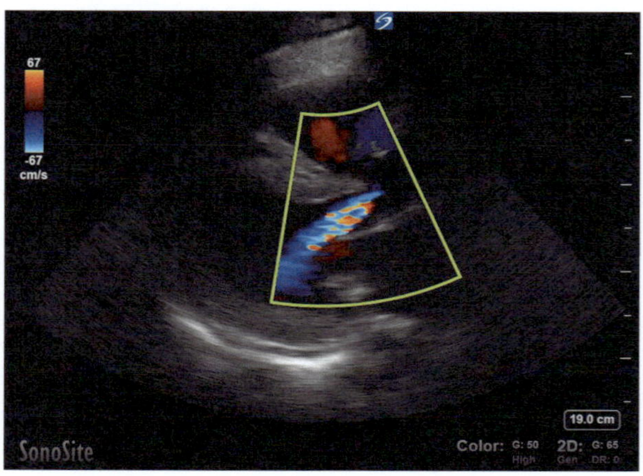

Fig. 4.15 Aortic regurgitation demonstrated by a color flow jet away from the aortic valve during diastole

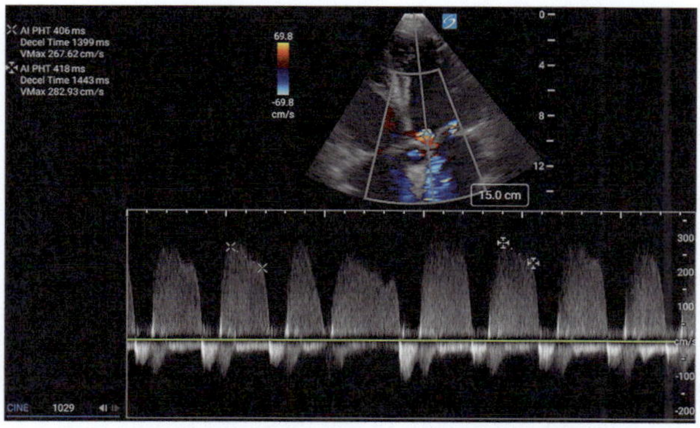

Fig. 4.16 Grading of aortic regurgitation severity demonstrated by measurement of pressure half time. The regurgitant jet is identified by color flow. Continuous wave Doppler is placed through the regurgitant jet. Using a calculation package, pressure half-time is calculated by measuring the time it takes for the velocity of the regurgitant jet to decrease by half

    - Grading of AR using this method is as follows:
      - Mild: <0.25
      - Moderate: 0.25–0.45
      - Moderate to severe: 0.45–0.65
      - Severe: >0.65 [16]
  - Another qualitative method for measuring AR is pressure half-time
    - How to perform:
      - Obtain the apical five-chamber view of the heart
      - Place color flow over the mitral valve to identify the maximal AR jet
      - Place continuous wave Doppler through the AR jet
      - Measure the time it takes for the regurgitant jet to decrease by half
        - Figure 4.16
    - Grading of AR using this method is as follows:
      - Mild: >500 ms
      - Moderate: 500–200 ms
      - Severe: <200 ms [16]
      - Note: significantly increased LV end diastolic pressure may lead to overestimation of AR by this method as increased LV end diastolic pressure can independently shorten the pressure half time.

Mitral Valve

- When evaluating the mitral valve, it is important to identify both mitral stenosis and mitral regurgitation. While there are many methods and measurements for these conditions, we will focus on the simplest and most accessible methods for ease of implementation.

- When considering whether mitral valve assessment is needed, it is helpful to evaluate the size of the left atrium. Usually, if the left atrium appears much larger than expected, it may be a hint that significant mitral valve pathology is present.
- Mitral stenosis
  - Mitral stenosis can be evaluated qualitatively and quantitatively
  - Qualitative evaluation in the parasternal long axis view:
    - Look for "doming" of the anterior mitral valve leaflet in the parasternal long-axis view.
    - Look for a "hockey stick" appearance of the anterior mitral valve leaflet.
      - Video 4.11
      - Figure 4.17 [17]
    - Look for anterior movement of the posterior mitral valve.
  - Quantitative evaluation using planimetry of the mitral valve.
    - How to perform this measurement:
      - Obtain a parasternal short axis view and visualize the mitral valve leaflets opening and closing.
      - Freeze the image in the early diastole phase where the valve is maximally opened.
      - Trace the area of the mitral valve orifice opening
        - Figure 4.18 [17]
    - Important value cutoffs are as follows:
      - Normal: 4–6 cm^2
      - Mild stenosis: 1.5–4 cm^2
      - Moderate stenosis: 1–1.5 cm^2
      - Severe stenosis: <1 cm^2 [18]
    - Limitations:
      - Poor image quality
      - Inaccurate plane of imaging
      - Calcified valve causing dropout
      - Atrial fibrillation

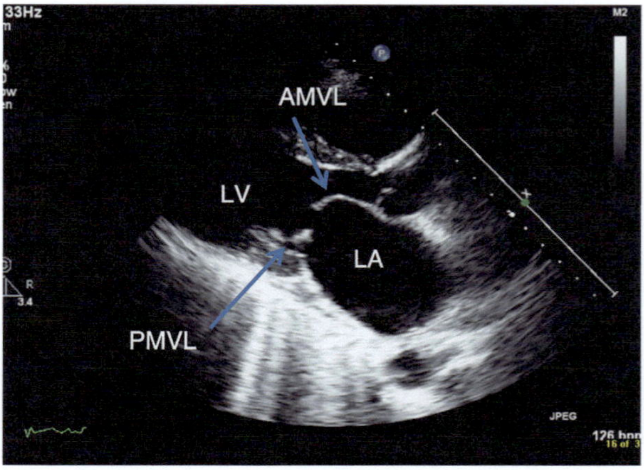

Fig. 4.17 "Hockey stick" appearance of mitral valve, demonstrating mitral stenosis [17]

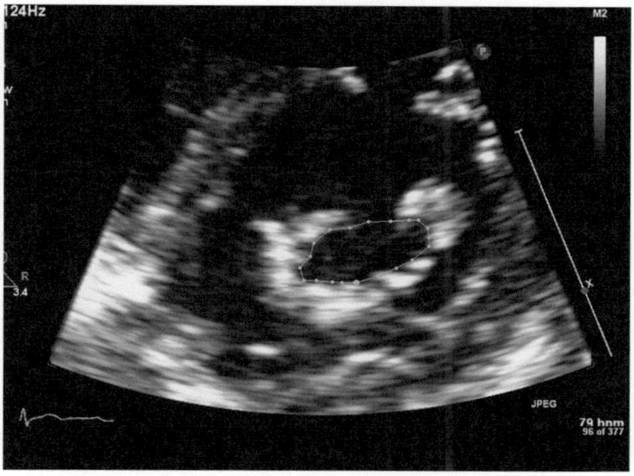

Fig. 4.18 2D planimetry measurement of the mitral valve in the parasternal short-axis view, demonstrating mitral stenosis [17]

  - Quantitative evaluation using pressure gradient across the mitral valve
    - How to perform this measurement:
      - Obtain an apical four-chamber view.
      - Obtain a continuous wave spectral Doppler tracing of the velocity of blood inflow across the mitral valve.
        - It is recommended to apply color Doppler first to visualize with color where the peak velocity is most likely to occur.
      - Trace the Doppler spectrum of the inflow and calculate peak velocity.
      - Using Bernoulli equation, your machine will calculate the mean pressure gradient across the mitral valve.
      - Also use pressure half-time to assist in calculation of mitral valve area.
        - Figure 4.19 [17]
    - Important value cutoffs for mitral stenosis gradients are as follows:
      - Mild: <5 mmHg
      - Moderate: 5–10 mmHg
      - Severe: >10 mmHg [18]
      - Note: gradients can be higher in the setting of mitral regurgitation
- Mitral regurgitation
  - Mitral regurgitation (MR) can be evaluated qualitatively, semi-quantitatively, and quantitatively. For simplicity, the simplest, most accessible methods will be presented here.
  - Qualitative evaluation of MR:
    - Evaluate the mitral valve in the parasternal long axis and apical four-chamber view
    - Look for poor coaptation of the valve
    - Look for evidence of flail leaflet or mitral valve prolapse
      - Video 4.12
    - Look for secondary evidence of MR, such as an enlarged left atrium
  - Semi-quantitative evaluation by percentage of color filling the left atrium.

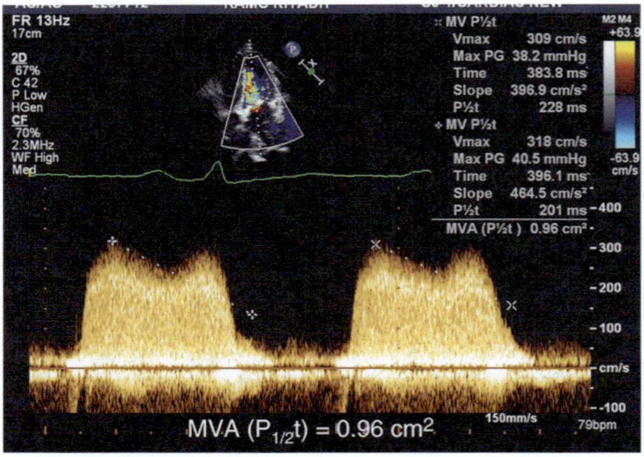

Fig. 4.19 Measurement of peak gradient across the mitral valve and calculation of pressure half time across the mitral valve by continuous wave Doppler in the apical four-chamber view to demonstrate calculation of mitral valve area [17]

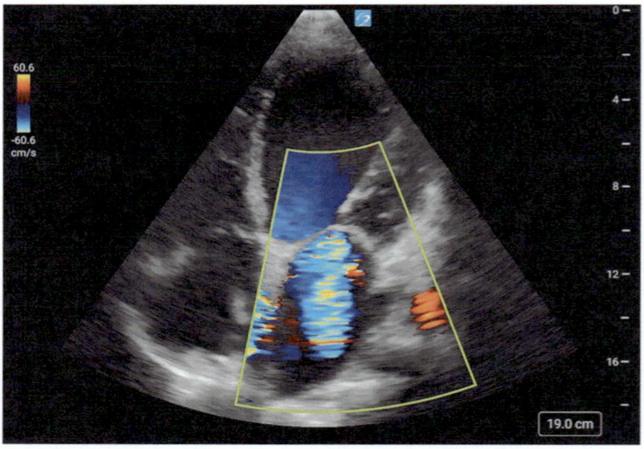

Fig. 4.20 Severe mitral regurgitation demonstrated by the regurgitant jet into the left atrium covering >70% of the left atrial area during systole

- How to perform this measurement:
  - Obtain the apical four-chamber view of the heart
  - Place color Doppler over the mitral valve, filling the entire left atrium
  - Estimate the percentage of the left atrium area that is filled with regurgitant color flow
    - Video 4.13
    - Figure 4.20
- Grading of MR using this method is as follows:
  - Mild: <20%
  - Moderate: 20–40%
  - Severe: >40% [16]

- Semi-quantitative evaluation of MR by vena contracta width.
  - How to perform this measurement:
    - Obtain the apical four-chamber view of the heart
    - Place color Doppler over the mitral valve, filling the entire left atrium.
    - Freeze the image at the maximum jet
    - Measure the vena contracta (narrowest width) just distal to the mitral valve leaflets
  - Grading of MR using this method is as follows:
    - Mild: <0.3 cm
    - Moderate: 0.3–0.7 cm
    - Severe: >0.7 cm [19]

Vegetations

- Vegetations should be considered in the clinical context, most commonly in a patient that is febrile, tachycardic, and with factors that might put the patient at higher risk.
- They will appear as thickened, irregular collections on the valves that are often mobile.
  - Video 4.14
  - Figure 4.21
- Be sure to evaluate the tricuspid, mitral, and aortic valves for evidence of vegetations.
- Consider adding color flow to the valve to evaluate flow dynamics.

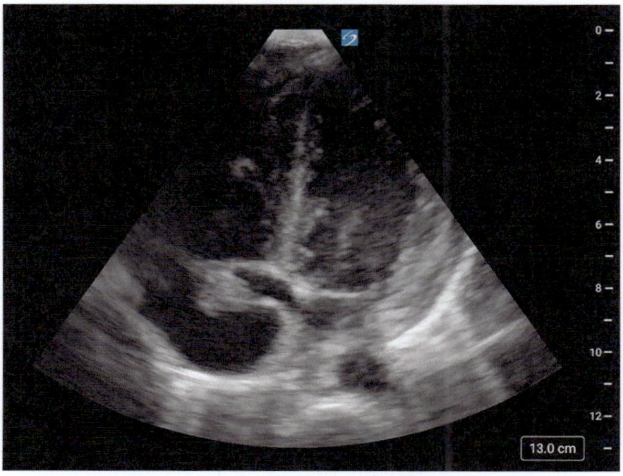

Fig. 4.21 Vegetation of the tricuspid valve demonstrated by the hyperechoic structure tethered to the tricuspid valve leaflets

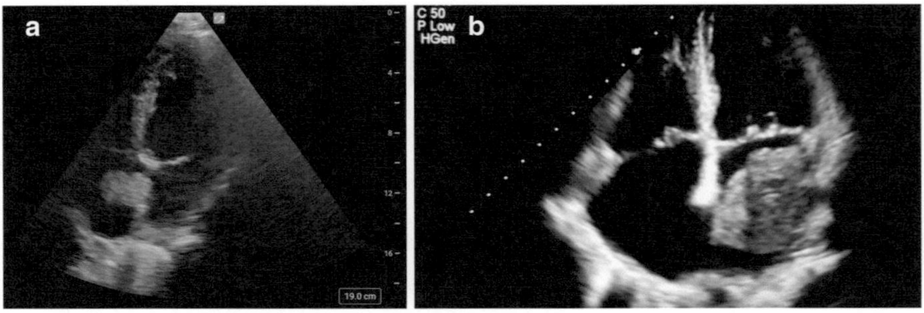

Fig. 4.22 (**a**) Right atrial myxoma demonstrated by hyperechoic, circumscribed structure tethered to the intra-atrial septum. (**b**) Left atrial myxoma demonstrated by hyperechoic, circumscribed structure tethered to the left atrium [21]

Myxoma

- Myxomas are the most common primary cardiac tumor [20].
- The most commonly occur in the atria [20].
  - Video 4.15
  - Figure 4.22a, b [21]
- They will appear as hyperechoic, round, mobile structures.

Pulmonary Embolism

- There are multiple qualitative and quantitative methods for evaluating patients with suspected pulmonary embolism (PE). These measurements are also useful for risk stratification.
- Qualitative findings:
  - Enlarged right ventricle
    - Abnormal "rule of threes"
      - This can be evaluated in the parasternal long-axis view.
      - The RV, LVOT, and LA should all approximately be of equal size.
      - If the RV appears significantly larger than the LVOT and LA, this may lead one to suspect PE.
        - Video 4.16
        - Figure 4.23
    - Septal "D" Sign
      - This can be evaluated in the parasternal short-axis view.
      - The RV, if under abnormally high pressure, can become enlarged and push into the lumen of the LV.
      - This can cause the LV to appear like a "D" with a flattened septum.
        - Video 4.17
        - Figure 4.24

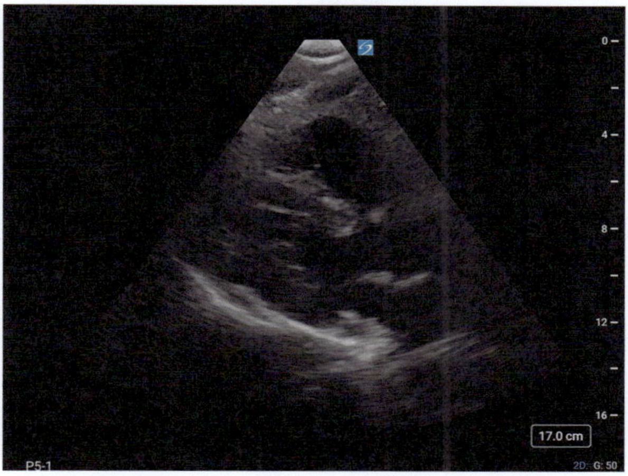

Fig. 4.23 Right ventricular enlargement seen on parasternal long axis view demonstrated by the right ventricle being much larger in size than the aortic outflow trace and left atrium, violating the "rule of threes"

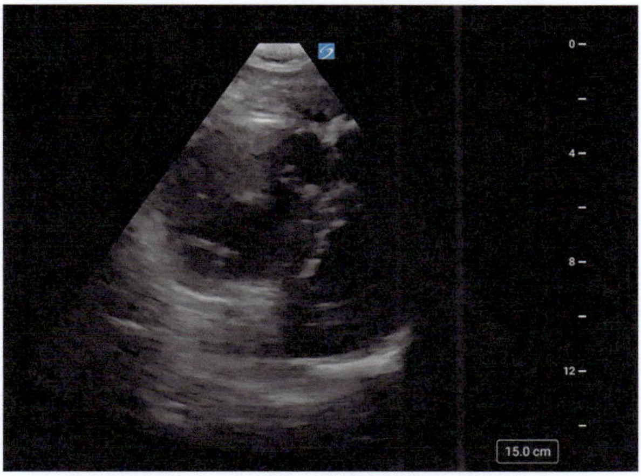

Fig. 4.24 "D sign" demonstrated by flattening of the ventricular septum secondary to elevated pressure in the right ventricle

- Enlarged RV:LV ratio
  - This can be evaluated in the apical four-chamber view.
  - If the RV is enlarged, it will cause the ratio of the RV:LV to be enlarged as well.
  - Normal RV:LV ratio is 0.7.
  - An RV:LV ratio of 1 or greater is suggestive of elevated RV pressure [22, 23].
    - Video 4.18
    - Figure 4.25

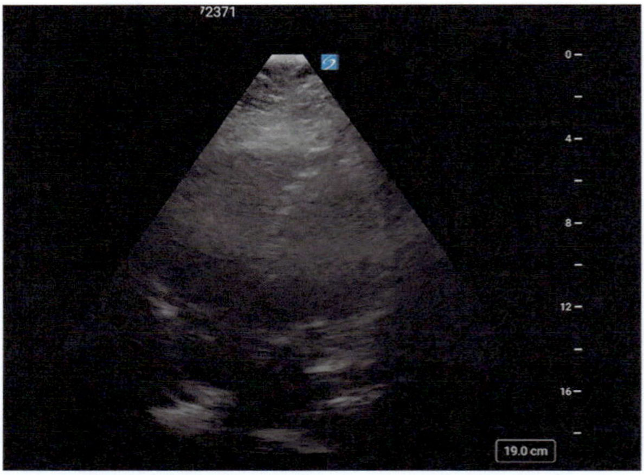

Fig. 4.25 Enlarged RV:LV ratio, suggestive of right heart strain

  - McConnel's sign is a sign that can indicate right heart strain [24].
    - This is evaluated in the apical four-chamber view
    - It is a sign describing abnormal motion of the right ventricle in the setting of acute RV strain.
      - There is hypokinesis of the midventricular RV free wall
      - There is relative hyperkinesis of the RV apex [23]
        - Video 4.19
        - Figure 4.26
- Quantitative findings:
  - Tricuspid annular plane systolic excursion (TAPSE)
    - How to obtain this measurement:
      - Obtain the apical four-chamber view with the tricuspid annulus in view
      - Place the M-mode cursor through the lateral tricuspid annulus
      - Record the M-mode tracing
      - Measure the vertical distance from peak to trough of the M-mode tracing of the lateral tricuspid annulus as a surrogate of the longitudinal contraction of the right ventricle
        - Figure 4.27
    - Measurement cutoffs are varied in the literature, but suggested cutoffs are as follows:
      - Normal: 20 mm or greater [22]
      - Abnormal: 15 mm or less [22]
      - A lower TAPSE has been shown to be an indicator of a poor prognostic factor in patients with acute PE [25].
  - Right ventricular systolic pressure (RVSP)
    - If a patient has an acute PE, their right ventricle will increase its pressure in an attempt to overcome the obstruction.

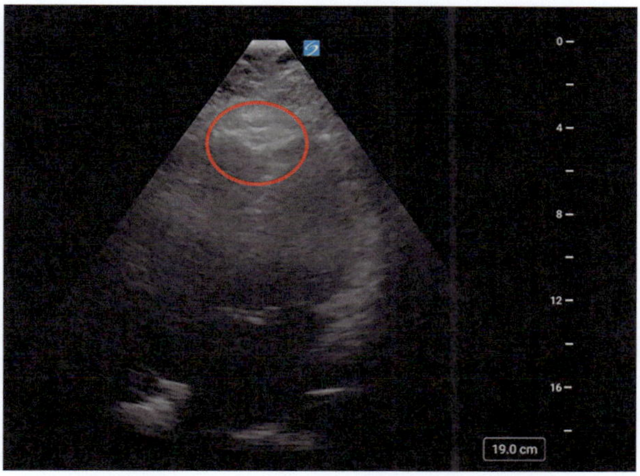

Fig. 4.26 McConnell's sign demonstrated by hyperkenetic movement at the apex of the right ventricular in the apical four-chamber view

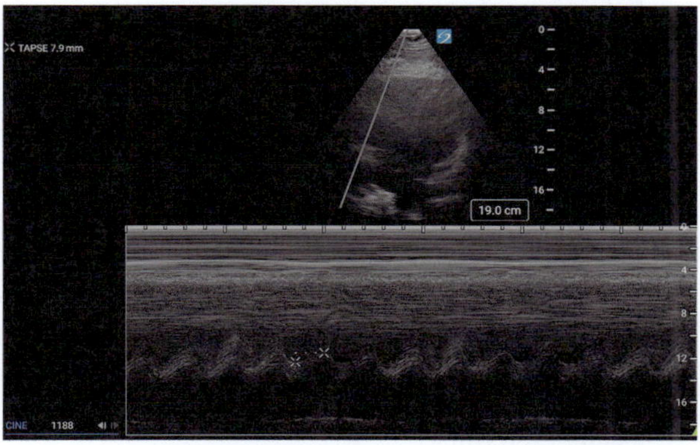

Fig. 4.27 Tricuspid annular plane systolic excursion (TAPSE) measurement calculated by obtaining a M-mode tracing of the lateral tricuspid annulus during multiple cardiac cycles. TAPSE is measured by obtaining the vertical distance between the peak and trough of the tricuspid annular movement. A TAPSE of 7.9 as measured here indicates abnormal right ventricular function

- How to obtain this measurement:
  - Obtain the apical four-chamber view with the tricuspid annulus in view
  - Place a color flow box over the right ventricle to identify the maximal tricuspid regurgitant jet
  - Place continuous wave Doppler through the maximal tricuspid regurgitant jet and obtain a spectral Doppler tracing.
  - Measure the maximum velocity of the tricuspid regurgitant jet and use Bernoulli's equation to convert that to the peak gradient.
    - Video 4.20
    - Figure 4.28

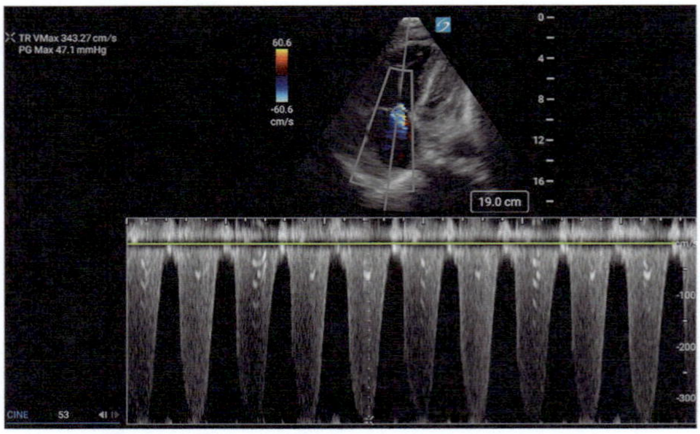

Fig. 4.28 Calculation of maximum velocity of tricuspid regurgitant jet which is converted to a peak gradient using Bernoulli's equation

- Add the right atrial pressure to obtain the total RVSP
  - Right atrial pressure can be estimated by evaluating the IVC
    - IVC <2.1 cm with >50% collapse: 3 mmHg
    - IVC <2.1 cm with <50% collapse: 8 mmHg
    - IVC >2.1 cm with >50% collapse: 8 mmHg
    - IVC >2.1 cm with <50% collapse: 15 mmHg [26]
- Measurement cutoffs are as follows:
  - Normal RVSP: <25 mmHg [22]
  - Abnormally high RVSP (likely acute): 30–60 mmHg [22]
  - Chronically elevated RVSP: >60 mmHg [22]
  - It is important to note that some patients will have chronically elevated RVSP measurements. It is unlikely that a patient can reach a pressure of greater than 60 mmHg in an acute setting. Always take clinical context into account.

- Pulmonary acceleration time
  - How to obtain this measurement:
    - Obtain the right ventricular outflow tract view of the heart.
      - First obtain the parasternal short-axis view.
      - Slide toward the base of the heart to see the "Mercedes-Benz" sign of the aortic valve.
      - Visualize the RVOT wrapping around the aortic valve in the near field of the screen.
    - Place pulse wave Doppler in the RVOT just proximal to the pulmonary valve
    - Obtain the pulse wave Doppler tracing
    - Measure the time it takes to reach peak velocity
      - Figure 4.29
  - Measurement cutoffs are as follows:
    - Normal time to peak is >60 ms [23]
    - Abnormal time to peak is <60 ms [23]
    - "Early systolic notching" may also be present [23]

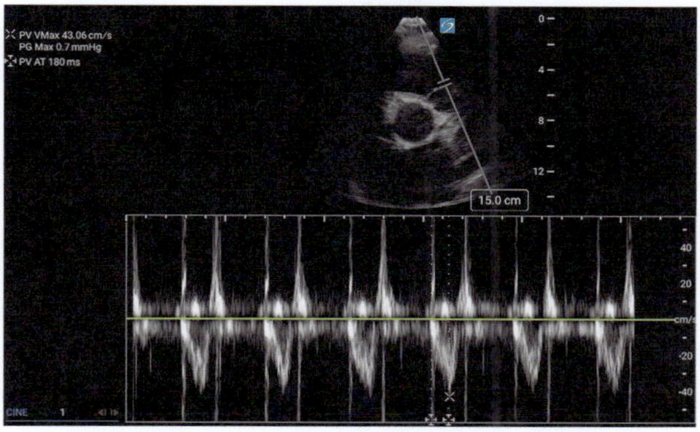

Fig. 4.29 Calculation of peak pulmonary velocity and pulmonary acceleration time in the parasternal short-axis view

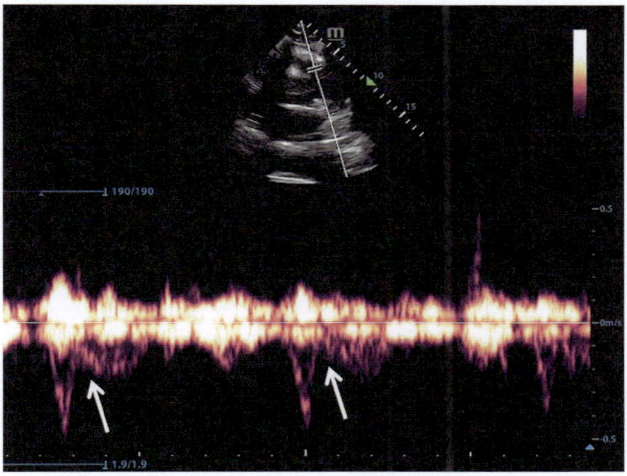

Fig. 4.30 Example of early systolic notching. Arrow points to early notch, which is abnormal compared to a normal pulmonary artery waveform [23]

  - This is when there is a notch during early systole in the RVOT pulse wave Doppler
  - This indicates significant obstruction of the RVOT.
  - Figure 4.30 [23]
- Combine right ventricular systolic pressure (RVSP) with pulmonary acceleration time (PAT) to evaluate for 60/60 sign
  - RVSP <60 mmHg
  - PAT <60 ms
  - Studies have demonstrated a 13–51% sensitivity and a 69–98% specificity of the 60/60 sign for PE [22].

Key Points

- For advanced evaluation of systolic function, use EPSS (abnormal greater than 10 mm) and MAPSE (abnormal less than 7 mm).
- For evaluating valvular stenosis, look for restricted movement or hyperechoic calcifications on valve leaflets and perform additional measurements with Doppler for confirmation.
- For valvular regurgitation, use color Doppler to confirm regurgitation, and perform additional measurements after confirmation.
- For evaluating right heart strain, use RV:LV ratio, TAPSE (abnormal less than 15 mm), and RVSP (abnormal greater than 25).

References

1. Massie BM, Schiller NB, Ratshin RA, Parmley WW. Mitral-septal separation: new echocardiographic index of left ventricular function. Am J Cardiol. 1977;39(7):1008–16. https://doi.org/10.1016/S0002-9149(77)80215-4.
2. Elnoamany MF, Abdelhameed AK. Mitral annular motion as a surrogate for left ventricular function: correlation with brain natriuretic peptide levels. Eur J Echocardiogr. 2006;7(3):187–98. https://doi.org/10.1016/j.euje.2005.05.005.
3. Simonson JS, Schiller NB. Descent of the base of the left ventricle: an echocardiographic index of left ventricular function. J Am Soc Echocardiogr. 1989;2(1):25–35. https://doi.org/10.1016/S0894-7317(89)80026-4.
4. Shams P, Goyal A, Makaryus AN. Left ventricular ejection fraction. In: StatPearls. StatPearls Publishing; 2025. http://www.ncbi.nlm.nih.gov/books/NBK459131/. Accessed 17 July 2025.
5. Otterstad JE, Froeland G, St. John Sutton M, Holme I. Accuracy and reproducibility of biplane two-dimensional echocardiographic measurements of left ventricular dimensions and function. Eur Heart J. 1997;18(3):507–13. https://doi.org/10.1093/oxfordjournals.eurheartj.a015273.
6. Villavicencio C, Leache J, Marin J, et al. Basic critical care echocardiography training of intensivists allows reproducible and reliable measurements of cardiac output. Ultrasound J. 2019;11:5. https://doi.org/10.1186/s13089-019-0120-0.
7. Patel N, Durland J, Awosika AO, Makaryus AN. Physiology, cardiac index. In: StatPearls. StatPearls Publishing; 2025. http://www.ncbi.nlm.nih.gov/books/NBK539905/. Accessed 14 July 2025.
8. Gibbons RC, Smith D, Feig R, Mulflur M, Costantino TG. The sonographic protocol for the emergent evaluation of aortic dissections (SPEED protocol): a multicenter, prospective, observational study. Acad Emerg Med. 2024;31(2):112–8. https://doi.org/10.1111/acem.14839.
9. Sobczyk D, Nycz K. Feasibility and accuracy of bedside transthoracic echocardiography in diagnosis of acute proximal aortic dissection. Cardiovasc Ultrasound. 2015;13:15. https://doi.org/10.1186/s12947-015-0008-5.
10. Okura H, Yoshida K, Hozumi T, Akasaka T, Yoshikawa J. Planimetry and transthoracic two-dimensional echocardiography in noninvasive assessment of aortic valve area in patients with valvular aortic stenosis. J Am Coll Cardiol. 1997;30(3):753–9. https://doi.org/10.1016/S0735-1097(97)00200-3.
11. Ramaraj R, Sorrell VL. Degenerative aortic stenosis. BMJ. 2008;336(7643):550–5. https://doi.org/10.1136/bmj.39478.498819.AD.
12. Otto C. Textbook of clinical echocardiography. 5th ed. Elsevier; 2013.
13. Hlaing M, Panzer O. New diagnostic capabilities of ultrasound in the intensive care unit. Curr Anesthesiol Rep. 2015;5(4):370–9. https://doi.org/10.1007/s40140-015-0128-3.

14. Vahanian A, Otto CM. Risk stratification of patients with aortic stenosis. Eur Heart J. 2010;31(4):416–23. https://doi.org/10.1093/eurheartj/ehp575.
15. Finegold JA, Manisty CH, Cecaro F, Sutaria N, Mayet J, Francis DP. Choosing between velocity-time-integral ratio and peak velocity ratio for calculation of the dimensionless index (or aortic valve area) in serial follow-up of aortic stenosis. Int J Cardiol. 2013;167(4):1524–31. https://doi.org/10.1016/j.ijcard.2012.04.105.
16. Zoghbi WA, Adams D, Bonow RO, et al. Recommendations for noninvasive evaluation of native valvular regurgitation: a report from the American Society of Echocardiography developed in collaboration with the Society for Cardiovascular Magnetic Resonance. J Am Soc Echocardiogr. 2017;30(4):303–71. https://doi.org/10.1016/j.echo.2017.01.007.
17. Omran AS, Arifi AA, Mohamed AA. Echocardiography in mitral stenosis. J Saudi Heart Assoc. 2011;23(1):51–8, ISSN 1016-7315. https://doi.org/10.1016/j.jsha.2010.07.007.
18. Baumgartner H, Hung J, Bermejo J, et al. Echocardiographic assessment of valve stenosis: EAE/ASE recommendations for clinical practice. Eur J Echocardiogr. 2009;10(1):1–25. https://doi.org/10.1093/ejechocard/jen303.
19. El-Tallawi KC, Messika-Zeitoun D, Zoghbi WA. Assessment of the severity of native mitral valve regurgitation. Prog Cardiovasc Dis. 2017;60(3):322–33. https://doi.org/10.1016/j.pcad.2017.11.005.
20. Islam AKMM. Cardiac myxomas: a narrative review. World J Cardiol. 2022;14(4):206–19. https://doi.org/10.4330/wjc.v14.i4.206.
21. Admin. Atrial myxoma: case presentation and review. J Med Sci | “Medicinos mokslai”. ISSN: 2345-0592. Email: info@medicsciences.com. 2021. https://medicsciences.com/atrial-myxoma-case-presentation-and-review/. Accessed 17 July 2025.
22. Fields JM, Davis J, Girson L, et al. Transthoracic echocardiography for diagnosing pulmonary embolism: a systematic review and meta-analysis. J Am Soc Echocardiogr. 2017;30(7):714–723.e4. https://doi.org/10.1016/j.echo.2017.03.004.
23. Alerhand S, Sundaram T, Gottlieb M. What are the echocardiographic findings of acute right ventricular strain that suggest pulmonary embolism? Anaesth Crit Care Pain Med. 2021;40(2):100852. https://doi.org/10.1016/j.accpm.2021.100852.
24. McConnell MV, Solomon SD, Rayan ME, Come PC, Goldhaber SZ, Lee RT. Regional right ventricular dysfunction detected by echocardiography in acute pulmonary embolism. Am J Cardiol. 1996;78(4):469–73. https://doi.org/10.1016/S0002-9149(96)00339-6.
25. Alerhand S, Hickey SM. Tricuspid Annular Plane Systolic Excursion (TAPSE) for risk stratification and prognostication of patients with pulmonary embolism. J Emerg Med. 2020;58(3):449–56. https://doi.org/10.1016/j.jemermed.2019.09.017.
26. Aduen JF, Castello R, Lozano MM, et al. An alternative echocardiographic method to estimate mean pulmonary artery pressure: diagnostic and clinical implications. J Am Soc Echocardiogr. 2009;22(7):814–9. https://doi.org/10.1016/j.echo.2009.04.007.

Resuscitative Transesophageal Echocardiography

5

Jordan Tozer and Lindsay Taylor

Transesophageal echocardiography (TEE) is an advanced and technical clinical application of echocardiography that can be learned once transthoracic image acquisition and interpretation competence has been achieved. Rather than the more widely applicable TTE, transesophageal echocardiography has a narrow application: typically limited to shock, cardiac arrest, or procedural guidance [1]. It is important to note that TEE can only be performed in this setting once a definitive airway has been achieved via endotracheal intubation. There are many detailed cardiac and valvular views that can be obtained using TEE, but this chapter will focus on the standard "resuscitative" TEE views, that is, cardiac views most likely to be helpful in a critically ill or unstable patient.

Clinical Application and Indications

- Evaluate cardiac activity in the critically ill patient; typically to determine causes of cardiac arrest or shock [2, 3].
- To guide resuscitation efforts depending on underlying cardiac pathology [2].
- An alternative approach to transthoracic echo, when views may not be able to be obtained due to ongoing resuscitative efforts or the patient's body habitus [3].
- The patient must be intubated in the critical care setting to perform resuscitative TEE.

Supplementary Information The online version contains supplementary material available at https://doi.org/10.1007/978-3-032-27643-8_5.

J. Tozer (✉) · L. Taylor
Department of Emergency Medicine, Virginia Commonwealth University Health, Richmond, VA, USA
e-mail: jordan.tozer@vcuhealth.org; Lindsay.Taylor@vcuhealth.org

A. Lindsay et al. (eds.), *Clinical Ultrasound*,
https://doi.org/10.1007/978-3-032-27643-8_5

Normal Cardiac Anatomy

- See Cardiac Ultrasound Chapter

Image Acquisition

- Transducer Selection
  - Transesophageal transducer.
  - Specialized transducer that must be attached to your ultrasound machine.
  - Selecting this transducer on the machine will automatically adapt the machine settings.
- Transducer Anatomy
  - Figure 5.1—Transducer design
  - Video 5.1—Transducer movements
  - Transducer design
    - Snake-like device with transducer shaft length approximately 1 m.
    - Transducer elements embedded into distal probe face.
  - Wheels
    - Two wheels are located on the transducer grip handle.
    - The larger bottom wheel controls anterior–posterior flexion.
    - The smaller wheel controls side-to-side flexion.
  - Omniplane
    - Figure 5.2—Omniplane image
    - Video 5.2—Omniplane moving
    - Two buttons on grip handle control the electronic beam steering, creating rotation into different imaging planes.

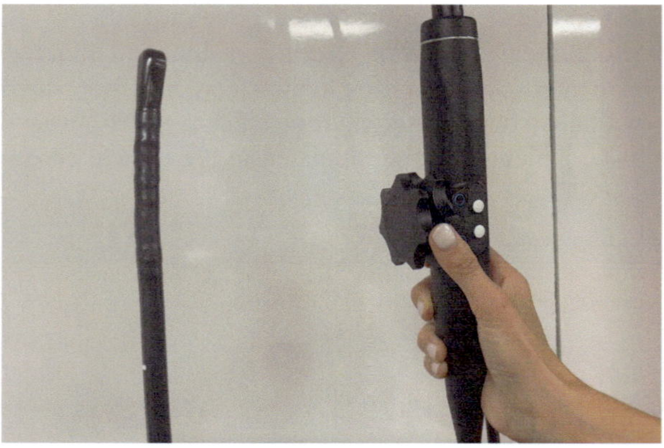

Fig. 5.1 TEE transducer design showing the two large wheels (left/right, anterior/posterior flexion) and the white omniplane buttons

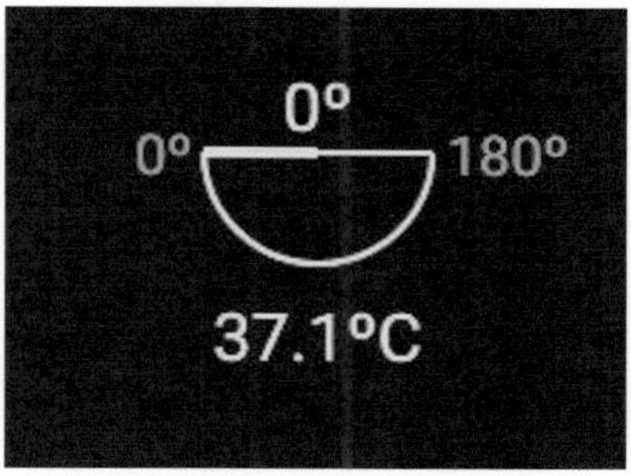

Fig. 5.2 The omniplane indicator will usually be in the upper left portion of the screen when using TEE. The angle indicates how much rotation has been selected using the omniplane buttons

- Patient Position and Procedure
  - The patient must have an endotracheal tube in place.
  - The patient should be supine.
  - ETT tube secured but out of the way of probe insertion.
- Standard Resuscitative Exam Views
  - Mid-esophageal 4-chamber (ME4C)
  - Mid-esophageal 2-chamber (ME2C)
  - Mid-esophageal long axis (ME LAX)
  - Transgastric short axis (TG SAX)
  - Midesophageal Bicaval (ME Bicaval)
- Transducer Introduction
  - Transducer insertion into the esophagus is often the most difficult part of obtaining TEE images.
  - The ETT cannot be secured, and care must be taken not to dislodge it during TEE probe insertion.
  - Carefully slide the probe behind the ETT tube and down into the esophagus.
    - Lift the ETT with a Mac blade
    - Gentle anterior flexion of the TEE tip
    - Gentle forward pressure with the transducer tip

Mid-esophageal Four-Chamber

This view is ideal for assessing LV/RV size and function, pathology of the pericardium, regional wall motion abnormalities (RWMA), and myocardial activity during resuscitation.

- Transducer Placement
  - Once the transducer has been successfully inserted into the esophagus, advance the probe 30–40 cm until the heart is visualized.
  - Rotate the probe left or right to center the heart in the image.
  - Gently retroflex the probe tip by rotating the larger bottom wheel counterclockwise with the thumb to elongate the heart.
  - The omniplane should remain at 0°.

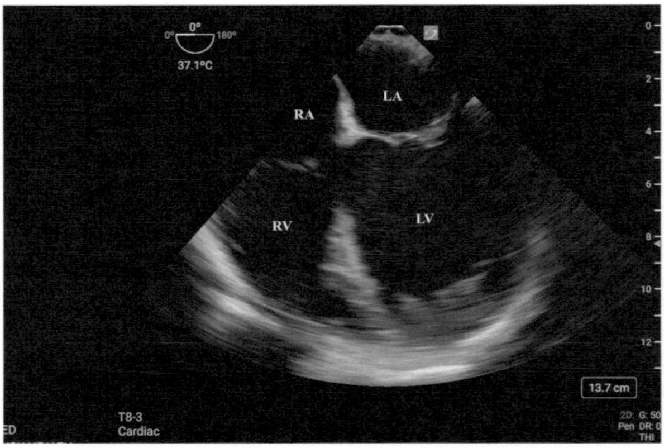

Fig. 5.3 Mid-esophageal 4-chamber image showing all four cardiac chambers (labelled) in this post-arrest heart with dilated cardiomyopathy. Note the omniplane is at 0 deg for ME4C imaging

- Ultrasound Anatomy
  - Figure 5.3—ME4C
  - Video 5.3—ME4C
  - Anatomic Orientation:
  - In contrast to the TTE apical four-chamber view, the apex will be at the bottom of the screen.
  - The left atrium will be closest to the transducer face and therefore displayed at the top of the screen, toward screen right.
  - The right atrium with be slightly below and toward screen left.
    - Rotate the probe toward patient right to see more of the right atrium.
  - The ventricles will be located toward the bottom of the screen, with the larger left ventricle on screen right.
    - Retroflexion of the transducer tip can improve the foreshortening of the ventricles that often occurs with standard insertion.

Mid-esophageal 2-Chamber

This view is ideal for assessing LA pathology, mitral valve pathology, LV function, regional wall motion abnormalities (RWMA), and myocardial activity during resuscitation.

- Transducer Placement
  - No movement of the transducer is necessary to achieve the ME2C view.
  - Simply "omniplane" to 90°.
  - Rotate the transducer toward the patients left if the ventricle is not centered.
- Ultrasound Anatomy
  - Figure 5.4—ME2C
  - Video 5.4—ME2C
  - Anatomic Orientation:

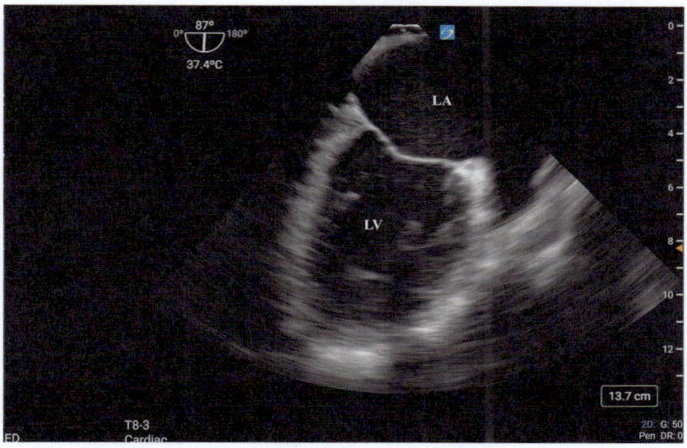

Fig. 5.4 Mid-esophageal 2 chamber image showing the left heart chambers (labelled) in this post-arrest heart with dilated cardiomyopathy. Note the omniplane is near 90 deg for ME2C imaging

- The left atrium should dominate the top of the screen with the left ventricle below it.
- In contrast to the ME4C view, this view allows visualization of the infero-posterior wall of the LV (screen left) and anterior wall (screen right).
- The corresponding mitral valve leaflets and portions of associated papillary muscles will also be visualized.

Mid-esophageal Long Axis

This view is ideal for assessing LV function, chest compression location in CPR (area of maximal compression), pathology of mitral valve, pathology of the pericardium, and aortic outflow tract size and morphology.

- Transducer Placement
  - No movement of the transducer is necessary to achieve the MELAX view.
  - Simply "omniplane" to 120–140°.
  - Rotate the transducer toward the patients left if the ventricle is not centered.
- Ultrasound Anatomy
  - Figure 5.5—MELAX
  - Video 5.5—MELAX
  - Anatomic Orientation:
    - The left atrium should dominate the top of the screen with the left ventricle below toward the screen left and the left ventricular outflow tract (LVOT) below toward the screen right.
    - Below the LVOT is the right ventriculе.
    - The mitral valve is located between the LA and LV.
    - The aortic valve is located between the LV and ascending aorta.

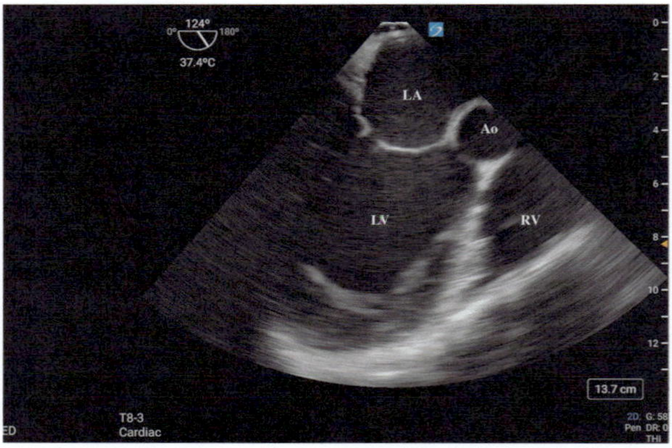

Fig. 5.5 Mid-esophageal long axis image showing the left heart chambers (labelled) and aortic outflow (Ao) in this post-arrest heart with dilated cardiomyopathy. Note the omniplane is near 120 deg for ME2C imaging

Transgastric Short Axis

This view displays a circular cross-section of the LV and is helpful for evaluating global and regional systolic function as well as pathology to the pericardium.

- Transducer Placement
  - Advance the probe into the stomach while maintaining a neutral omniplane (0°).
  - Once in the stomach, gently anteflex the probe tip using the large bottom wheel until the left ventricle appears in short axis.
  - Rotate the probe as needed to center the LV in the image.
- Ultrasound Anatomy
  - Figure 5.6—TG SAX
  - Video 5.6—TG SAX
  - Anatomic orientation:
    - Papillary muscles (at mid-LV level)
    - Interventricular septum (screen left)
    - LV free wall (screen right)
    - Advance or withdrawal the transducer or anteflex the transducer tip to view other levels of the LV, such as:
      - Basal (mitral valve level)
      - Mid-papillary (most common)
      - Apical (closest to LV apex)

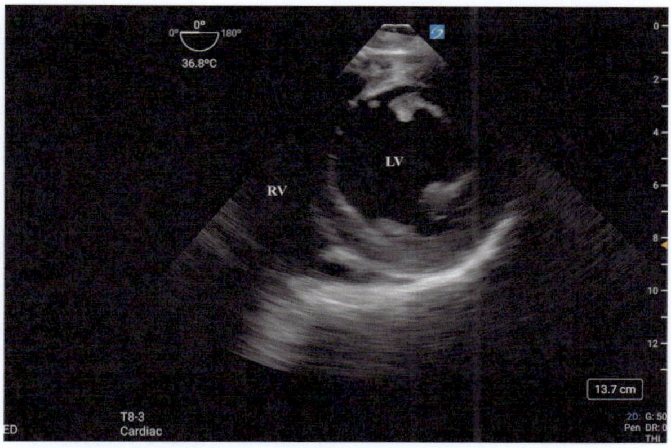

Fig. 5.6 Transgastric short-axis image showing the LV and RV in cross-section. Contrasting from TTE, the inferior wall is closest to the probe in this TEE image. Note that the omniplane is at 0 deg for the TGSAX image

Mid-esophageal Bicaval View

This view is ideal for assessing right atrial volume, catheter placement (e.g., ECMO, transvenous pacemaker placement, and central venous lines), and atrial septal abnormalities.

- Transducer Placement
  - Start from the mid-esophageal position and increase the omniplane angle to approximately 90–110°.
  - Rotate the transducer until both cavae are visible entering the right atrium.
  - Slight transducer advancement will increase visualization of the (IVC) on screen left.
  - Slight transducer withdrawal may be needed to optimize the alignment of the superior vena cava (SVC) on screen right.
- Ultrasound Anatomy
  - Figure 5.7—ME Bicaval
  - Video 5.7—ME Bicaval
  - Anatomic orientation:
    - Right atrium: center of the screen
    - IVC: enters from screen left
    - SVC: enters from screen right

Resuscitation Specific Pathologies

- See "Cardiac" chapter for basic pathologies that can also be seen in TEE

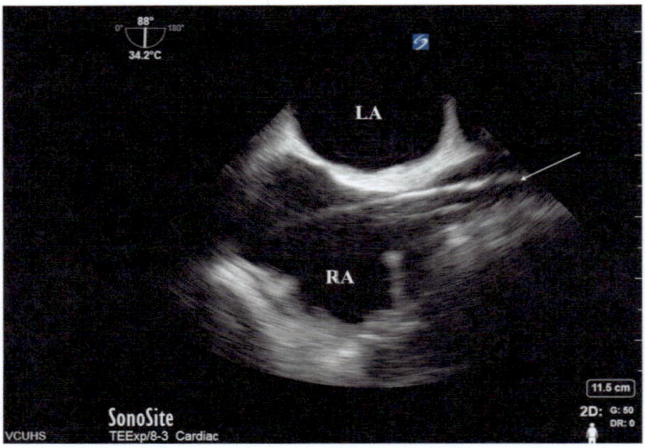

Fig. 5.7 This bicaval image taken during ECMO cannula placement shows the left atrium (LA) closest to the probe and the cannula (arrow) entering the right atrium (RA) from the SVC (near arrow)

Asystole

- Video 5.8—TEE asystole
- No organized movement of the cardiac chambers.
- Typically, there will be no associated valve openings as even agonal contractions will not generate the force necessary to move blood forward.

Ventricular Fibrillation

- Video 5.9—TEE vfib.
- Can be seen as a quivering of the ventricular muscle wall and valve leaflets.
- Coarse fibrillation may be easier to see than fine fibrillation.
- TEE-detected fibrillation may be incongruent with the ECG tracing, but suspected fibrillation should be defibrillated during cardiac arrest.
- Check with your transducer manufacturer regarding defibrillation with the probe in situ.

RV Dilation

- TEE provides more optimal visualization of the RV than TTE.
- During cardiac standstill or ventricular fibrillation, the RV will naturally dilate in the absence of forward flow.
- Care must be taken to distinguish this from pathological dilation due to obstructive pathology such as a pulmonary embolism (PE).
  - Figure 5.8—RV dilation without a definitive PE
  - Video 5.10—Large RV during CPR
- Clot in transit is a definitive sign
  - Figure 5.9—Clot in transit
  - Video 5.11—Clot in transit

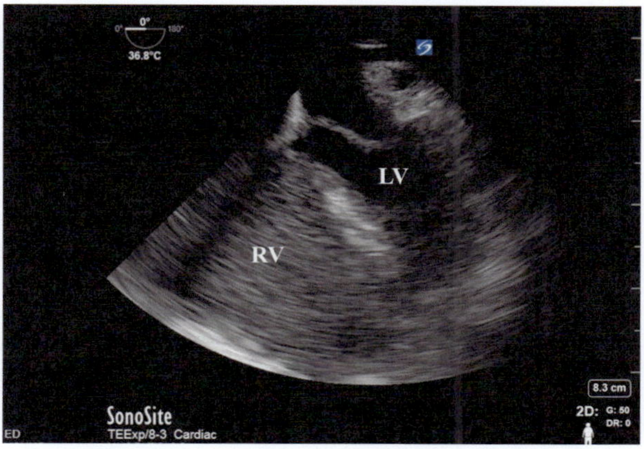

Fig. 5.8 Mid-esophageal 4 chamber image taken during cardiac arrest showing a dilated RV with poor forward flow noted by the swirling "smoke" opacifying the chamber

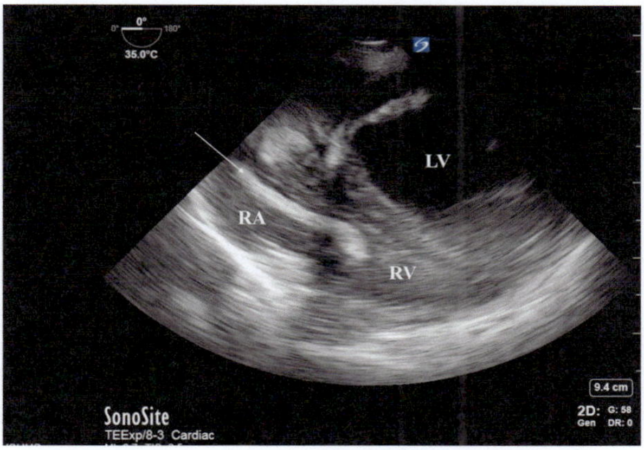

Fig. 5.9 Mid-esophageal 4 chamber image taken during cardiac arrest that shows a large thrombus (arrow) floating between the RA and RV

CPR

- Figure 5.10—CPR before compression
- Figure 5.11—CPR bad compression
- Figure 5.12—CPR good compression
- Video 5.12—CPR bad compression
- Video 5.13—CPR good compression
- The MELAX view should be used to evaluate the location of maximum compression during CPR
- The ideal location should be over the mid-portion of the LV
  - During compression, the aortic valve should be visualized as opening, without compression over the valve or ascending aorta
  - If compression is noted to be over the LV outflow tract, instructions should be given to change location of compression, usually leftward

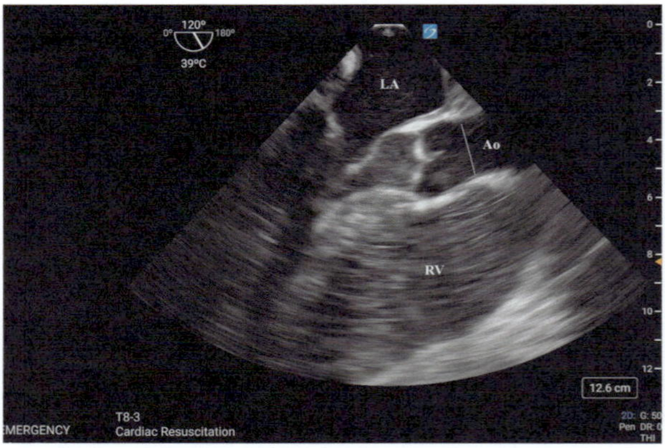

Fig. 5.10 Mid-esophageal long-axis image taken during ongoing CPR just prior to the compression phase. Note the white line indicating the open aortic (Ao) outflow channel

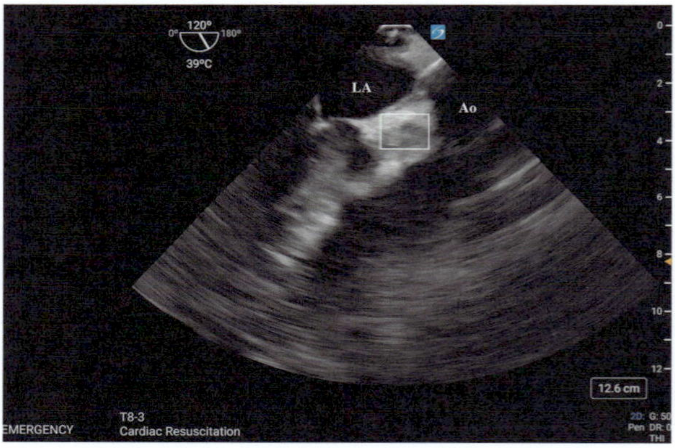

Fig. 5.11 Mid-esophageal long-axis image taken during ongoing CPR during the compression phase. Note the complete obliteration (white box) of the aortic (Ao) outflow channel. Little to no blood can move out of the heart during the compression phase if the aortic outflow is being compressed

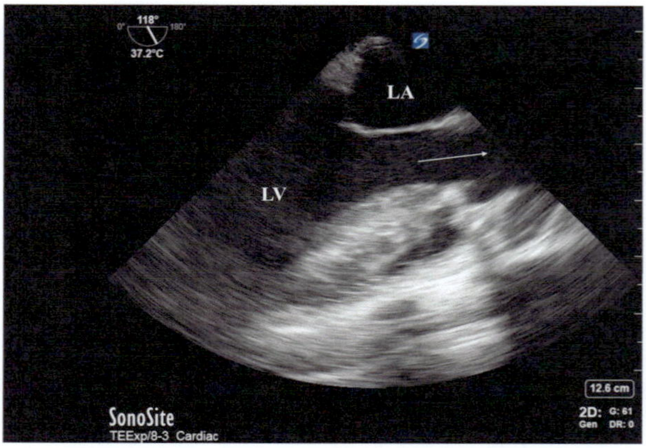

Fig. 5.12 Mid-esophageal long-axis image taken during ongoing CPR during the compression phase. Compression is being done over the base of the LV. Note the open aortic (Ao) outflow channel

Limitations/Complications

- Fundamental knowledge of transthoracic echocardiography should be achieved before attempting.
- The patient must have a secured airway.
- Risk for airway and esophageal injury [7].

Key Points

- TEE is a unique ultrasound modality that can provide critical information for medical decision-making during critical care resuscitation [4].
- It can be performed simultaneously with CPR [5].
- Use the mid-esophageal four-chamber view to assess for most cardiogenic pathologies including asystole, severely reduced EF, enlarged RV, pericardial effusion, and ventricular fibrillation [6].
- Use the mid-esophageal long axis view to evaluate CPR effectiveness, ensuring there is no compression over the left ventricular outflow tract that would obstruct blood flow [3].

References

1. American College of Emergency Physicians. Use of transesophageal echocardiography in the ED for shock, cardiac arrest, and procedural guidance. Approved June 2023. Available from: https://www.acep.org/emultrasound/newsroom/oct2024/acep-newsletter-tee-and-area-of-maximal-compression
2. Fair J, Mallin MP, Mallemat H, Seif D, Mohr NM, Nomura JT, et al. Transesophageal echocardiography: guidelines for point-of-care applications in cardiac arrest resuscitation. Ann Emerg Med. 2018;71(2):201–7.
3. American College of Emergency Physicians. Critical care updates: Two views to save lives—transesophageal echocardiography for peri-arrest and cardiac arrest patients. ACEP Newsroom. 2019. Available from: https://www.acep.org/emultrasound/newsroom/jun2019/critical-care-updates-two-views-to-save-lives-transesophageal-echocardiography-for-peri-arrest-and-cardiac-arrest-patients
4. American College of Emergency Physicians. TEE and area of maximal compression. ACEP Newsroom. 2024. Available from: https://www.acep.org/emultrasound/newsroom/oct2024/acep-newsletter-tee-and-area-of-maximal-compression
5. O'Neil M. How to perform resuscitative transesophageal echocardiography in the emergency department. ACEP Now. 2020. Available from: https://www.acepnow.com/article/how-to-perform-resuscitative-transesophageal-echocardiography-in-the-emergency-department
6. Chen EH. TEE in the ED: a new frontier in emergency ultrasound. EMRA. 2022. Available from: https://www.emra.org/emresident/article/tee-in-the-ed
7. American College of Emergency Physicians. Coding for echocardiography in the emergency department. ACEP Newsroom. 2022. Available from: https://www.acep.org/emultrasound/newsroom/january-2022/coding-for-echocardiography-in-the-emergency-department

6 Thoracic Ultrasound

Elizabeth Morrison, Lindsay Taylor, Angela Lindsay, and Michael Joyce

Patients commonly seek medical evaluation for shortness of breath. Thoracic ultrasound is a tool that has improved our diagnostic capability to rapidly determine the cause of their symptomatology and guide management, which is specifically advantageous in patients with respiratory distress. It can diagnose conditions such as pneumothorax, pulmonary edema, pleural effusion, or pneumonia. Importantly, thoracic ultrasound can help differentiate between chronic obstructive pulmonary disease exacerbations and decompensated heart failure, a common conundrum. These two conditions can appear similar, be quite severe, and require vastly different treatment. Thoracic ultrasound is relatively easy to learn, quick to employ, and most importantly, can be lifesaving for patients. This chapter will review indications, basic anatomy, image acquisition, normal ultrasound anatomy, and interpretation of pathology.

Supplementary Information The online version contains supplementary material available at https://doi.org/10.1007/978-3-032-27643-8_6.

E. Morrison (✉)
Emergency Department, Bon Secours Mercy Health St. Rita's Medical Center, Lima, OH, USA
e-mail: eamorrison@mercy.com

L. Taylor · A. Lindsay · M. Joyce
Department of Emergency Medicine, Virginia Commonwealth University Health, Richmond, VA, USA
e-mail: lindsay.taylor@vcuhealth.org; angela.creditt@vcuhealth.org; john.joyce@vcuhealth.org

A. Lindsay et al. (eds.), *Clinical Ultrasound*,
https://doi.org/10.1007/978-3-032-27643-8_6

Indications/Clinical Application

- Evaluate the etiology of acute dyspnea including pneumothorax, pleural effusion, consolidation, pulmonary contusion, and pulmonary edema.
- Guidance for thoracentesis or thoracostomy tube placement.
- Guidance for intercostal nerve block.

Normal Thoracic Anatomy

- Chest wall is composed of 12 ribs on either side; ribs 1–7 are true ribs, 8–10 false ribs, and 11–12 floating ribs.
- There are two lungs within the thoracic cavity, with the right lung larger than the left lung due to the heart taking up space on the left.
  - Right lung has three lobes: upper, middle, and lower.
  - Left lung has two lobes: upper and lower.
    - The left lung also has a lingula between the upper and lower lobes, which may be referred to as an additional lobe.
- The lungs are enclosed by the pleurae, which are made up of the parietal pleura and visceral pleura.
  - Between these two pleurae is a potential space, which is called the pleural cavity and will normally contain less than 20 mL of pleural fluid.
- Terminology of Thoracic Ultrasound
  - A-lines: reverberation artifact due to the reflection of ultrasound waves from the pleura, seen as multiple echogenic horizontal lines (repetitions of the pleural line) separated by a distance equal to the thickness of the chest wall [1, 2].
    - A-lines will typically be seen throughout normal lung parenchyma; they are often absent in the setting of interstitial disease, consolidation, and pleural effusions.
    - Figure 6.1—A-lines
  - B-lines: ray-like or "comet-tail" vertical lines extending from the pleural line down to the bottom of the screen without fading [2, 3].
    - B-lines will move synchronously with lung sliding.
    - B-lines are artifacts generated by alveoli [2].
    - It is normal to have up to two B-lines in one field of view.
    - Three or more B-lines within a rib space is considered abnormal and can be seen with pulmonary edema and conditions that cause thickened inter-alveolar soft tissue such as pulmonary fibrosis [4].
    - Figure 6.2—B-lines
    - Video 6.1—B-lines

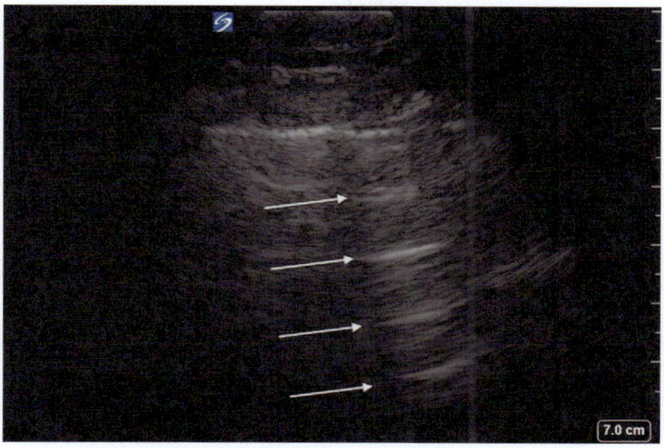

Fig. 6.1 A-lines: Normal lung findings include horizontal A-lines (arrows) throughout the lung caused by reverberation artifacts from the pleural line

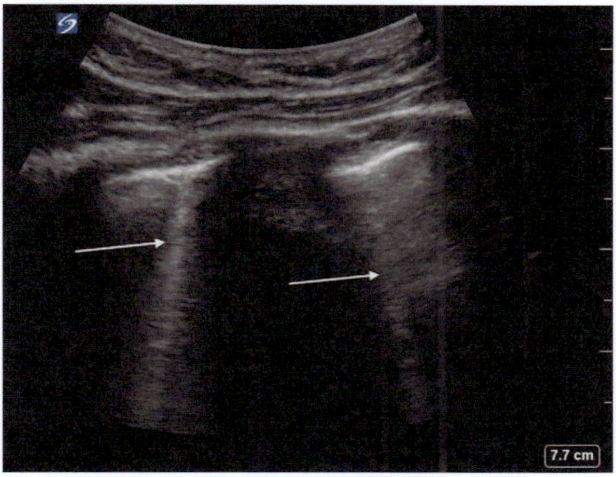

Fig. 6.2 B-lines: B-lines extend from the pleural line down to the bottom of the screen without fading. Up to three B-lines per lung field is considered normal

- E-lines: similar to B-lines but arise from the chest wall, not the pleural line; sometimes also called Z-lines or false B-lines
  - A type of reverberation artifact that occurs due to subcutaneous emphysema [2, 5].
- Hepatization: increased density and alteration of lung tissue creating an appearance similar to liver tissue.
  - Due to consolidation from disease processes such as pneumonia or contusions [6].
  - Figure 6.3—Hepatization
  - Video 6.2—Hepatization

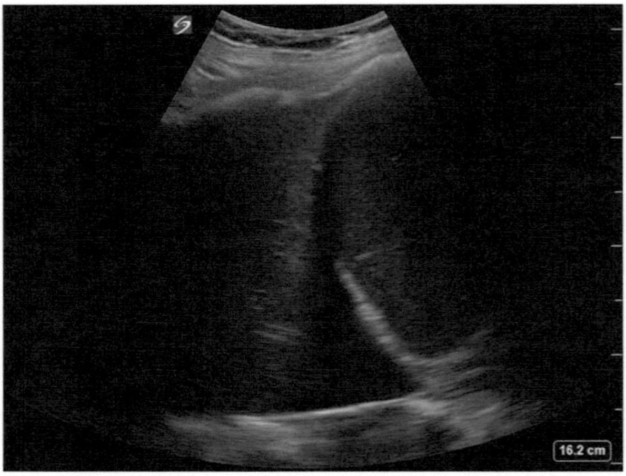

Fig. 6.3 Hepatization: Lung tissue above the diaphragm (left side) appears similar to liver tissue below the diaphragm (right side). Also noted is a pleural effusion

Image Acquisition

- Transducer Selection
  - Linear array: allows best visualization of the pleura and superficial lung fields.
  - Curvilinear: allows visualization of multiple rib spaces at once, best for viewing deep lung fields.
  - Phased array: allows the ability to image between rib spaces and view deeper lung fields.
- Patient Position
  - Ideally, the patient should be imaged while sitting upright to obtain optimal views, especially to evaluate for pleural effusion.
  - If the patient is unable to sit up, such as in the setting of trauma assessment, they can be imaged supine for anterior and lateral views and in a lateral recumbent position for posterior views, as needed.
- Standard Exam Views
  - A complete lung scan includes at least eight zones:
    - Anterior, lateral, posterior, and costophrenic angles bilaterally.
    - If there is concern for effusion, you can obtain similar views on the posterior and lateral aspects to better visualize fluid.
  - Figure 6.4—Lung zones

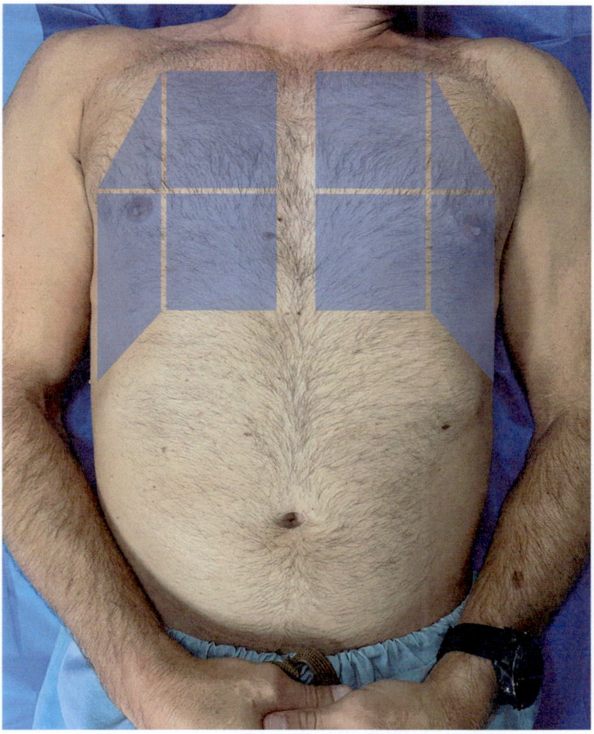

Fig. 6.4 Lung zones: Anterior and lateral lung zones are outlined here. When imaging the lung, it is important to evaluate multiple zones for completeness

Image Acquisition

(a) Lung Fields
- Place the transducer vertically with the marker pointed cephalad.
- Begin by evaluating for lung sliding.
  - Lung sliding occurs when the visceral pleura slides against the parietal pleura during normal respirations.
  - Adjust the depth and gain so that the lung pleura is optimally visualized in the middle of the screen; decreasing the gain can help better visualize the pleura.
  - Visualize at least two ribs with a hyperechoic horizontal line between them representing the pleural line.
    - Figure 6.5—Normal pleural line view
  - Lung sliding will appear as two thin hyperechoic lines moving horizontally against each other in a to-and-fro movement.
    - Video 6.3—Lung sliding

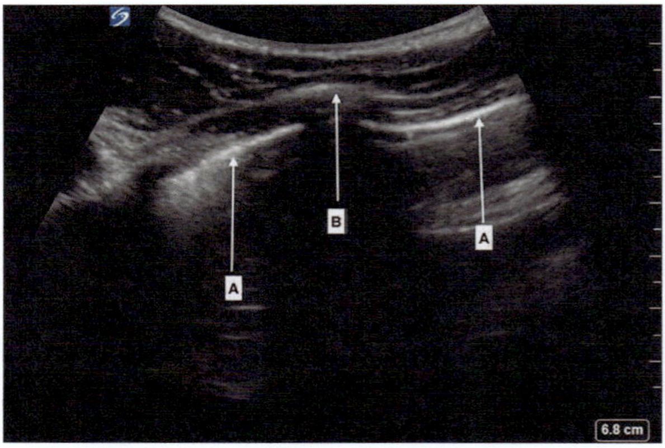

Fig. 6.5 Normal pleural line: Normal pleural line is hyperechoic and linear (A) located between rib shadows (B)

- If unable to determine if the pleura is sliding, utilize M-mode for further evaluation.
  - Place the M-mode line between two ribs so it crosses perpendicularly over the pleura.
    - Figure 6.6—M-mode with correct spike position
  - Horizontal lines represent the static chest wall [3].
  - Granular or wave-like pattern represents alveolar movement beyond the pleural line [3].
    - Figure 6.7—Normal sliding lung M-mode "seashore sign"
- Next, increase the depth to obtain views of the entire lung, or at least 15 cm.
  - Image each lung field (see above for recommended scanning locations).
  - Evaluate for A-lines, B-lines, and signs of pathology such as consolidation or effusion.
    - Figure 6.8—Lung fields with depth increased

(b) Costophrenic Angles

- Place the transducer inferiorly and posterolaterally where the diaphragm meets the liver or spleen with the transducer marker pointed cephalad.
  - Figure 6.9—Photo of transducer location and orientation for costophrenic angle imaging
- Visualize the hyperechoic diaphragm superior to the liver or spleen as it interfaces with the adjacent lung.
- Evaluate for consolidation, B-lines, or pleural effusion.
- The lung parenchyma is seen superior to the diaphragm.
  - Figure 6.10—Right costophrenic angle
  - Figure 6.11—Left costophrenic angle

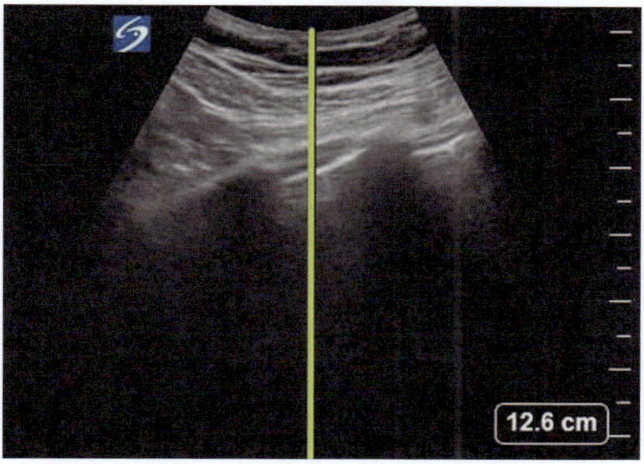

Fig. 6.6 M-mode with correct spike position: The M-mode spike should be placed between the two rib shadows overlying the hyperechoic pleural line

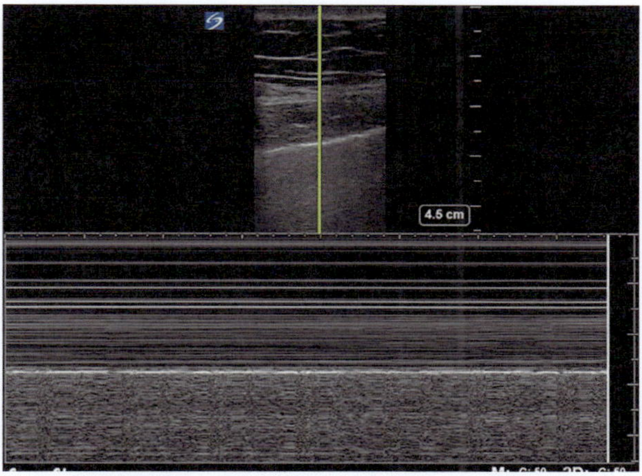

Fig. 6.7 Normal sliding lung M-mode "seashore sign": M-mode ultrasonography of a normal lung demonstrates the static chest wall in the top half of image and wavelike movement of the lungs in the bottom half consistent with normal respiration. This is sometimes referred to as "seashore" sign

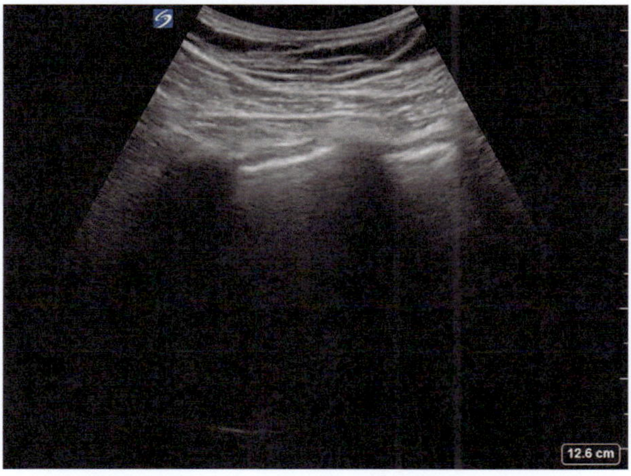

Fig. 6.8 Lung fields: Depth is increased for better visualization of the entire lung field, at least 15 cm

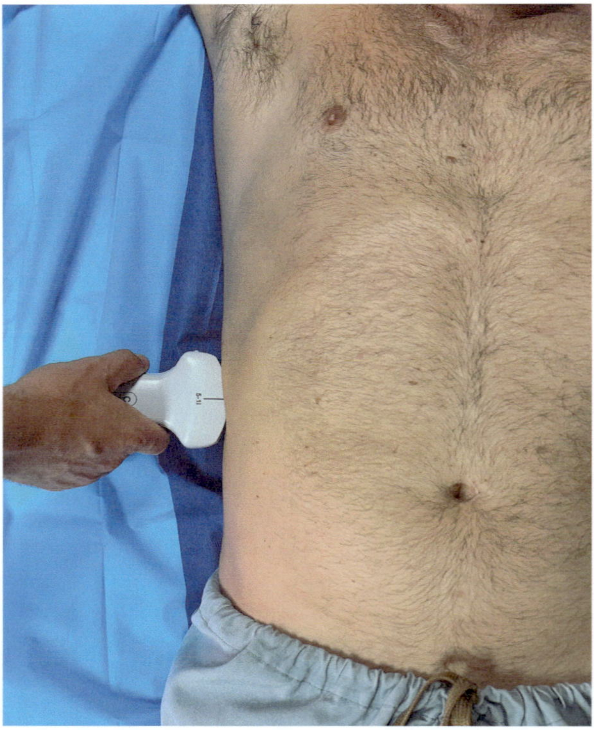

Fig. 6.9 Transducer location for right costophrenic angle: The transducer should be placed at each costophrenic angle bilaterally

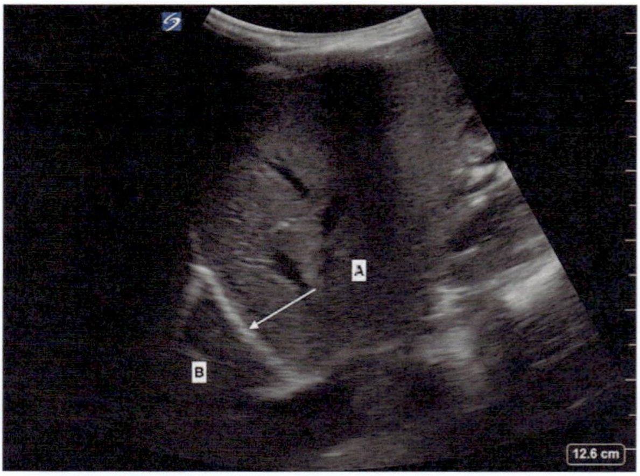

Fig. 6.10 Right costophrenic angle: The hyperechoic diaphragm (arrow) is seen separating the liver (A) and lung tissue (B) at the costophrenic angle

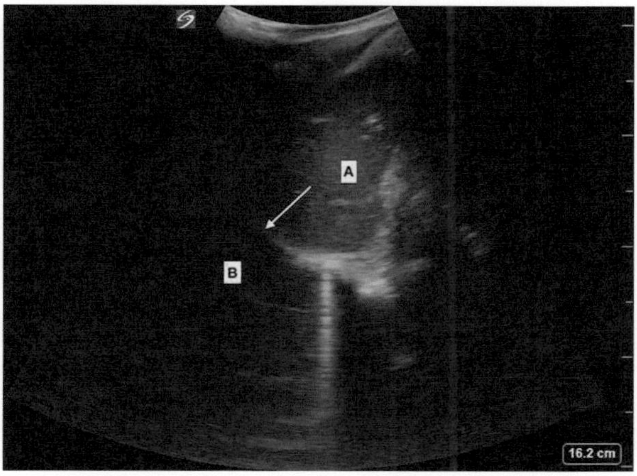

Fig. 6.11 Left costophrenic angle: The hyperechoic diaphragm (arrow) is seen separating the spleen (A) and lung tissue (B) at the costophrenic angle

Thoracic Pathology

- Pneumothorax
  - Caused by separation of the lung visceral pleura away from the chest wall parietal pleura, resulting in a collapsed lung.
  - Often spontaneous, traumatic, or iatrogenic.
  - On ultrasound, there is absent lung sliding due to separation of the visceral pleura from the parietal pleura [3].
    - Typically best seen in anterior and superior lung fields.
    - Video 6.4—Pneumothorax
  - Ultrasound for the evaluation of lung sliding has a negative predictive value of approximately 99.2–100%; therefore, the presence of lung sliding on ultrasound rules out pnemuothorax in most cases [3].
  - If lung sliding is absent, move the transducer superior or inferior to locate the lung point sign.
    - Lung point sign is the transition point between normal lung sliding and a pneumothorax with the absence of lung sliding.
    - Video 6.5—Lung point sign
    - Lung point sign is 100% specific for pneumothorax; however, it may not always be present, especially with a large pneumothorax when the lung is fully collapsed [3]
  - Use M-mode to confirm absence of sliding, as described above
    - M-mode will demonstrate no movement of the lungs, sometimes referred to as a barcode sign due to the horizontal lines throughout the entire image [3].
    - Figure 6.12—Barcode sign

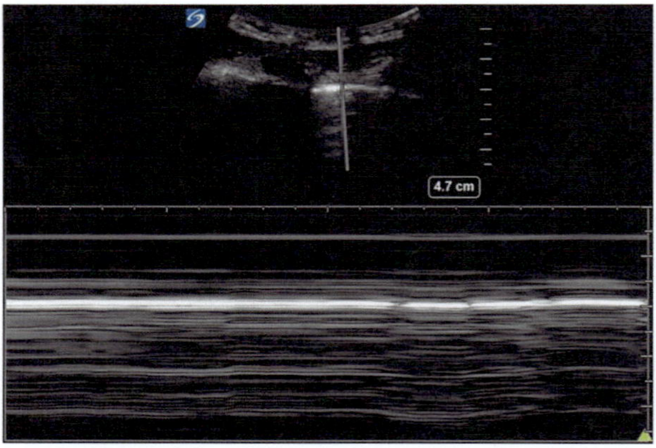

Fig. 6.12 Barcode sign: M-mode through the pleural line demonstrates no movement as evidenced by the steady horizontal lines in the bottom half of the image. This is sometimes referred to as the barcode sign given the similar appearance to retail barcodes

- Pulmonary Edema
  - Abnormal presence of fluid in the interstitium or alveoli of the lung.
  - Can be seen in patients with heart failure, acute respiratory distress syndrome (ARDS), fluid overload, hypertensive emergency, kidney failure, or liver failure.
  - On ultrasound, pulmonary edema is defined by the presence of three or more B-lines in two or more lung fields bilaterally [1, 7].
    - Figure 6.13—Pulmonary edema
    - Video 6.6—Pulmonary edema
- Pneumonia
  - Infection of a focal area or multiple areas of the lung tissue.
  - Identified as local consolidation on ultrasound in the presence of clinical signs and symptoms of pneumonia.
  - Consolidation is identified by an area of hypoechoic heterogeneous echotexture.
    - Consolidation can appear similar to the liver, called hepatization [6]
    - The margin of the consolidation can be blurred and irregular, sometimes referred to as shred or fractal sign [8].
    - Posterior to the consolidation, B-lines may be seen.
    - Figure 6.14—Consolidation
    - Video 6.7—Consolidation
  - Unilateral and focal B-lines are strongly suggestive of pneumonia even if consolidation is not seen.
  - Air bronchograms and fluid bronchograms may also be identified [1].
    - Air-filled bronchi can be identified as echogenic tubular structures within the consolidation [1, 8].
    - Fluid bronchograms are identified as anechoic tubular structures within the consolidation [1].

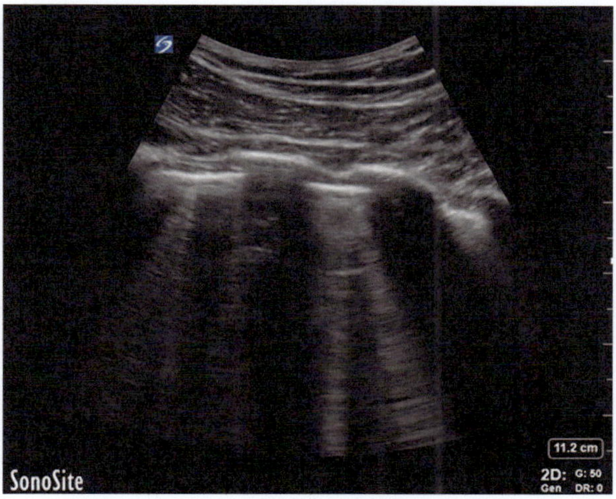

Fig. 6.13 Pulmonary edema: Diffuse B-lines taking up the entire lung field suggest pulmonary edema in the right clinical setting.

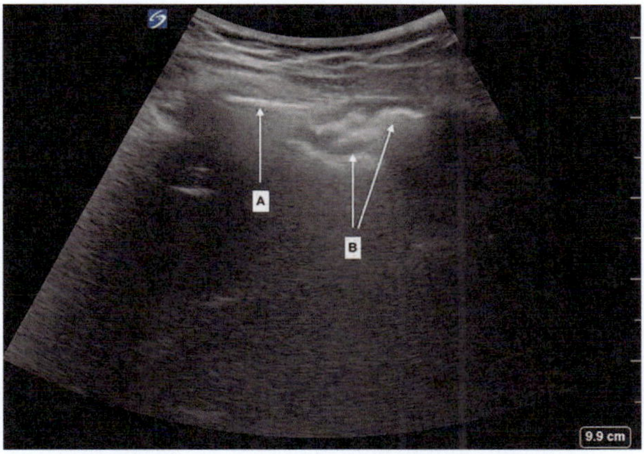

Fig. 6.14 Consolidation: Disruption of the pleural line (A) shows consolidation (B) of the lung tissue

- Pulmonary Contusion
  - Caused by blunt trauma to the lung parenchyma
  - Initially, trauma can cause alveolar disruption, which can be identified on ultrasound as B-lines due to developing interstitial edema [1]
  - As contusions evolve, alveolar bleeding displaces air from the affected parenchyma, causing hepatization of pulmonary tissue and subpleural consolidation [1]
  - Figure 6.15—Pulmonary contusion
  - Video 6.8—Pulmonary contusion
- Pleural Effusion
  - Abnormal collection of fluid between the two pleural layers.
  - Acute effusion is seen in dependent areas of the lung due to gravity.

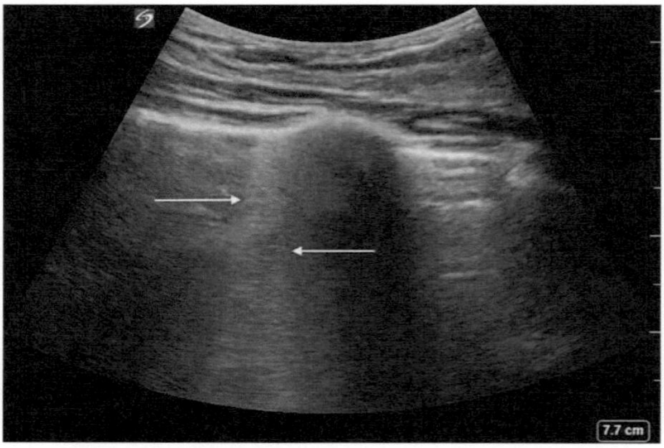

Fig. 6.15 Pulmonary contusion: In the setting of trauma, isolated B-lines suggest pulmonary contusion

    - Long-standing effusions can become organized or loculated and be visualized in nondependent areas.
  - On ultrasound, a pleural effusion is identified as an anechoic or hypoechoic area between the visceral and parietal pleura.
    - Accumulates posteriorly if the patient is supine.
    - Accumulates inferiorly between the diaphragm and lung in an upright patient.
    - Can often visualize the spine through the pleural effusion, where not visible through the lung, referred to as spine sign.
    - Figure 6.16—Pleural effusion
    - Video 6.9—Pleural effusion
  - Transudative effusion is typically anechoic without internal echoes [2, 9].
  - With exudative or hemorrhagic effusions, internal echoes will often be identified, sometimes referred to as plankton sign when scattered heterogenous echogenicity or hematocrit sign for gravity-dependent layering from blood settling and clotting [2, 9].
  - Curtain, jellyfish, or flag sign are terms to describe the lung sliding into the effusion during respirations [4].
    - Figure 6.17—Floating lung

Key Points

- Lung sliding may be absent or difficult to visualize in other disease processes, such as acute respiratory distress syndrome (ARDS), consolidation, right mainstem intubation [3], and shallow breathing.
- The presence of B-lines is strong evidence against a pneumothorax [2].
- Diffuse bilateral B-lines can be present in conditions other than pulmonary edema, such as ARDS, interstitial lung disease, and multifocal pneumonia [7].
- Typical pneumonia will appear as consolidation, but atypical pneumonia will not have focal findings.

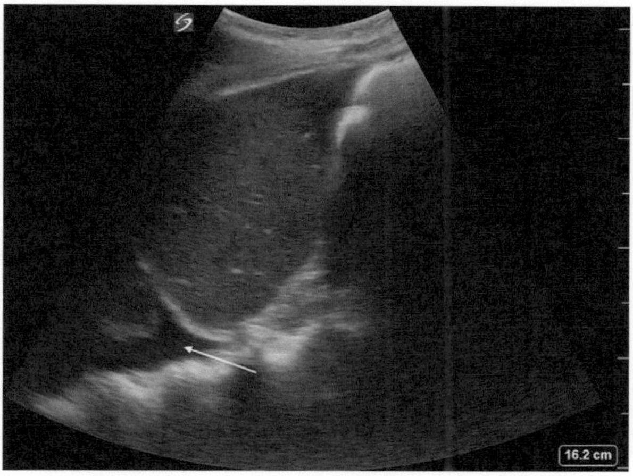

Fig. 6.16 Pleural effusion: A small pleural effusion (arrow) is noted above the diaphragm. Also, the spine is able to be visualized, called spine sign

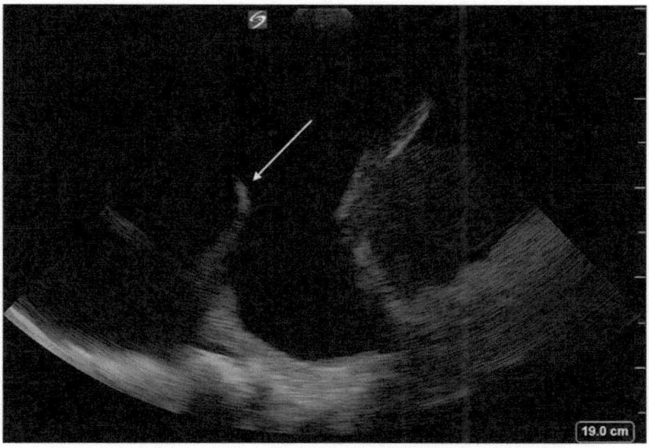

Fig. 6.17 Floating lung: With large pleural effusions, the lung will appear to be floating in the fluid, creating what looks like a flag flapping in the wind (flag/curtain/jellyfish sign)

References

1. Silva FR, Mills LD. Chapter 7: Pulmonary. In: Ma OJ, Mateer JR, Reardon RF, Joing SA, editors. Emergency ultrasound. 3rd ed. China: McGraw-Hill Education; 2014. p. 169–90.
2. Saraogi A. Lung ultrasound: present and future. Lung India. 2014;32(3):250–7. https://www.ncbi.nlm.nih.gov/pmc/articles/PMC4429387/. Accessed 25 Apr 2017 (Lung)
3. Husain LF, Hagopian L, Wayman D, Baker WE, Carmody KA. Sonographic diagnosis of pneumothorax. J Emerg Trauma Shock. 2012;5(1):76–81. https://www.ncbi.nlm.nih.gov/pmc/articles/PMC3299161/. Accessed 26 Apr 2017
4. Bhoil R, Ahluwalia A, Chopra R, Surya M, Bhoil S. Signs and lines in lung ultrasound. J Ultrasonogr. 2021;21(86):e225–33.
5. Francisco Neto MJ, Rahal Junior A, Vieira FAC, da Silva PSD, de Funari GMB. Advances in lung ultrasound. Einstein (São Paulo). 2016;14(3):443–8.

6. Durant A, Nagdev A. Ultrasound detection of lung hepatization. West J Emerg Med. 2010;11(4):322–3. https://www.ncbi.nlm.nih.gov/pmc/articles/PMC2967681/. Accessed 26 Apr 2017 (US Detect)
7. Martindale JL, Wakai A, Collins SP, Levy PD, Diercks D, Hiestand BC, Fermann GJ, deSouza I, Sinert R. Diagnosing acute heart failure in the emergency department: a systematic review and meta-analysis. Acad Emerg Med. 2016;23(3):223–42.
8. Lee FCY. Lung ultrasound – a primary survey of the acutely dyspneic patient. J Intensive Care. 2016;4(1):57. https://www.ncbi.nlm.nih.gov/pmc/articles/PMC5007698/. Accessed 26 Apr 2017
9. Prina E, Torres A, Roberto C, Carvalho R. Lung ultrasound in the evaluation of pleural effusion. J Bras Pneumol. 2014;40(10):1–5. https://www.ncbi.nlm.nih.gov/pmc/articles/PMC4075927/. Accessed 26 Apr 2017

Head and Neck Ultrasound 7

Zackary Funk, Jordan Tozer, Angela Lindsay, and Michael Joyce

Using point-of-care ultrasound to evaluate head and neck pathology is a relatively new and evolving entity. One of the more routine but common indications to perform this exam is to assess for and assist with incision and drainage of a peritonsillar abscess. However, there are other areas of interest such as the thyroid gland, parotid gland, and carotid artery. In addition, assessing for proper endotracheal tube location can be done immediately following intubation using ultrasound techniques. While head and neck ultrasound may be intimidating to the novice sonographer, the technical skills needed to obtain and interpret these images are quite simple due to superficial and easy-to-identify structures. Therefore, with minimal practice, one can become an expert in head and neck ultrasound. This chapter will review indications to perform a head or neck ultrasound, basic anatomy, image acquisition, normal ultrasound anatomy, and interpretation of pathology.

Supplementary Information The online version contains supplementary material available at https://doi.org/10.1007/978-3-032-27643-8_7.

Z. Funk
Department of Emergency Medicine, Virginia Commonwealth University Medical Center, Richmond, VA, USA
e-mail: zackary.funk@vcuhealth.org

J. Tozer · A. Lindsay (✉) · M. Joyce
Department of Emergency Medicine, Virginia Commonwealth University Health, Richmond, VA, USA
e-mail: jordan.tozer@vcuhealth.org; angela.creditt@vcuhealth.org; john.joyce@vcuhealth.org

A. Lindsay et al. (eds.), *Clinical Ultrasound*,
https://doi.org/10.1007/978-3-032-27643-8_7

Tonsillar Ultrasound

(a) Clinical Application and Indications
- Asymmetrical tonsillar enlargement
- Evaluate for peritonsillar abscess

(b) Tonsillar Anatomy
- Paired lymphatic structures located in the posterior oropharynx

(c) Transducer Selection
- Endocavitary transducer for intraoral approach
- Linear transducer for submandibular approach

(d) Patient Position
- Have the patient sit upright with the back of their head supported by the head of the bed [1]

(e) Standard Exam Views
- Insert the transducer into the patient's mouth
- Place the head of the transducer against the affected tonsil
- Very slowly fan the transducer to evaluate for signs of a fluid collection indicating peritonsillar abscess or cobblestoning indicating tonsillar edema
- Compared to the unaffected side
- Identify the carotid artery posterior to the tonsil
  - Figure 7.1—Carotid artery posterior to the tonsil
  - Video 7.1—Carotid artery posterior to the tonsil

(f) Peritonsillar Abscess
- Walled-off bacterial infection resulting in a collection of purulent fluid next to a tonsil, usually due to sequelae of bacterial pharyngitis.
- Will appear as a hypoechoic fluid collection next to an asymmetrically enlarged tonsil.
  - Can contain complex fluid with internal echoes and debris
  - Figure 7.2—Peritonsillar abscess
  - Video 7.2—Peritonsillar abscess
- Measure the size of the abscess

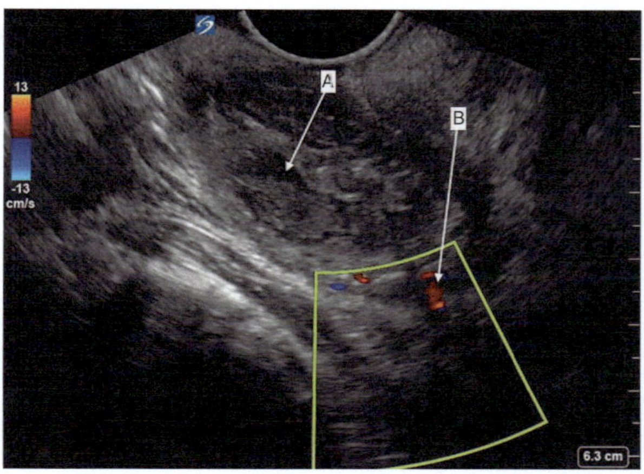

Fig. 7.1 Carotid artery posterior to tonsil: The carotid artery (B) can be visualized posterior to the tonsil. A peritonsillar abscess can be seen in this image (A)

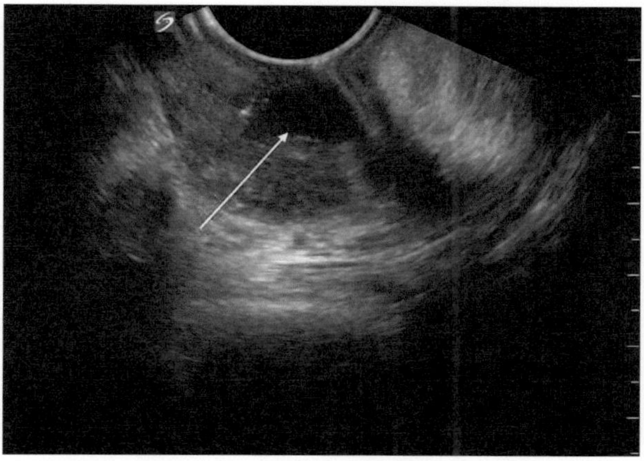

Fig. 7.2 Peritonsillar abscess: A large area of hypoechoic fluid (arrow) represents a peritonsillar abscess

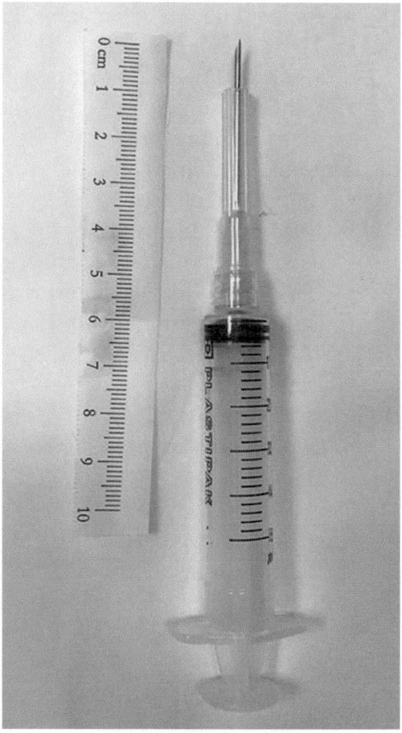

Fig. 7.3 Needle with plastic cap cut: To avoid entering too far into the peritonsillar space, a needle cap can be cut to only allow a set amount of needle to enter

- Measure the depth of the abscess cavity from the transducer [1]
  - Based on this measurement, choose the appropriate needle length
  - Place the plastic cap on the needle and cut the cap a distance back from the needle tip that is just longer than this measurement.
    - Figure 7.3—Needle with plastic cap cut
  - This will ensure the needle does not enter the tonsil too far putting the carotid artery at risk for injury.

- Perform incision and drainage of the abscess using landmarks or direct ultrasound guidance.
- Reimage the area to evaluate for improvement of the fluid collection

Key Points

- When evaluating for a peritonsillar abscess, the patient may have limited ability to open the mouth secondary to trismus.
- Have the patient hold their tongue down themselves with a tongue depressor or even a laryngoscope as they will know their own gag reflex.

Thyroid Ultrasound

(a) Clinical Application and Indications
- Evaluation of a palpable neck mass [2]
- Thyroid enlargement
- Abnormal thyroid function labs
- Further evaluation of an incidental finding on other imaging studies such as thyroid nodule or cyst [2]

(b) Thyroid Anatomy
- Superficial endocrine organ in the neck that overlies the trachea.
- Isthmus of the thyroid is the connection between the right and left lobes and usually lies over the second or third tracheal ring.
- Each lobe is located anterior and lateral to the trachea, with the carotid artery and internal jugular veins located posteriorly.

(c) Transducer Selection
- Linear array transducer

(d) Patient Position
- The patient should be supine or in a semi-recumbent position with their neck extended.

(e) Standard Exam Views
- Begin by imaging the thyroid gland in a transverse plane.
- Place the transducer below the laryngeal prominence with the marker pointed toward the patient's right.
  - Figure 7.4—Transducer position
- Scan inferiorly until the isthmus of the thyroid is visualized
  - Thyroid gland will appear as a uniform, finely granular structure that is slightly more echogenic than the surrounding musculature [3].
  - Isthmus will be seen anterior to the hyperechoic trachea with the left and right lobes on either side, respectively.
  - Figure 7.5—Isthmus of the thyroid
- Move the transducer laterally to each side to image the right and left lobes of the thyroid.
  - Figure 7.6—Thyroid lobes

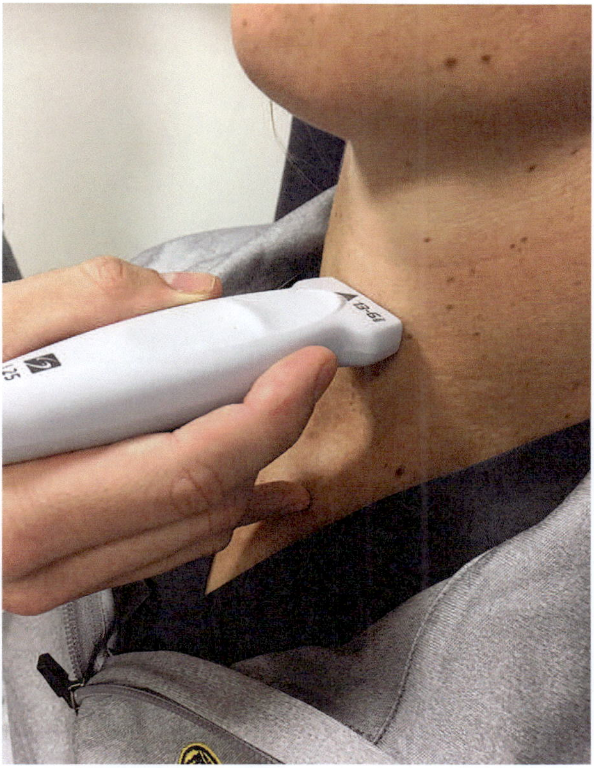

Fig. 7.4 Transducer position on neck: For thyroid ultrasound, having the patient sit in a supine position slightly recumbent can facilitate easy scanning of the neck

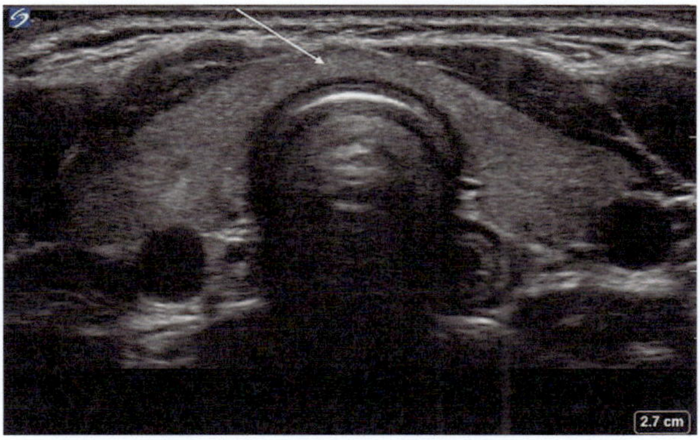

Fig. 7.5 Isthmus of thyroid: The isthmus of the thyroid (arrow) will be seen anterior to the hyperechoic trachea

- Lateral to each lobe will be the paired thick-walled anechoic and pulsatile carotid arteries followed by the thinner-walled internal jugular veins [4].
- The esophagus is often found posterior to the left thyroid lobe and anterior to the cervical vertebral body. It is visualized as an oval or flattened structure with alternating hypo- and hyperechogenicity [3].

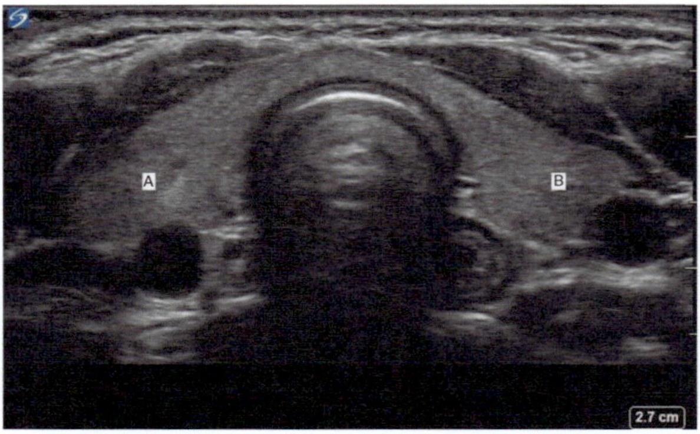

Fig. 7.6 Thyroid lobes: Right (A) and left (B) thyroid lobes

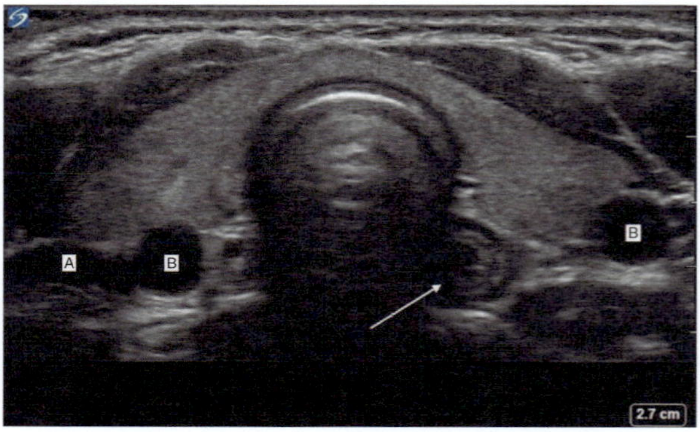

Fig. 7.7 Thyroid with surrounding structures: Lateral to each thyroid lobe will be the paired thick-walled anechoic and pulsatile carotid arteries (B) followed by the thinner-walled internal jugular veins (A). The esophagus (arrow) is often found posterior to the left thyroid lobe and anterior to the cervical vertebral body

  - Figure 7.7—Thyroid and surrounding structures
  - Video 7.3—Thyroid ultrasound
- Rotate the transducer clockwise 90° with the marker pointed cephalad. Image each lobe of the thyroid in a sagittal plane.
  - Figure 7.8—Thyroid in a sagittal plane
  - Video 7.4—Thyroid in sagittal plane
- Apply color Doppler to each area of the thyroid to evaluate vascular flow
  - Figure 7.9—Color Doppler of the thyroid gland
  - Video 7.5—Color Doppler of the thyroid gland

(f) Thyroid Pathology
- Thyroid nodule
  - Lesion within the thyroid gland caused by an overgrowth of thyroid cells.
  - Majority of thyroid nodules are benign with only about 5% malignant [5].
  - Common incidental findings on computed tomography or with ultrasound of the thyroid.
  - Will appear as a discrete lesion that distorts the normal thyroid echotexture [4].
  - Figure 7.10—Thyroid nodule

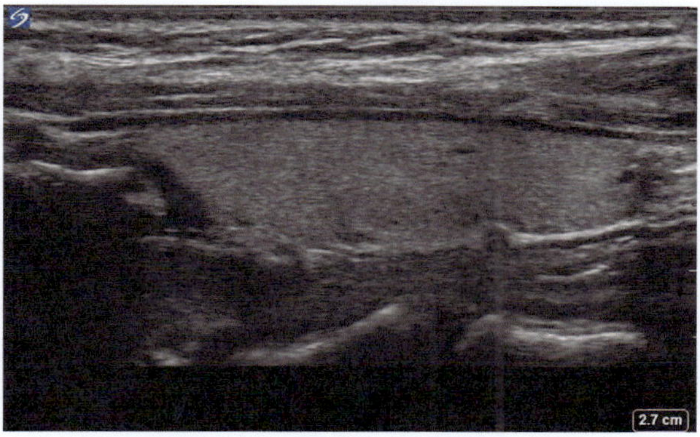

Fig. 7.8 Thyroid in a sagittal plane: Left lobe of the thyroid visualized in sagittal plane

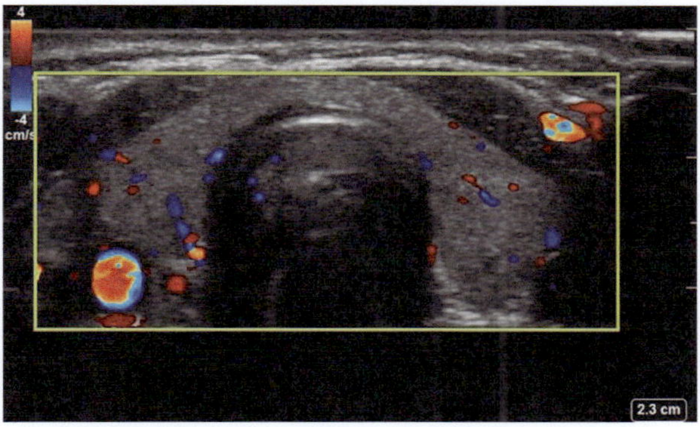

Fig. 7.9 Color Doppler of the thyroid gland: Normal vascular flow of the thyroid gland using color Doppler

- Thyroid Cyst
  - A type of benign thyroid nodule that can be simple, colloid, or hemorrhagic.
  - Simple cysts will appear as round, anechoic, or hypoechoic structures with posterior acoustic enhancement.
  - Figure 7.11—Thyroid cyst
  - Video 7.6—Thyroid cyst
- Thyroiditis
  - Inflammation of the thyroid gland.
  - Will appear as decreased echogenicity with increased vascularity resulting in increased flow with color Doppler [6].
  - Figure 7.12—Thyroiditis
  - Video 7.7 Thyroiditis

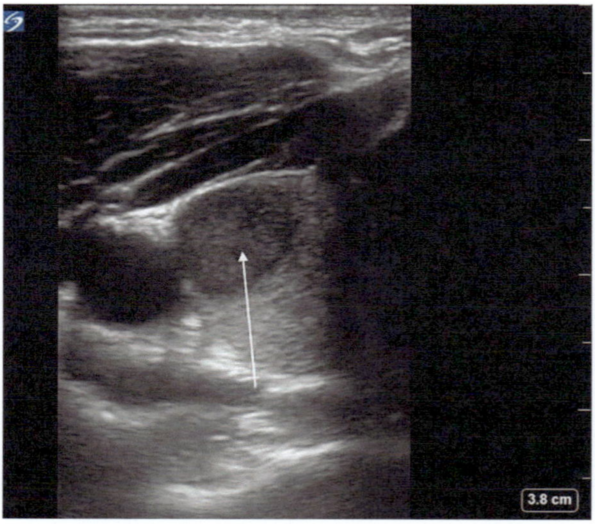

Fig. 7.10 Thyroid nodule: A thyroid nodule (arrow) is a distinct lesion within the thyroid that is formed by an overgrowth of thyroid cells

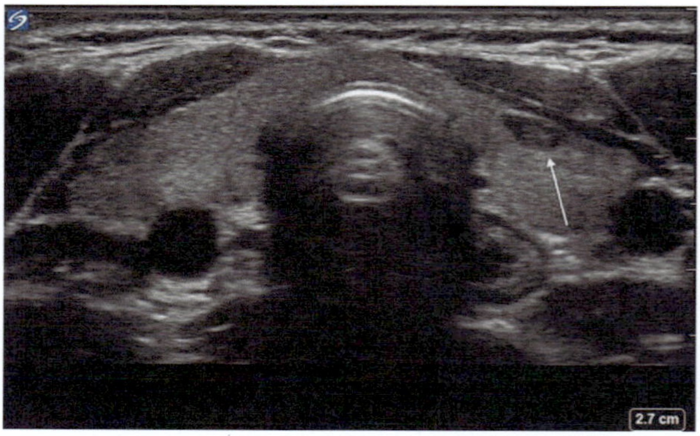

Fig. 7.11 Thyroid cyst: Thyroid cysts (arrow) are a type of benign nodule that can be simple, colloid, or hemorrhagic

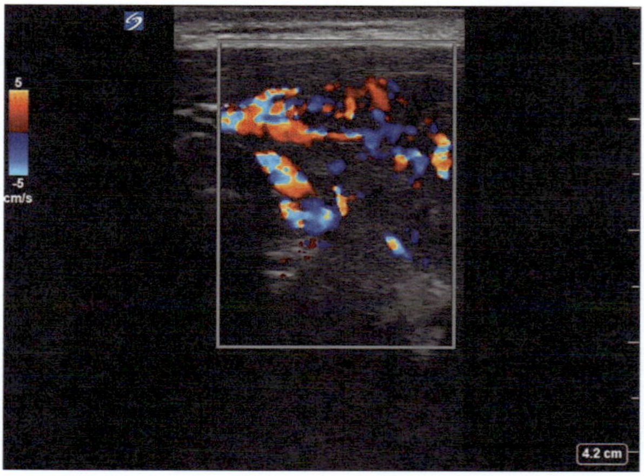

Fig. 7.12 Thyroiditis: With any inflammatory state of the thyroid, there will be increased vascular flow as evidenced here by placing color Doppler over the thyroid gland

Tracheal Ultrasound

- Clinical Application and Indications
  - Confirm endotracheal tube placement
- Trachea Anatomy
  - Located superficially in the anterior neck
  - Membranous tube that connects the pharynx and larynx to the lungs
  - Reinforced by anterior rings of cartilage
  - Cricothyroid membrane sits between the thyroid cartilage superiorly and cricoid cartilage inferiorly
- Transducer Selection
  - Linear array transducer
- Patient Position
  - This exam will typically be performed on an intubated patient; therefore, the patient should be supine or with the head of the bed elevated to 30°.
- Standard Exam Views
  - Place the transducer on the midline anterior neck in a transverse plane. The trachea will appear as an echogenic curved stripe with posterior acoustic shadowing.
    - Figure 7.13—Transducer placement over the trachea
    - Figure 7.14—Trachea
    - Video 7.8—Trachea

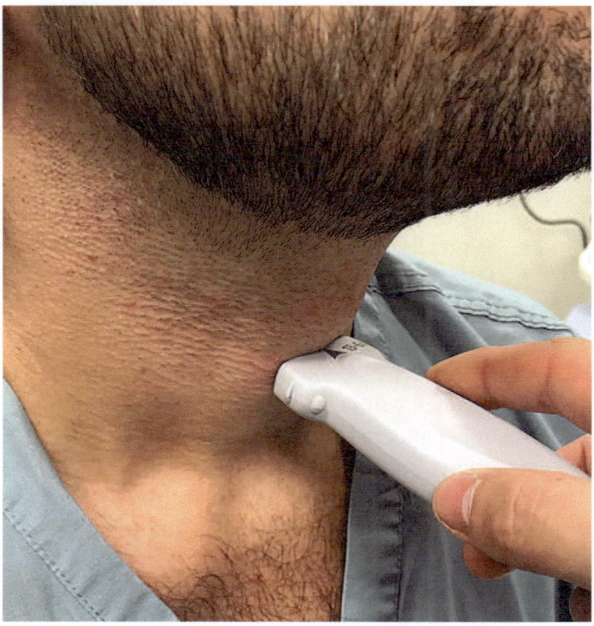

Fig. 7.13 Transducer placement over trachea: To visualize the trachea, place the transducer in a transverse orientation over the center of the neck

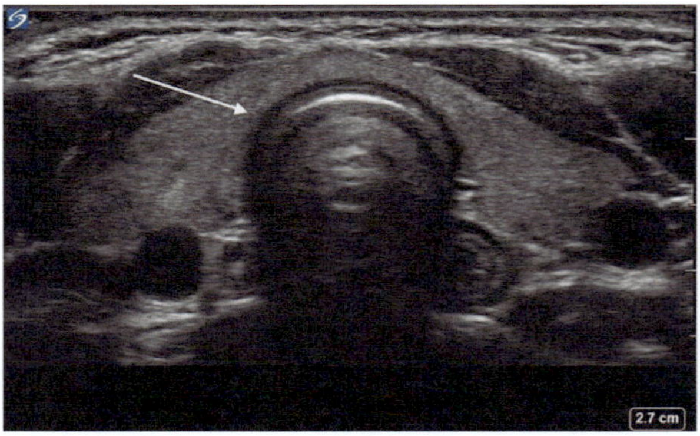

Fig. 7.14 Trachea: The trachea (arrow) will appear as an echogenic curved stripe with posterior acoustic shadowing

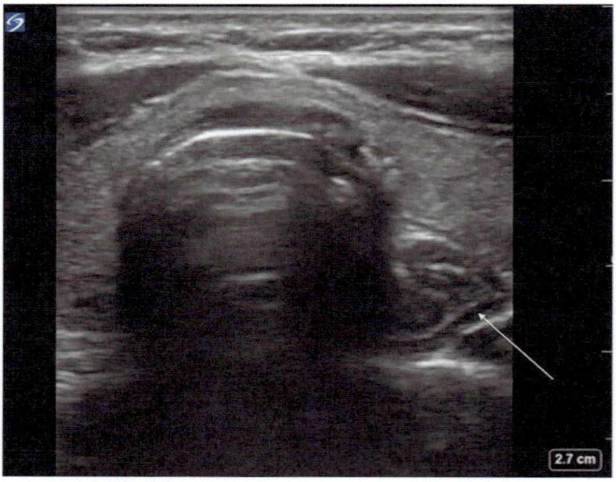

Fig. 7.15 Image of trachea with esophagus identified: Attempt to visualize the esophagus (arrow), which is located to the left of the trachea (on the right of the image) as seen here

  - Scan both cranially and caudally to evaluate the trachea.
  - Attempt to visualize the esophagus located to the left; this can be enhanced by asking the patient to swallow.
    - Typically found posterior to the left lobe of the thyroid gland.
    - Figure 7.15—The trachea and esophagus
- Confirmation of Endotracheal Tube Placement
  - Ultrasound the trachea as described above.
  - With correct placement of an endotracheal tube, two curved parallel echogenic lines will be seen [3] with more prominent posterior acoustic enhancement [7] and an increased amount of B-lines.
    - Figure 7.16—Correct ETT placement
    - Video 7.9—Correct ETT placement
  - Slight shaking or movement of the tube will demonstrate movement of the trachea on ultrasound.

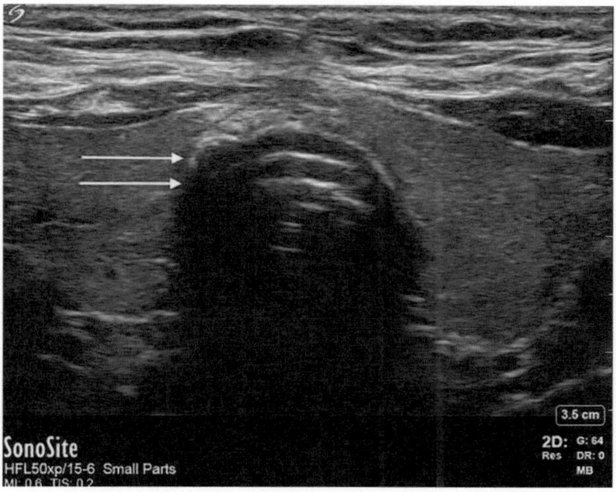

Fig. 7.16 Correct ETT placement: With correct placement of an endotracheal tube, two curved parallel echogenic lines (arrows) will be seen

- Esophageal Intubation
  - Incorrect placement of an endotracheal tube will be visualized as an echogenic curved line with posterior acoustic shadowing posterior and lateral to the trachea [7].
    - Usually posterior to the left lobe of the thyroid gland [3].
    - Occasionally referred to as "double trachea sign" [7].

Key Points

- Endotracheal tube confirmation can also be performed in real time by visualizing the tube [7] in long [3] or short axis as the tube is placed.
- Using ultrasound to confirm endotracheal tube placement has been found to have a sensitivity and specificity of 98% [8].

Carotid Artery Ultrasound

- Clinical Application and Indications
  - Evaluate for carotid artery dissection
- Carotid Artery Anatomy
  - Right carotid artery is a branch of the brachiocephalic artery.
  - Left carotid artery branches directly off the arch of the aorta.
  - Splits into the external and internal carotid arteries at the level of the fourth cervical vertebrae, just distal to the carotid bulb.
- Transducer Selection
  - Linear array transducer
- Patient Position
  - Have the patient lay supine or in a semi-recumbent position with their neck extended and head facing away from the side being imaged.

- Standard Exam Views
  - Place the transducer in a transverse plane, just above the clavicle to obtain a short-axis view of the carotid artery.
  - Scan cranially to evaluate the entire length of the carotid artery.
    - Figure 7.17—Short axis of the carotid artery
  - Switch to long axis by rotating the transducer marker toward the patient's head and scan cranially to evaluate the carotid bulb.
    - Figure 7.18—Long axis with carotid bulb
- Carotid Artery Dissection
  - Separation of the inner wall of the carotid artery creating a false lumen.
  - Appears as a hyperechoic linear stripe within the lumen of the carotid artery.

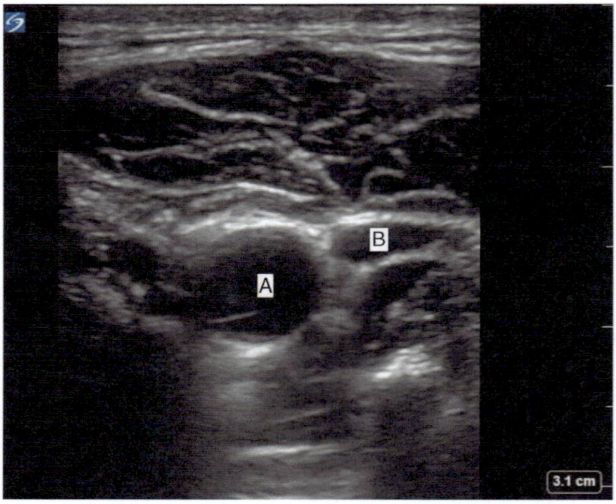

Fig. 7.17 Short axis of the carotid artery: In a transverse plane, the carotid artery will be imaged in short axis appearing as a thick-walled anechoic vessel (A) next to the thin and collapsible vein (B)

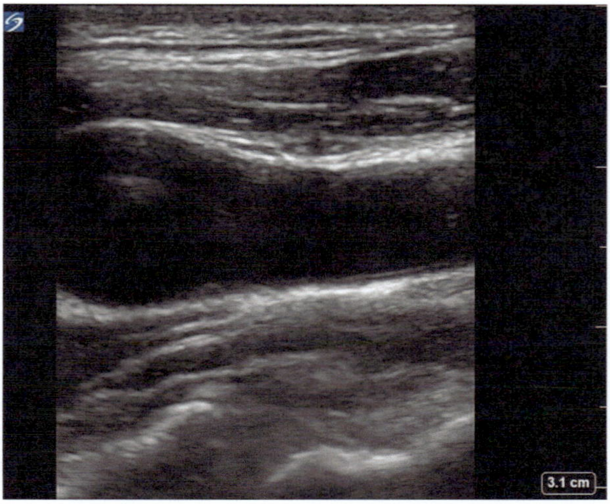

Fig. 7.18 Long axis with carotid bulb labeled: In long axis, with the transducer oriented so the marker is pointed toward the patient's head, the carotid artery will appear as an anechoic tube with the carotid bulb locater more superior

Salivary Gland

(a) Clinical Application and Indications
  - Preauricular pain and/or swelling

(b) Basic Anatomy
  - Parotid gland
    - Located anterior to the ear bilaterally with the upper portion nearly in line with the external auditory meatus [3]
    - Parotid gland duct courses from the anterior surface of the gland through buccal fat and buccinator muscle. It enters the mouth adjacent to the second upper molar as the parotid papilla [3]
  - Submandibular gland
    - Triangular shaped within the submandibular triangle [3] inferior to the mandible
    - Submandibular duct courses medially and superiorly where it enters the mouth as a papilla near the lingual frenulum [3]

(c) Transducer Selection
  - Linear array transducer

(d) Patient Position
  - Place the patient in a position of comfort; they can be supine, semi-recumbent, or sitting up with the back of their head supported.
  - When imaging the submandibular gland, it may be helpful to tilt the patient's head up.

(e) Standard Exam Views
  - Parotid gland
    - Begin by imaging the parotid gland in a sagittal plane with the transducer marker pointed superiorly.
      - Figure 7.19—Transducer position parotid gland
    - Parotid gland will have a homogeneous, finely granular echotexture [3].
      - Figure 7.20—Parotid gland
      - Video 7.10—Parotid gland
    - Scan through the gland looking for any abnormalities.
    - Rotate the transducer counterclockwise with the transducer marker pointed toward the patient's right to image the parotid duct in a transverse plane.
    - Line the transducer up with the earlobe near mid-cheek to identify the duct as two thin hyperechoic lines close together and parallel [3].
      - Figure 7.21—Parotid duct
  - Submandibular gland
    - Place the transducer within the submandibular space anterior to the angle of the mandible.
      - Figure 7.22—Transducer placement submandibular gland
    - Identify the gland just beneath the subcutaneous tissue as a homogeneous structure with intermediate echogenicity [9], similar to the parotid gland.

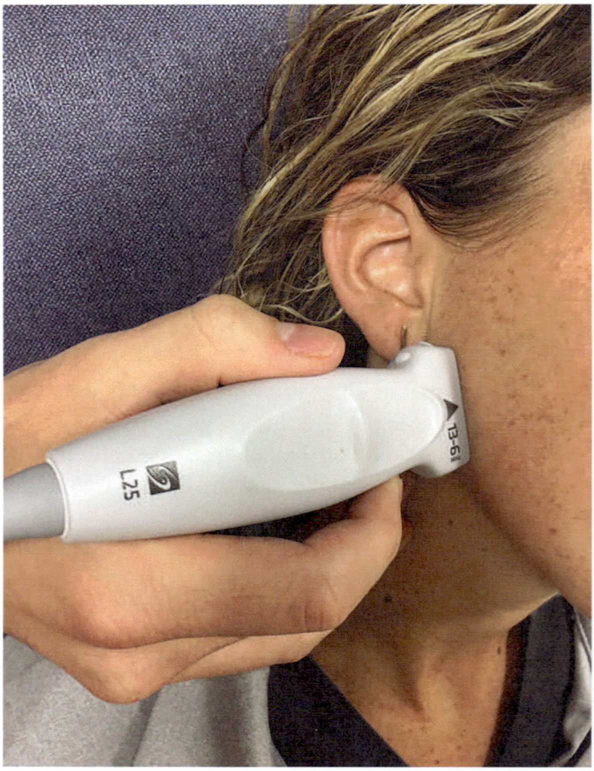

Fig. 7.19 Transducer position parotid gland: Place the transducer near the angle of the jaw with the marker pointed superiorly

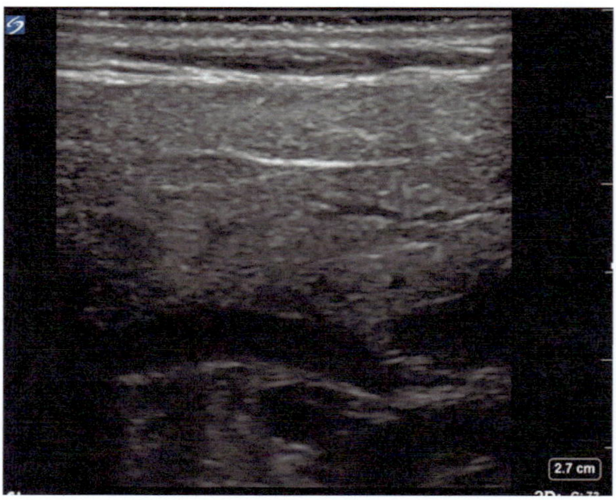

Fig. 7.20 Parotid gland: The parotid gland is seen just below the skin with a homogenous, finely granular echotexture

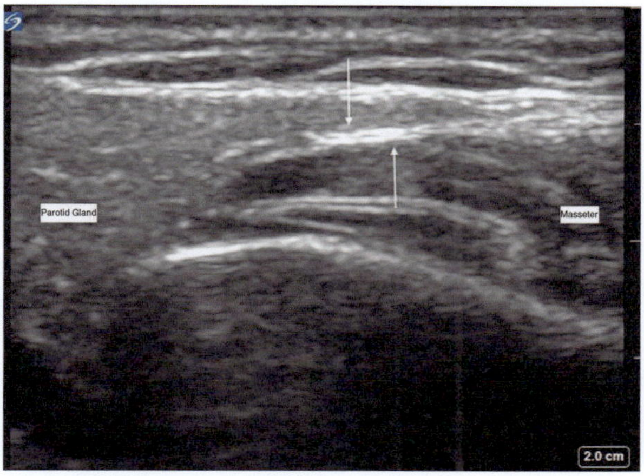

Fig. 7.21 Parotid duct: The parotid duct will appear as two thin parallel hyperechoic lines coursing over the masseter muscle (arrows)

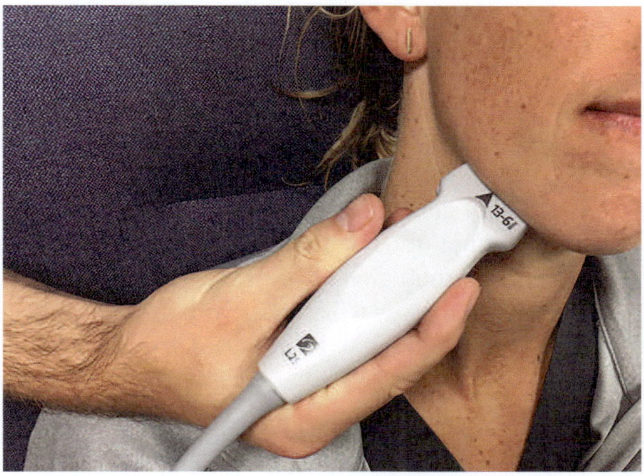

Fig. 7.22 Transducer placement submandibular gland: Place the transducer inferior to the mandible within the submandibular space to visualize the submandibular gland

- Figure 7.23—Submandibular gland
- Video 7.11—Submandibular gland

– The facial artery and vein will be seen near the gland [9].

(f) Salivary Gland Pathology

- Sialolithiasis
  – Stone within a salivary gland or duct.
  – Found within the parotid gland and, more commonly, the submandibular gland [3] or duct.
  – Visualized as echogenic foci with posterior acoustic shadowing [3], similar to gallstones or renal stones.
  – If obstructed, the duct will become dilated representing a small anechoic tube leading to an echogenic stone [3].

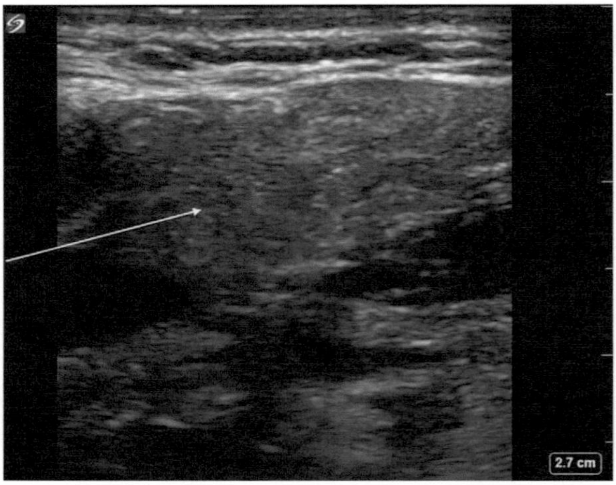

Fig. 7.23 Submandibular gland: Submandibular gland (arrow) appears as a homogenous structure, similar to the parotid gland, just deep to the subcutaneous tissue

- Sialadenitis
  - Inflammation or infection of a salivary gland.
  - Gland will appear enlarged with a more heterogeneous, echogenic architecture as compared with normal salivary gland tissue [3].
  - Can also see increased blood flow on color Doppler [3].
- Salivary gland mass
  - Benign (most common) or malignant lesion of a salivary gland, usually the parotid gland [3].
  - Solid masses will appear with mixed echogenicity with some hypoechoic areas; there may be posterior acoustic enhancement [3].
  - Cystic masses will typically appear similar to cysts elsewhere as an anechoic lesion [3].

Lymph Nodes

(a) Clinical Application and Indications
  - Evaluation of an area of painful or painless swelling to determine next best step in management or evaluation.
    - E.g., determining if axillary swelling is due to an enlarged lymph node, which should not undergo incision and drainage, or an abscess, for which incision and drainage is typically the most appropriate management.

(b) Basic Anatomy
  - Well-circumscribed homogeneously hypoechoic structure with color Doppler signal over vascular hyperechoic hilum [10].
    - Some liken the gross appearance with color Doppler as similar in appearance to the kidney
      - Figure 7.24—Lymph node anatomy

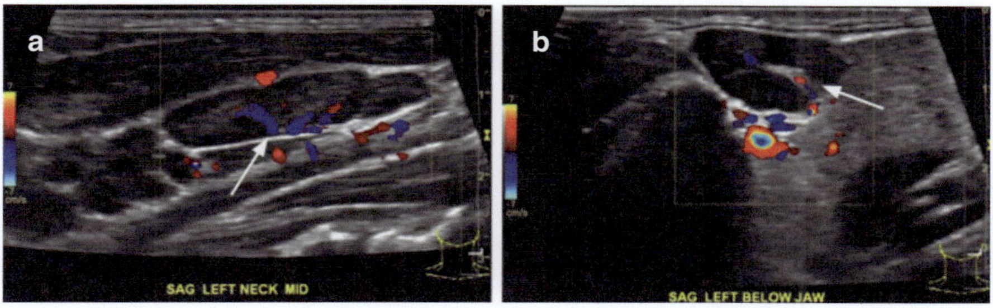

Fig. 7.24 Lymph node anatomy: Ovoid-shaped structure with hypoechoic cortex and hyperechoic vascular hilum. The arrows in Figures (**a**) and (**b**) demonstrate the hyperechoic vascular hilum with color flow

(c) Transducer Selection
  - Linear array transducer

(d) Patient Position
  - Place the patient in a position of comfort that allows for adequate evaluation of the area of interest.

(e) Standard Exam Views
  - B mode Imaging
    - Ideally, the site of interest should be surveyed in two orthogonal planes (i.e., transverse and sagittal planes).
    - When possible, sliding or fanning from normal appearing tissue through the area of interest is recommended to both delineate margins of involvement and provide contrast between normal and affected tissues.
  - Color Doppler
    - The application of color Doppler is essential when evaluating encapsulated structures.
      - Absence or abnormality of the vascular hilum may suggest processes such as abscess, cyst, or malignancy.
        - Video 7.12—Lymph node color Doppler

(f) Lymph Node Pathology
  - Lymphadenopathy
    - Hypertrophy of lymph node cortex due to lymph tissue hyperproliferation.
    - Typically preserve the normal hypoechoic cortex, hyperechoic hilum, and overall ovoid of a lymph node.
    - Not necessarily a pathologic finding but can be indicative of other disorders.
      - Figure 7.25—Lymphadenopathy
  - Lymphadenitis
    - Painful enlargement of lymph nodes typically reactive to infection.
    - Bilateral lymphadenitis (e.g., cervical chain lymphadenitis) is typically suggestive of a viral etiology, whereas unilateral lymphadenitis could be more suggestive of a bacterial etiology.

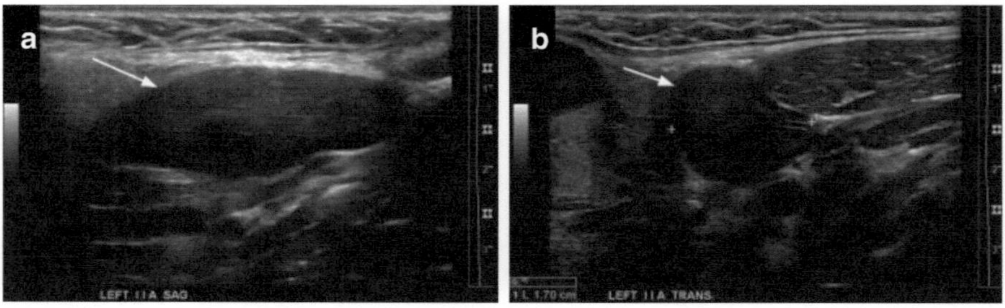

Fig. 7.25 Lymphadenopathy: Enlargement of the hypoechoic cortex with overall preservation of lymph node architecture. The arrows in Figure (**a**) and (**b**) demonstrate the lymph nodes with features characteristic of lymphadenopathy with enlargement of the hypoechoic cortex with overall preservation of lymph node architecture

  - Features of uncomplicated lymphadenitis include:
    - Overall preservation of normal lymph node architecture with ovoid shape but with potential loss of the clear hyperechoic hilum [10].
    - Homogenous parenchyma with low echogenicity [10].
    - Increased vascularity on color Doppler [10].
      - Figure 7.26—Lymphadenitis
  - Complications of lymphadenitis can occur, such as:
    - Suppurative lymphadenitis
      - Bacterial infection of lymph node
      - Potential features on ultrasound include
        - Increased heterogenicity of normally homogenous hypoechoic echotexture [10].
        - Hilar atrophy and decreased vascularity, as well as cobblestoning or subcutaneous fluid surrounding the lymph node [10].
          - Figure 7.27—Suppurative lymphadenitis
    - Abscess formation
      - Formation of encapsulated fluid-filled structure or cavitation within lymph node structure.
      - Increased peripheral vascularity of lymph node [10].
        - Figure 7.28—Lymph node abscess
- Malignancy
  - Features which may suggest a lymph node may be malignant include:
    - Larger size and heterogeneous echotexture [11].
    - A progression toward a more rounded lymph node shape rather than the typical ovoid appearance is thought to be highly suggestive of malignancy [11].
    - Nodal matting, i.e., the coalescence of several lymph nodes into an ill-defined structure [11].
    - Distortion/edema of surrounding structures [11].

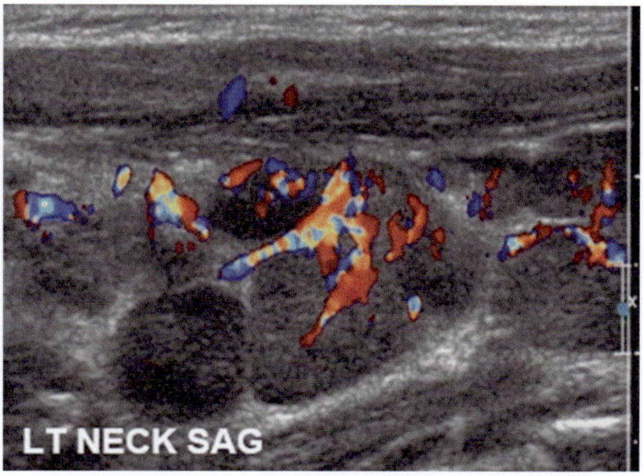

Fig. 7.26 Lymphadenitis: Enlarged lymph nodes with increased vascularity but overall preserved architecture that are tender to palpation on exam

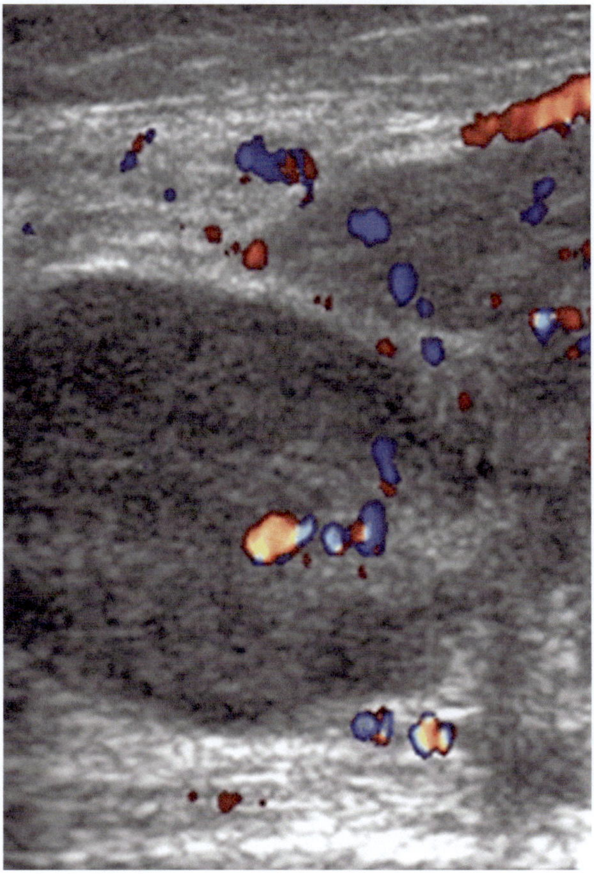

Fig. 7.27 Suppurative lymphadenitis: Increased vascularity and loss of the normally more clearly delineated hyperechoic vascular hilum

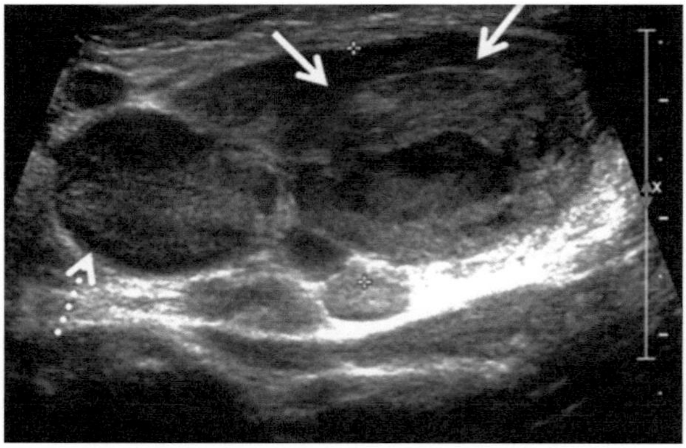

Fig. 7.28 Lymph node abscess: Formation of a cavitation within the otherwise homogenous lymph node tissue with associated increased peripheral vascularity

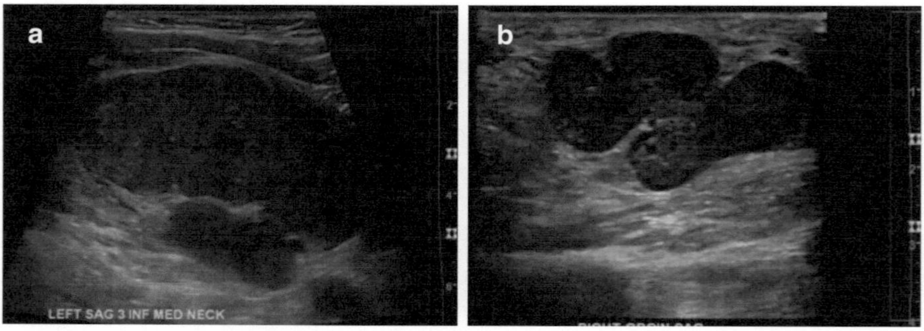

Fig. 7.29 Nodal matting: Coalescence of adjacent lymph nodes often suggestive of malignant process. Figures (**a**) and (**b**) demonstrate the coalescence of adjacent lymph nodes often suggestive of malignant process

    - Figure 7.29—Nodal matting
- Color Doppler ultrasound exams may also demonstrate signs of malignant lymph nodes.
    - Aberrant course or location of hilar or capsular/peripheral vessels [11].
    - Heterogeneous vascularity/areas of absent signal suggesting avascularity [11].
        - Figure 7.30—Malignant lymph node

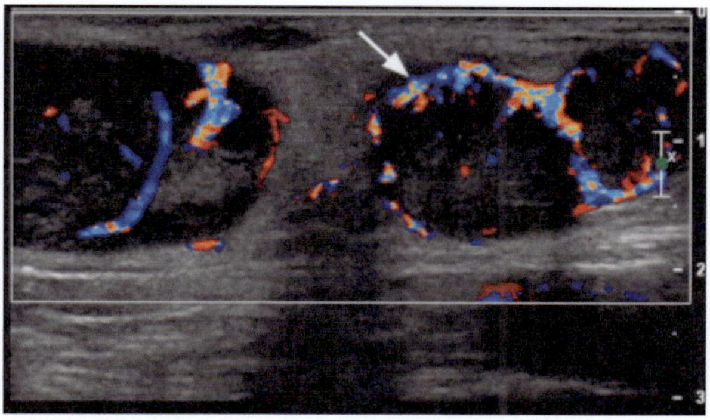

Fig. 7.30 Malignant lymph node: More circular lymph nodes with increased peripheral vascularity or otherwise abnormal vascular signal pattern

References

1. Mallin M, Dawson M. Introduction to bedside ultrasound: volume 2. United States of America: emergency ultrasound solutions; 2013. iBook. https://itun.es/us/ueELM.l
2. American Institute of Ultrasound in Medicine. Thyroid and Parathyroid Ultrasound Examination. 2003. AIUM Practice Parameter Website. http://www.aium.org/resources/guidelines/thyroid.pdfn. Updated 2007 and 2013. Accessed 1 May 2017.
3. Dewitz A. Chapter 18: Musculoskeletal, soft tissue, and miscellaneous applications. In: Ma OJ, Mateer JR, Reardon RF, Joing SA, editors. Emergency ultrasound. 3rd ed. China: McGraw-Hill Education; 2014. p. 503–68.
4. Xie C, Cox P, Taylor N, LaPorte S. Ultrasonography of thyroid nodules: a pictorial review. Insights. Imaging. 2016;7(1):77–86. https://www.ncbi.nlm.nih.gov/pmc/articles/PMC4729706/. Accessed 1 May 2017
5. Yeung MJ, Serpell JW. Management of the solitary thyroid nodule. The Oncologist. 2008;13(2):105–12. http://theoncologist.alphamedpress.org/content/13/2/105.full.pdf+html. Accessed 1 May 2017
6. Shah C, Johnson PT. Diffuse thyroiditis. Sonoworld Website. https://sonoworld.com/CaseDetails/Diffuse_thyroiditis.aspx?CaseId=50. Accessed 1 May 2017.
7. Chao A, Gharahbaghian L. Tips and tricks: airway ultrasound. ACEP Website. https://www.acep.org/content.aspx?id=102309. Accessed 1 May 2017.
8. Das SK, Choupoo NS, Haldar R, Lahkar A. Transtracheal ultrasound for verification of endotracheal tube placement: a systematic review and meta-analysis. Can J Anesth. 2015;62(4):413–23. http://link.springer.com/article/10.1007%2Fs12630-014-0301-z. Accessed 1 May 2017
9. Dahiya N, Dogra VS. Small parts and superficial structures. Philadelphia: Elsevier Inc.; 2014. https://books.google.com/books?id=3lXOAwAAQBAJ&printsec=frontcover#v=onepage&q&f=false. Accessed 1 May 2017
10. Bansal AG, Oudsema R, Masseaux JA, Rosenberg HK. US of Pediatric Superficial Masses of the Head and Neck. Radiographics: a review Publication of the Radiological Society of North America, Inc [Internet]. 2018 [cited 2021 Jun 14];38(4):1239–63. Available from: https://pubmed.ncbi.nlm.nih.gov/29995618/
11. Prativadi R, Dahiya N, Kamaya A, Bhatt S. Chapter 5 Ultrasound characteristics of benign vs malignant cervical lymph nodes. Semin Ultrasound CT MRI. 2017;38(5):506–15.

Musculoskeletal Ultrasound

8

Michael Joyce and Angela Lindsay

Utility of ultrasound in musculoskeletal has rapidly evolved and become an essential tool for point-of-care ultrasound practitioners. Ultrasound is a quick, noninvasive way to assess for many different musculoskeletal ailments such as dislocated joints, tendinopathies, knee effusions, fractures, and nerve inflammation. It gives providers the ability to efficiently diagnose pathology and subsequently start patients on the appropriate treatment to achieve recovery. In addition, with information gained using ultrasound, procedures to reduce pain, such as a hematoma block or nerve block (covered in Chap. 20), can be performed to improve patient comfort. This chapter will review indications for performing a musculoskeletal ultrasound, basic anatomy, image acquisition, normal ultrasound anatomy, and interpretation of pathology.

Clinical Application and Indications

- Dislocated joints
- Tendinopathies
- Knee effusion
- Bone Fractures
- Median nerve inflammation (Carpal Tunnel Syndrome)

Supplementary Information The online version contains supplementary material available at https://doi.org/10.1007/978-3-032-27643-8_8.

M. Joyce · A. Lindsay (✉)
Department of Emergency Medicine, Virginia Commonwealth University Health, Richmond, VA, USA
e-mail: john.joyce@vcuhealth.org; angela.creditt@vcuhealth.org

A. Lindsay et al. (eds.), *Clinical Ultrasound*,
https://doi.org/10.1007/978-3-032-27643-8_8

Normal Musculoskeletal Anatomy

- Bone
  - Can be divided into long bones, short bones, flat bones, and irregular bones.
    - Long bones: clavicles, humeri, radii, ulnae, metacarpals, femurs, tibiae, fibulae, metatarsals, and phalanges
    - Short bones: carpal bones, tarsal bones, patellae, sesamoid bones
    - Flat bones: skull, mandible, scapulae, sternum, and ribs
    - Irregular bones: vertebrae, sacrum, coccyx, and hyoid
  - Outermost surface is the periosteum, which covers the bone and provides nutrients.
  - Next is cortical bone, which provides strength; this layer is thick and protects the layers beneath it.
  - Cancellous bone and bone marrow make up the inside of the bone, but are not visualized on ultrasound.
- Tendons
  - Band of fibro-elastic connective tissue that connects muscle to a bone.
  - Tendons transmit force from muscle to the bone and can withstand a large amount of tension.
- Ligaments
  - Similar to tendons, however, connect one bone to another bone.
- Nerves
  - Make up the Peripheral Nervous System (PNS), allowing various parts of the body to communicate with the brain and spinal cord, or Central Nervous System (CNS).
  - Each nerve has an outer layer of dense connective tissue called the epineurium that surrounds fascicles or bundles of nerve axons.
  - Deep to the epineurium is the perineurium, which is a delicate sheath of connective tissue that forms a sleeve around a fascicle of nerve axons.
  - The endoneurium surrounds each individual nerve axon.
- Shoulder Joint
  - Ball and socket joint with articulation between the head of the humerus and glenoid fossa of the scapula.
- Knee Joint
  - A hinge joint composed of two different articulations.
    - Patella and femur
    - Femur and tibia
  - The fibula courses lateral to the tibia, and while it articulates with the tibia, it is not part of the knee joint.

Image Acquisition

- Transducer Selection
  - Linear array transducer
  - May need Curvilinear transducer for deeper structures
- Patient Position
  - Dependent on the structure to be imaged
  - Shoulder Joint
    - Patient should sit upright on edge of bed facing away from operator.
    - Figure 8.1—Shoulder patient position
  - Tendons
    - Achilles tendon
      - Ideally, the patient should lay prone with their forefoot off the edge of the bed [1] to allow for a relaxed position of the Achilles tendon.
      - Figure 8.2—Achilles tendon patient position
    - Patellar and Quadriceps Tendons
      - Have the patient lay supine or seated with their knees flexed to 90 degrees.
      - Figure 8.3—Quadriceps tendon patient position
      - Figure 8.4—Patella tendon patient position
    - Finger Tendons
      - To image flexor tendons, position the patient's hand in supination with their fingers in as much extension as patient will allow.
      - Utilize a water bath for better image acquisition.

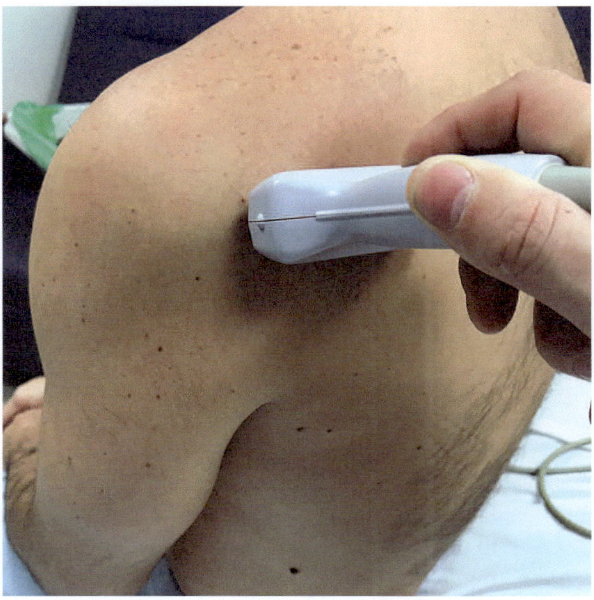

Fig. 8.1 Shoulder patient position. Have the patient in a seated position with arm bent at 90 degrees, place the transducer with the transducer indicator laterally

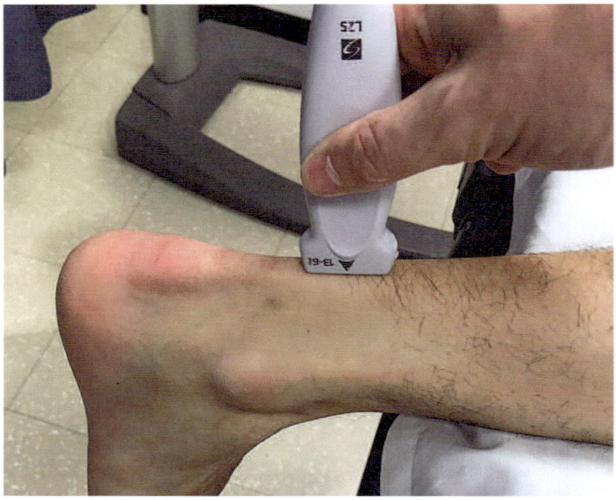

Fig. 8.2 Achilles tendon patient position. If possible, having the patient in the prone position allows for easy visualization of the Achilles tendon

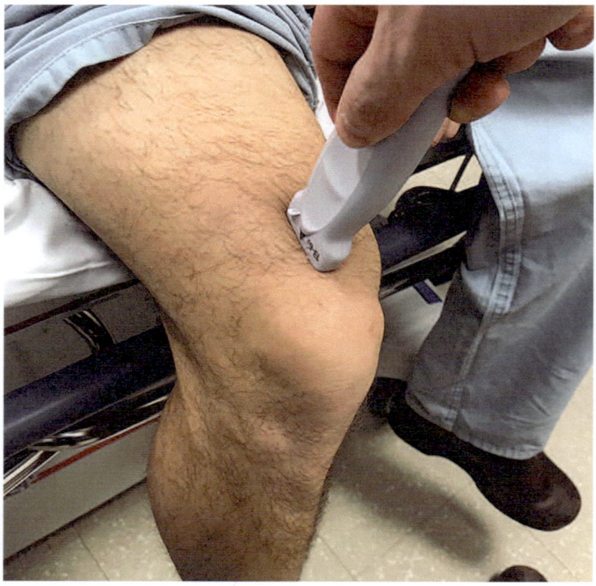

Fig. 8.3 Quadriceps tendon patient position. Have the patient lay supine or seated with their knee flexed to 90 degrees. Place the transducer proximal to the knee over the quadriceps tendon attachment site to the patella

    - Place area of interest within a basin filled with just enough water to submerge the area entirely, then place just the tip of the transducer into the water over the affected area.
    - Figure 8.5—Water bath example
- Knee Joint
  - Patient should lay supine with a towel rolled and placed under their knee to provide support and approximately 20 degrees of knee flexion.
  - Figure 8.6—Knee joint patient position

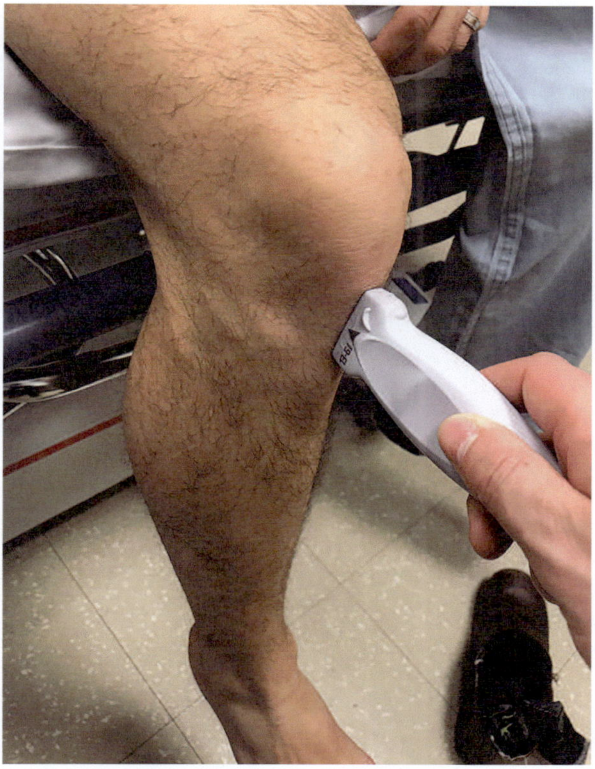

Fig. 8.4 Patella Tendon Position. With the patient's leg hanging over the side of the bed flexed at 90 degrees, place the transducer over the patella tendon attachment site inferior to the patella

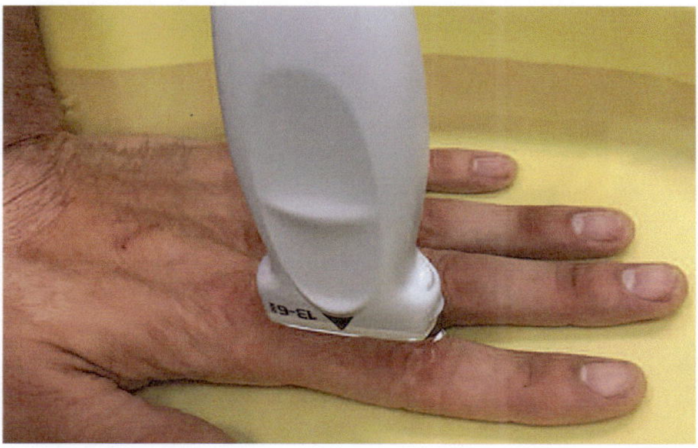

Fig. 8.5 Water bath example. To facilitate visualization of small parts, you can have the patient place the affected area in a container of water, and hover the probe over the area of interest

- Bone/Fractures
  - Dependent on which bone will be imaged.
  - Typically, the patient will be laying supine, in a position of comfort for lower extremity fractures.
- Median nerve
  - Position the forearm in supination and place on a flat surface
  - Figure 8.7—Median nerve patient position

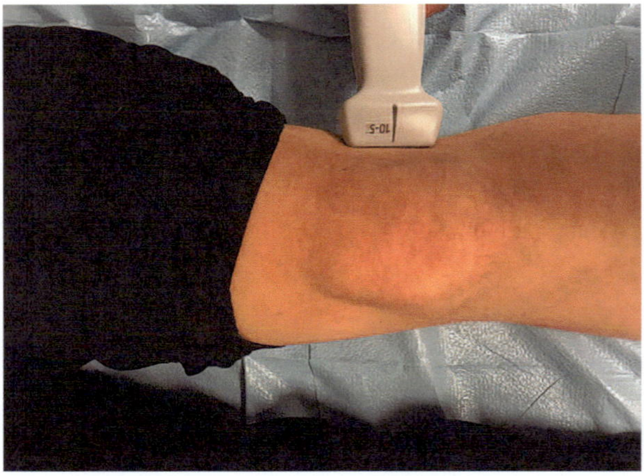

Fig. 8.6 Knee joint patient position. To view the knee joint, a lateral or medial approach is preferred. For patient comfort, a towel roll can be placed beneath the knee

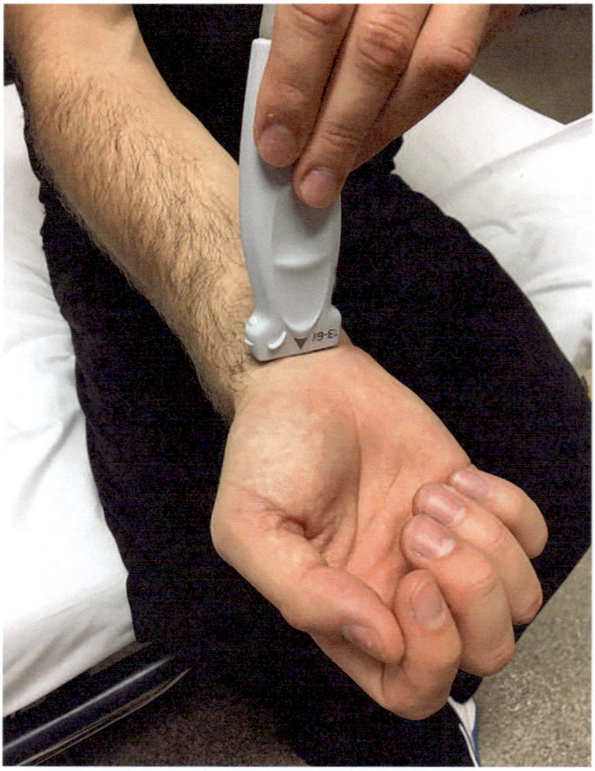

Fig. 8.7 Median nerve patient position. With the arm extended and in supination, place the transducer over the forearm to locate the median nerve, and then slide the transducer down the arm to the wrist while following the median nerve

Shoulder Joint

- Standard Exam Views
  - Begin by placing the transducer posteriorly on the proximal humerus in a transverse plane and trace it proximally to find the glenohumeral joint.
  - If the patient can range the joint, obtain a video clip of internal and external rotation.
- Ultrasound Anatomy
  - The bony cortex of humeral head and glenoid fossa will appear hyperechoic with posterior acoustic shadowing.
    - Figure 8.8—Normal shoulder on ultrasound
    - Video 8.1—Normal shoulder joint
  - Normally, the humerus will be 0.5 to 1.0 cm posterior to the glenoid [2].
    - Compare to contralateral side as needed.
  - Infraspinatus muscle can be seen as a hypoechoic band superior to the joint [1] attaching to the greater tuberosity of the humerus.
- Shoulder Pathology
  - Shoulder Dislocation
    - Studies have shown ultrasound to be 100% sensitive in detecting shoulder dislocations and nearly 100% sensitive with detecting complete reduction [3].
    - With anterior shoulder dislocations, which are most common, the humeral head will be anterior and inferior to the glenoid.
      - From a posterior approach as described above, the humeral head will be seen as a deeper structure on the ultrasound image.
      - Figure 8.9—Anterior shoulder dislocation
      - Video 8.2—Anterior shoulder dislocation

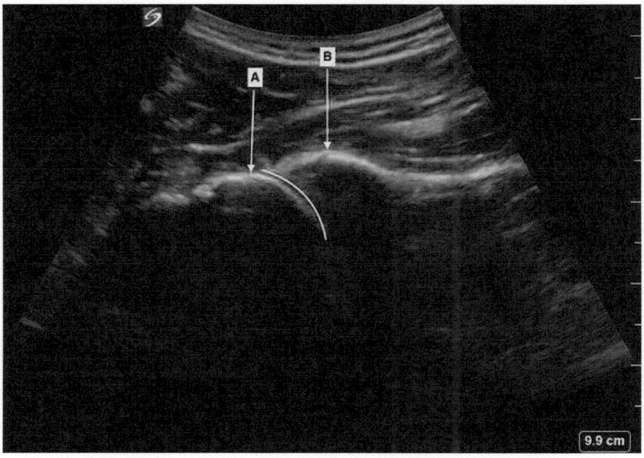

Fig. 8.8 Normal shoulder on ultrasound. In the normal shoulder, you can see the humeral head (A) sitting in the glenoid joint fossa (curved line) created by the scapula (B)

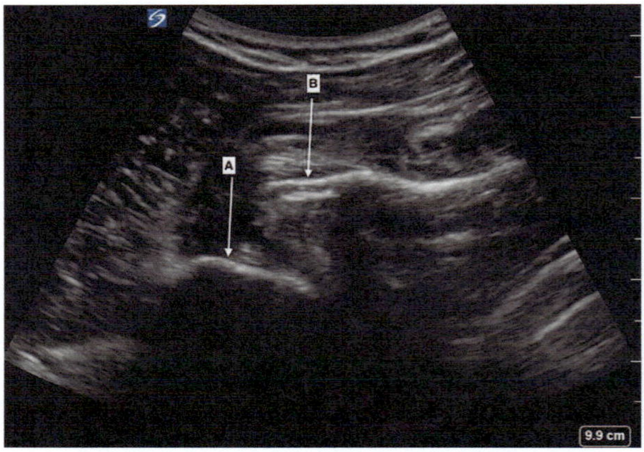

Fig. 8.9 Anterior shoulder dislocation. With an anterior dislocation, the humeral head (A) will be displaced anteriorly away from the scapula (B)

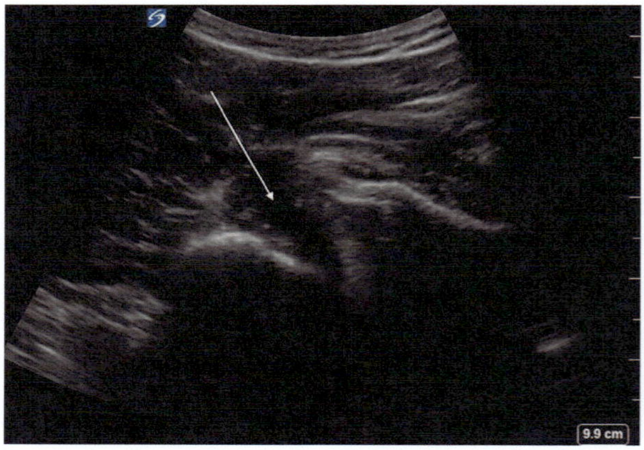

Fig. 8.10 Shoulder effusion. A shoulder effusion can be visualized as a hypoechoic area between the humeral head and scapula. Heterogeneous material may sometimes be visualized if blood has started to clot

  - In a posterior shoulder dislocation, which is much less common and typically only occurs due to seizure or electrocution, the humeral head will be posterior and inferior to the glenoid and appear more superficial on the ultrasound image.
  - A hypoechoic area may also be seen, which is indicative of a joint effusion.
    - Figure 8.10—Shoulder effusion
- After identifying shoulder dislocations, consider injecting lidocaine into the joint under ultrasound guidance. This may allow for reduction without procedural sedation.
  - Ultrasound guidance can also be used to facilitate arthrocentesis and hematoma blocks for fractures.

Tendons

- Standard Exam Views
  - Tendons should be imaged in both transverse or cross-sectional and longitudinal planes.
  - Be sure to scan through the entire length of the tendon to confirm the tendon is intact without tears or rupture.
  - Obtain similar views of contralateral tendon for comparison as needed.
- Ultrasound Anatomy
  - In a longitudinal plane, visualize the dense hyperechoic organized parallel fibers [1]; occasionally a surrounding sheath may also be seen.
    - Figure 8.11—Tendon in long axis
    - Video 8.3—Tendon in long axis
    - It is important to distinguish muscles from tendons.
      - Grossly, the location of the transducer can help with this.
      - On ultrasound, muscles appear as hypoechoic tissue separated by fine hyperechoic fibrillary septa with a striated appearance.
      - Figure 8.12—Muscle
  - In a transverse plane, tendons will appear as a circular or oval collection of hyperechoic, punctate structures.
    - Figure 8.13—Tendon in short axis
    - Video 8.4—Tendon in short axis
  - Tendons elicit a phenomenon called anisotropy, which can distinguish a tendon from nerves.
    - Anisotropy means that the echogenicity of tendons will change based on the angle of the transducer.
      - When the transducer is perpendicular to the tendon, it will appear hyperechoic [1] and organized.

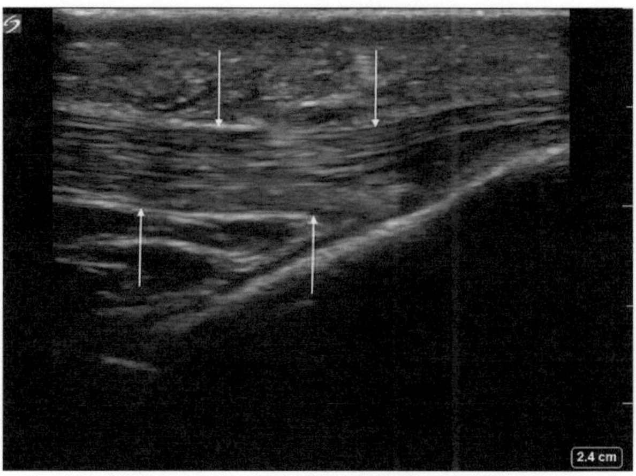

Fig. 8.11 Tendon in Longitudinal plane. A normal tendon appears with long fibular strands between a hyperechoic sheath (arrows)

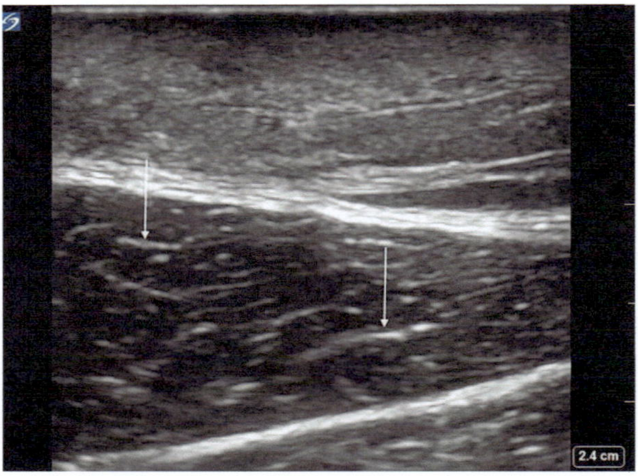

Fig. 8.12 Muscle. Muscle is more hypoechoic and less organized than tendons, with hyperechoic striations (arrows)

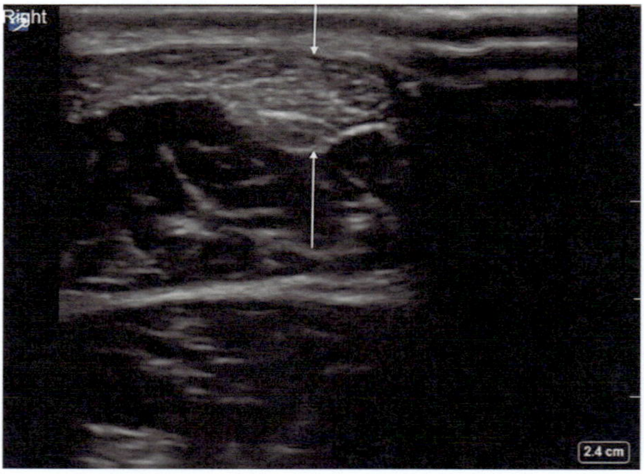

Fig. 8.13 Tendon in cross-section. In cross-section, tendons will have hyperechoic punctate structures

    - As the transducer moves away from a perpendicular plane and is angled down (e.g., at a 45-degree angle), the structure will become more hypoechoic [1]
    - Video 8.5—Anisotropy
- Tendon Pathology
  - Tendon rupture
    - Disruption of tendon fibers can be partial or complete.
    - Partial internal tears may just have hypo- or anechoic areas within the tendon [1] that lacks anisotropy.
      - Figure 8.14—Partial tendon tear
      - Video 8.6—Partial tendon tear
    - Complete rupture will be visualized as a complete disruption of the tendon fibers, usually with surrounding anechoic fluid due to hemorrhage and/or edema from inflammation [1].

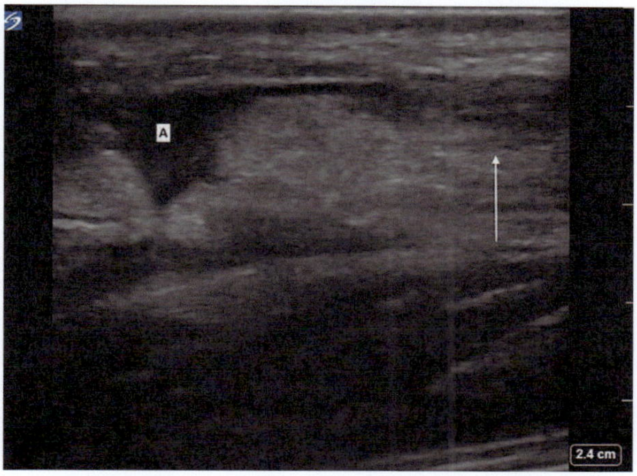

Fig. 8.14 Partial tendon rupture. The normal tendon (arrow) becomes edematous then has a noticeable defect (A) where it is torn. The hypoechoic area is blood filling the defect

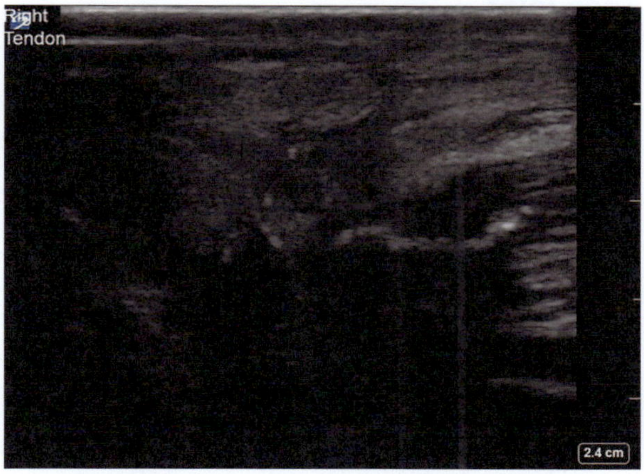

Fig. 8.15 Complete tendon rupture. With a complete tendon rupture there is complete loss of normal tendon architecture, as well as swelling of the tendon due to inflammation

  - Figure 8.15—Complete tendon rupture
  - Video 8.7—Complete tendon rupture short axis
  - Video 8.8—Complete tendon rupture long axis
- Flexor tenosynovitis
  - Acute inflammation usually due to infection within the flexor tendon sheath of a finger.
  - On a normal finger, the flexor tendon sheath is not visualized.
  - With flexor tenosynovitis, the tendon sheath will be thickened. Inside the sheath, the tendon will course through surrounding hypoechoic or anechoic fluid [1, 4].
  - Figure 8.16—Flexor tenosynovitis
  - Video 8.9—Flexor tenosynovitis

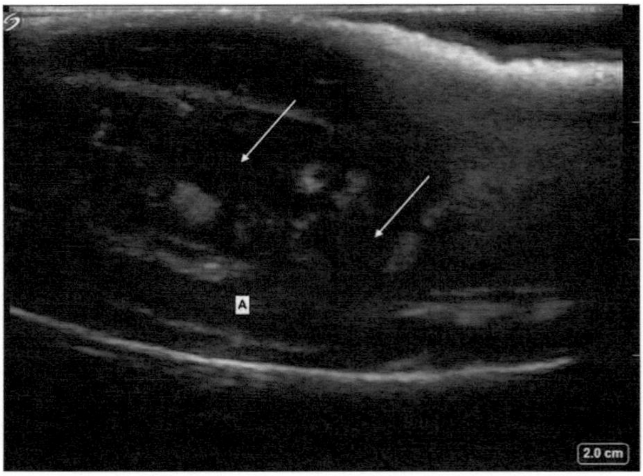

Fig. 8.16 Flexor tenosynovitis. The flexor tendon (A) is seen to have a thickened flexor tendon sheath with hypoechoic fluid surrounding the tendon (arrows)

Knee Joint

- Standard Exam Views
  - With the patient positioned appropriately, place the transducer anteriorly on the knee joint and scan through from the distal femur to the superior portion of the patella.
  - A transverse view in the appropriate location may facilitate ultrasound-guided arthrocentesis.
    - See the procedural chapter for more details.
- Ultrasound Anatomy
  - Visualize the hyperechoic cortex of the femur superior and deep with the patella more inferior and superficial.
  - Normal synovial fluid within the suprapatellar bursa will appear anechoic and will be less than 2 mm when measured [5].
  - The quadriceps tendon will be seen attaching to the patella in this view.
  - Figure 8.17—Normal knee
  - Video 8.10—Normal knee
- Knee Pathology
  - Knee Effusion
    - Excess fluid within or around the joint.
    - Typically, a fluid collection will be seen in the suprapatellar bursa [1].
      - This will appear as an anechoic or hypoechoic collection between the femur and patella.
      - Figure 8.18—Knee effusion
      - Video 8.11—Knee effusion

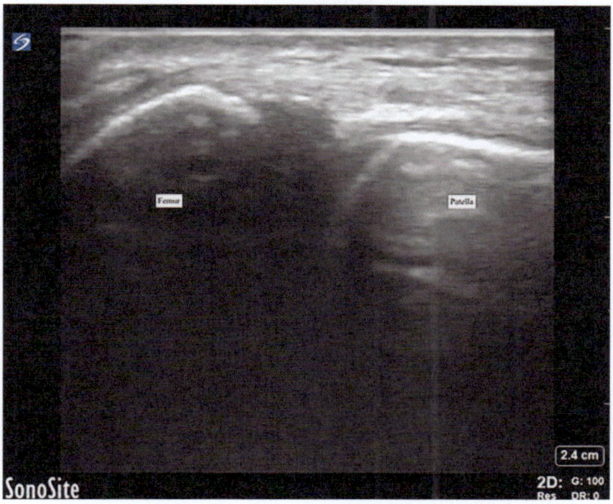

Fig. 8.17 Normal knee. Articulation of the femur and patella using a lateral transducer placement

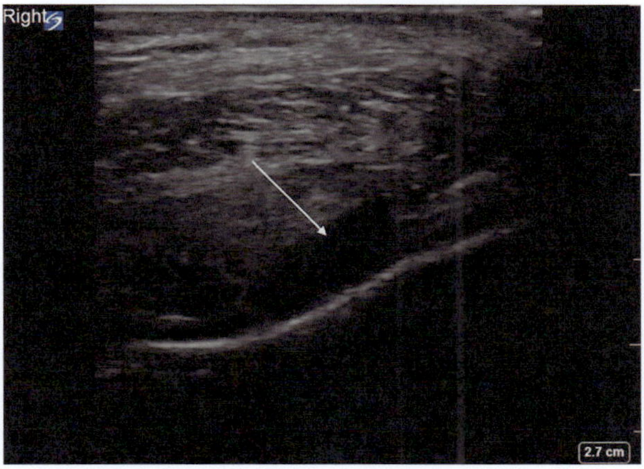

Fig. 8.18 Knee effusion. A small knee effusion (arrow)

- The echogenicity of the fluid collection can help to identify the type of fluid.
  - Simple fluid will appear anechoic [1].
  - Inflammatory fluid will be anechoic with loculations in the joint space [1].
  - Hemorrhagic fluid can appear anechoic initially, but typically will have increased echogenicity due to clot formation [1].
  - If there is debris within the effusion, consider infection, hemorrhage, and fat (lipohemarthrosis) [5].

Bone

- Standard Exam Views
  - Over the area of interest, obtain both transverse and longitudinal clips.
    - Begin by scanning in a transverse plane to identify bone and optimize the image on the screen by adjusting depth and gain [1].
    - Rotate the transducer to image the bone in a long axis and scan through to identify any irregularities representing a fracture [1].
  - Obtain similar views of contralateral bone for comparison as needed.
- Ultrasound Anatomy
  - Normal bones can be identified by a thick hyperechoic line representing the bony cortex with underlying posterior acoustic shadowing [1].
  - The cortex should be continuous without disruptions.
  - Figure 8.19—Normal bone
  - Video 8.12—Normal bone
- Bone Pathology
  - Fractures
    - Will appear as a disruption of the echogenic bony cortex [1] or with more displaced fractures, a step-off.
    - May see surrounding anechoic or hypoechoic collection suggestive of a hematoma.
    - Figure 8.20—Fracture
    - Video 8.13—Fracture

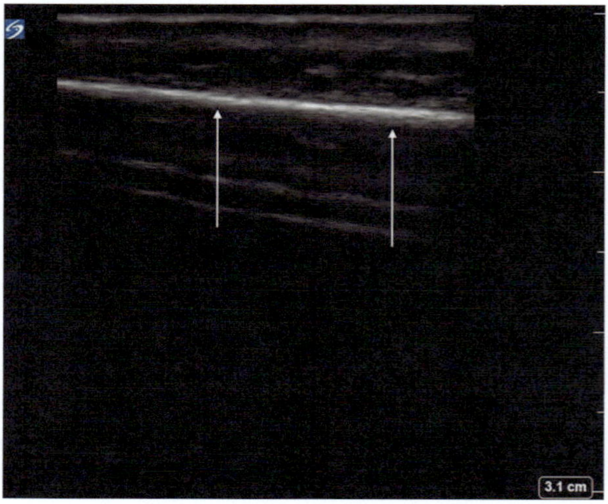

Fig. 8.19 Normal bone. Normal bone is hyperechoic with posterior shadowing

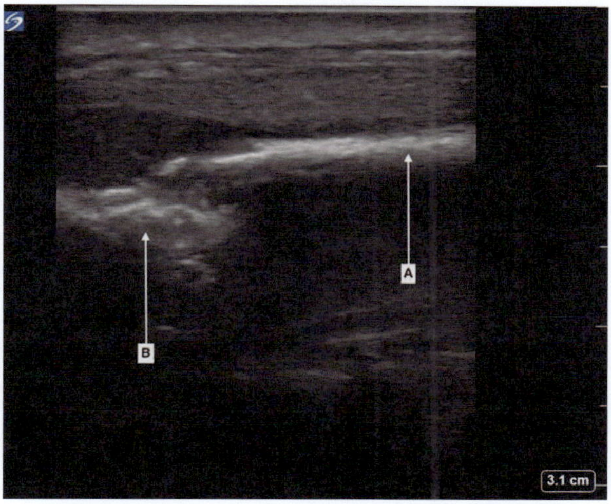

Fig. 8.20 Fracture. Bone (A) loses its typical appearance and will be seen as a disruption of the bony cortex at the site of the fracture (B)

Nerves

- Standard Exam Views
  - Identify the nerve of interest, place the transducer over this area with the patient in a position of comfort, then scan through the area.
    - Nerves are best visualized in a transverse plane.
  - For the median nerve, place the transducer over the flexor retinaculum. This can be found at the level of the scaphoid on the flexor surface of the wrist.
    - Measure the nerve to evaluate for inflammation.
- Ultrasound Anatomy
  - Nerves have a fascicular appearance with individual fascicles being hypoechoic and surrounded by hyperechoic connective tissue resembling a honeycomb [6].
    - Figure 8.21—Normal median nerve
    - Video 8.14—Normal median nerve
  - Nerves in a longitudinal axis appear as hyperechoic tubes with small parallel linear hypoechoic internal echoes [6].
  - Nerves can easily be mistaken for tendons; however, they do not exhibit anisotropy as tendons do.
- Nerve Pathology
  - Carpal Tunnel Syndrome
    - Compression of the median nerve within the carpal tunnel causes a range of symptoms depending on the severity of the condition.

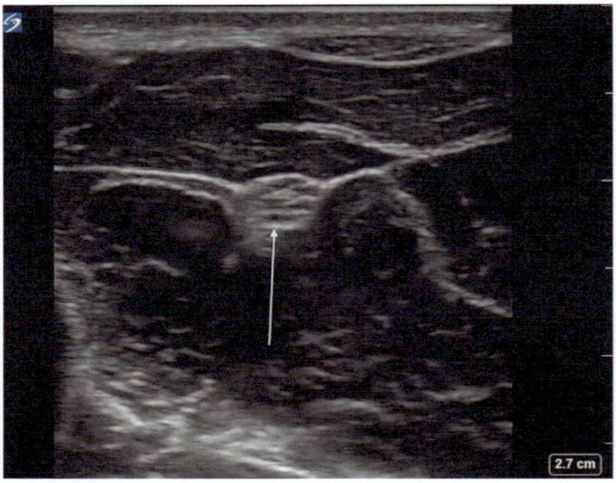

Fig. 8.21 Normal median nerve. Normal median nerves resemble a honeycomb with individual hypoechoic fascicles surrounded by a hyperechoic connective tissue border

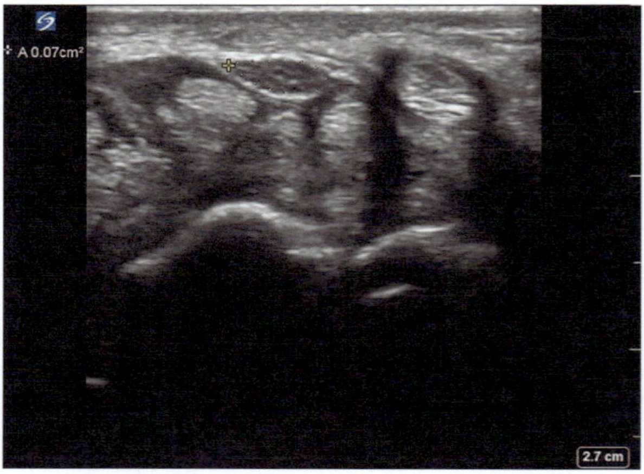

Fig. 8.22 Median nerve cross-sectional area. Normal cross-sectional area (CSA) measurement of the median nerve as it enters the carpel tunnel

- The median nerve within the carpal tunnel will appear enlarged [6] with some internal edema and an increased cross-sectional area of the nerve.
  - Measure the cross-sectional area (CSA) of the median nerve at the level of the scaphoid and pisiform.
    - Figure 8.22—Median nerve cross-sectional area
  - CSA >10 mm is suggestive of Carpal Tunnel Syndrome [6, 7].
    - Figure 8.23—Enlarged median nerve cross-sectional area
- Additionally, one may see flattening of the nerve distally and enlargement of the nerve proximally [6].

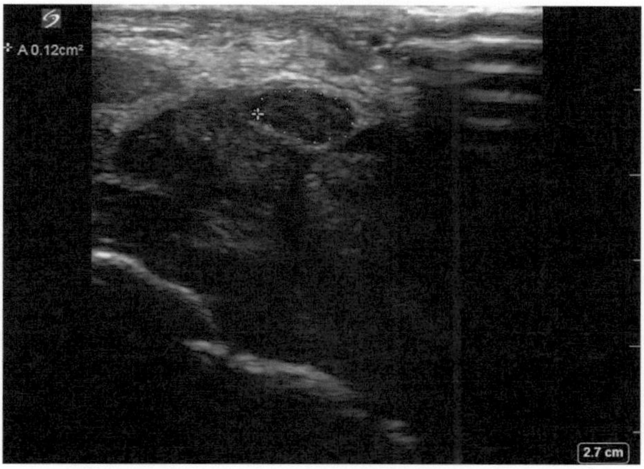

Fig. 8.23 Enlarged medical nerve cross-sectional area. Enlarged median nerve in the carpel tunnel with a cross-sectional area (CSA) measuring greater than 10 mm

Key Points
- When in doubt, compare to the contralateral side.
- Always use anisotropy to differentiate tendons from surrounding structures.
- Tendon pathology will be seen as a hypoechogenic defect. Because anisotropy can cause this appearance, it is important to determine if true pathology exists [1] by repositioning the transducer and imaging in both short and long axis.
- Light pressure may help reveal subtle fractures.

References

1. Dewitz A. Chapter 18: Musculoskeletal, soft tissue, and miscellaneous applications. In: Ma OJ, Mateer JR, Reardon RF, Joing SA, editors. Emergency ultrasound. 3rd ed. China: McGraw-Hill Education; 2014. p. 503–68.
2. Dawson M, Mallin M. Introduction to bedside ultrasound: Volumes 1 and 2. Lexington: Emergency Ultrasound Solutions; 2012.
3. Abbasi S, Molaie H, Hafezimoghadam P, et al. Diagnostic accuracy of ultrasonographic examination in the management of shoulder dislocation in the emergency department. Ann Emerg Med. 2013;62(2):170–5.
4. Padrez K, Bress J, Jonhnson B, Nagdev A. Bedside ultrasound identification of infectious flexor tenosynovitis in the Emergency Department. West J Emerg Med. 2015;16(2):260–2.
5. Razek AAKA, Founda NS, Elmetwaley N, Elbogdady E. Sonography of the knee joint. J Ultrasound. 2009;12(2):53–60. https://www.ncbi.nlm.nih.gov/pmc/articles/PMC3553228/. Accessed 27 Apr 2017
6. Lawande AD, Warrier SS, Joshi MS. Role of ultrasound in evaluation of peripheral nerves. Indian J Radiol Imaging. 2014;24(3):254–8. https://www.ncbi.nlm.nih.gov/pmc/articles/PMC4126140/. Accessed 27 Apr 2017
7. Wong SM, Griffith JF, Hui AC, et al. Carpal tunnel syndrome: diagnostic usefulness of sonography. Radiology. 2004;232(1):93–9.

Aortic Ultrasound

9

Ben Pastwik, Angela Lindsay, and Michael Joyce

Aortic abnormalities represent a potentially life-threatening condition depending on the size and characteristics of the pathology. Ultrasound is a useful modality to quickly assess the aorta for the presence of an aneurysm or arterial dissection, and to determine the relative risk of impending rupture. To do this, it is important for an ultrasonographer to learn how to accurately image and measure the diameter of the aorta and correctly identify aortic pathology. This chapter serves to educate the novice learner on how to take these measurements as well as how to overcome limitations to doing so. It will review indications for performing an aortic ultrasound, basic anatomy, image acquisition, normal ultrasound anatomy, and interpretation of pathology.

Clinical Application/Indications

- Evaluate the aorta as a cause for abdominal pain, flank pain, hypotension, syncope, or high-risk medical screening:
  - Common pathologies include abdominal aortic aneurysm (AAA), dissection, and thrombus.

Supplementary Information The online version contains supplementary material available at https://doi.org/10.1007/978-3-032-27643-8_9.

B. Pastwik
Department of Emergency Medicine, Virginia Commonwealth University Medical Center, Richmond, VA, USA
e-mail: benjamin.pastwik@vcuhealth.org

A. Lindsay (✉) · M. Joyce
Department of Emergency Medicine, Virginia Commonwealth University Health, Richmond, VA, USA
e-mail: Angela.creditt@vcuhealth.org; john.joyce@vcuhealth.org

A. Lindsay et al. (eds.), *Clinical Ultrasound*,
https://doi.org/10.1007/978-3-032-27643-8_9

Normal Aortic Anatomy

- The thoracic aorta begins at the aortic root, moves superiorly through the aortic arch, and then inferiorly along the descending aorta as it transitions from the thorax into the abdominal cavity.
- Thoracic aortic anatomy as it pertains to ultrasound.
  - Aortic root and ascending aorta visualized on parasternal long.
  - Aortic arch visualized on suprasternal notch.
  - Descending Aorta visualized on parasternal long.
- The abdominal aorta begins at the aortic hiatus of the diaphragm at the 12th thoracic vertebrae [4].
- It is a retroperitoneal structure that courses anterior to the spine until it bifurcates into the iliac arteries at the level of the umbilicus or second lumbar vertebrae.
- A normal aorta will have an anechoic lumen and a maximum diameter of less than 3.0 cm when measuring from outer wall to outer wall [1–3].
  - Average aortic diameter in males is 2.1 cm and in females is 1.8 cm [1].
- Near the iliac bifurcation, the aorta tapers and courses more anteriorly due to lumbar lordosis.
- Transverse Anatomy
  - The aorta lies to the left of midline, just anterior to the spine and adjacent to the more rightward inferior vena cava (IVC).
    - Figure 9.1—Transverse aorta
    - Video 9.1—Normal transverse aorta
  - Celiac artery is the first branch off the abdominal aorta.
    - Arises from the anterior wall of the aorta.
    - The celiac artery branches into the common hepatic artery on the right and the splenic artery on the left, known as "seagull sign" [3].
    - Figure 9.2—Celiac trunk with seagull sign
    - Video 9.2—Celiac trunk

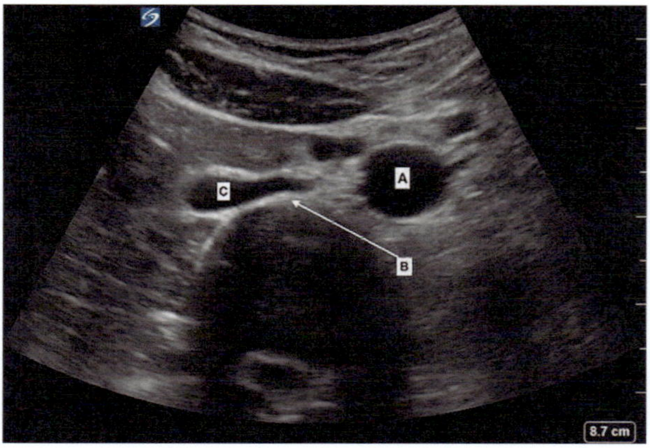

Fig. 9.1 Transverse aorta: The normal aorta in transverse will be a circular structure with hyperechoic walls and a hypoechoic center (A), usually located directly anterior to the vertebral body (B) or just lateral to it. The IVC, sometimes collapsed, will be visualized to the patient's right (C)

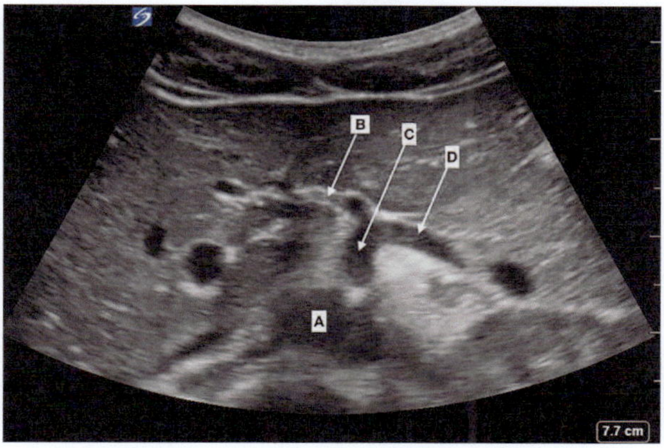

Fig. 9.2 Celiac trunk with seagull sign: Arising from the aorta (A) is the celiac trunk (C), branching into the hepatic artery (B) and splenic artery (D)

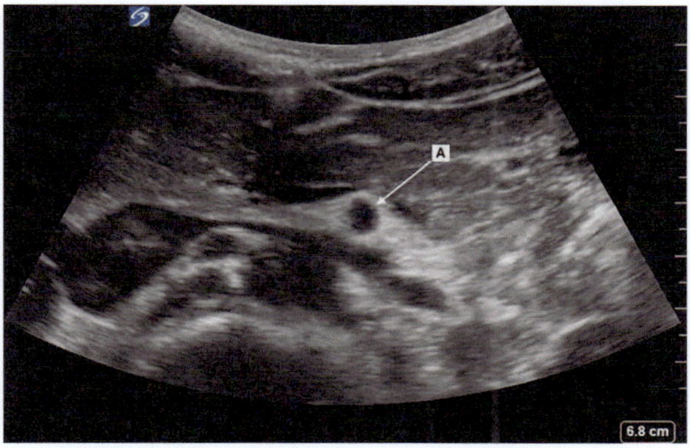

Fig. 9.3 Superior mesenteric artery: Superior mesenteric artery (A) is the second main branch from the abdominal aorta, just inferior to the celiac trunk

- Superior mesenteric artery (SMA) is the second branch from the aorta
  - Arises from the anterior wall of the aorta just inferior to the celiac artery.
  - The celiac artery and SMA may share a common trunk; this is a normal variant.
  - Figure 9.3—Superior mesenteric artery
  - Video 9.3—Superior mesenteric artery
- Renal arteries take off from each side of the aorta approximately 2 cm inferior to the SMA.
  - The right renal artery courses under the IVC.
  - Figure 9.4—Renal arteries
  - Video 9.4—Renal arteries
- Distal to the renal arteries are the gonadal arteries (testicular and ovarian) followed by the inferior mesenteric artery (IMA), each of which is difficult to image by ultrasound [1].
- The aorta bifurcates into the left and right common iliac arteries near the level of the umbilicus.

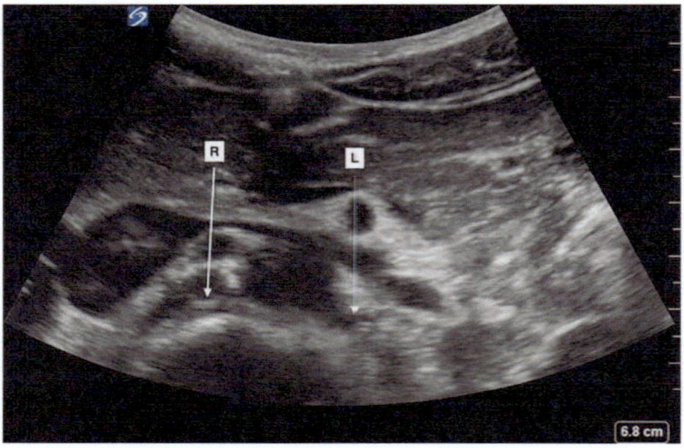

Fig. 9.4 Renal arteries: Left (L) and right (R) renal artery branches

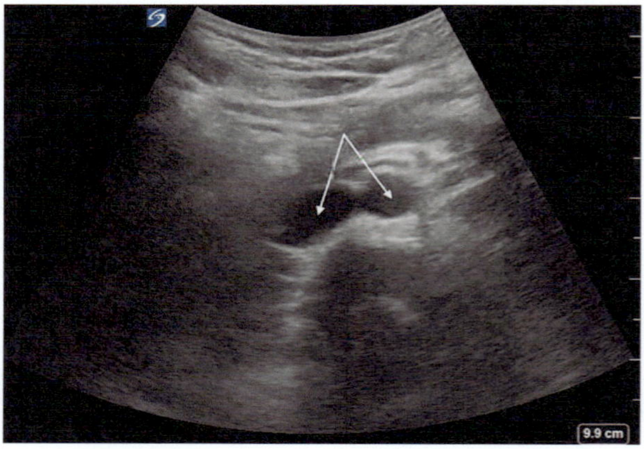

Fig. 9.5 Aortic bifurcation: Near the umbilicus, the aorta will bifurcate into the right and left iliac arteries (*arrows*)

  - Figure 9.5—Aortic bifurcation
  - Video 9.5—Bifurcation
- Sagittal Anatomy
  - The aorta can be viewed as a single continuous vessel in the sagittal plane, lying just anterior to the spinal column.
    - Figure 9.6—Sagittal aorta
    - Video 9.6—Sagittal aorta

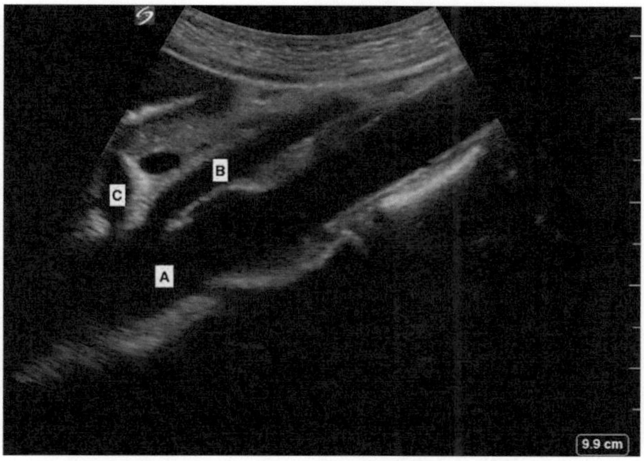

Fig. 9.6 Sagittal aorta: Sagittal view of the aorta (A) at the level of the superior mesenteric artery (B) and celiac artery (C)

Image Acquisition

(a) Transducer Selection
- Curvilinear
- Phased array

(b) Patient Position
- Place the patient in a supine position for optimal imaging of both the thoracic and abdominal aorta.
- A left lateral decubitus position can bring the heart closer to the chest wall and improve image acquisition of the thoracic aorta.
- If there is an excessive amount of bowel gas, a left or right lateral decubitus position can be utilized.

(c) Considerations to optimize imaging:
- Bowel gas can obscure all or part of the aorta.
  - To improve visualization:
    - Attempt to roll the patient.
    - Apply firm, increasing pressure to the abdomen to displace bowel gas.
    - Wait and rescan after a brief time to allow peristalsis to move bowel gas forward.
- Obesity can limit the evaluation of an abdominal aorta.
  - It may be helpful to place the patient in a right or left lateral decubitus position to move the pannus out of the way.
- Most abdominal aortic aneurysms are infrarenal; therefore, it is imperative to image the aorta all the way to the bifurcation [1].
  - In a sagittal plane, off-axis measurements can occur in which the image is not over the center of the vessel, resulting in an underestimation of the true diameter [3].

(d) Standard Exam Views
- Parasternal long-axis imaging to evaluate the thoracic aorta.
  - Place the transducer on the anterior chest at the second or third intercostal space to the left of the sternum with the transducer marker toward the patient's right shoulder; slide the transducer inferior or superior, one rib space at a time, to find the optimal cardiac window [5].
    - Figure 9.7—Parasternal long transducer placement
  - The aortic root can be found at the junction of the left ventricle and ascending aorta. Use the parasternal long axis view to see the aortic valve and the aortic root in a longitudinal plane by positioning the ultrasound probe slightly to the left of the patient's sternum with the probe marker facing the patient's right; this view provides the most accurate measurements of the aortic root diameter, and should be measured at end-diastole [5].
    - Figure 9.8—Aortic root and ascending aorta
  - The descending aorta is visualized immediately posterior to the echogenic pericardial sac.
    - Figure 9.9—Descending aorta
- Transverse or cross-sectional abdominal aorta imaging
  - Place the transducer over the epigastrium just inferior to the xiphoid with the transducer marker pointed toward the patient's right
  - Patient in supine position.
  - It is important to obtain measurements of the aortic diameter from outer wall to outer wall in both transverse and sagittal planes to ensure accuracy.
  - Normal Abdominal Aortic diameter: $\leq$3.0 cm [1–3].

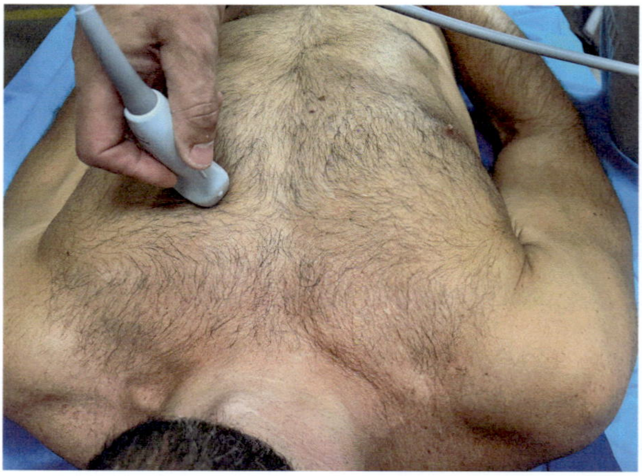

Fig. 9.7 Parasternal long transducer placement: Place the transducer on the anterior chest at the second or third intercostal space to the left of the sternum with the transducer marker toward the patient's right shoulder

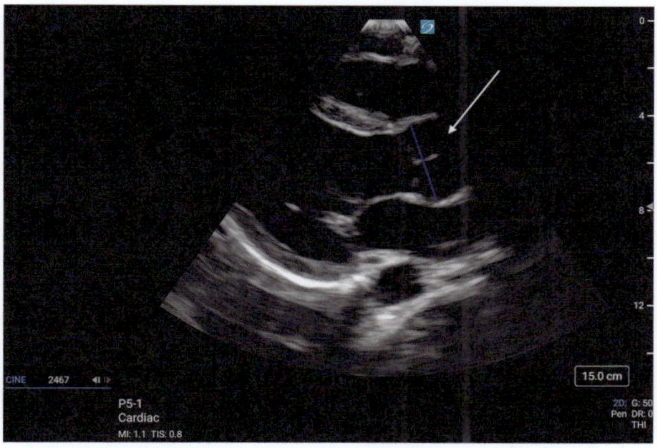

Fig. 9.8 Aortic root and ascending aorta: Aortic root (blue line) is located at the junction of the left ventricle and the ascending aorta (white arrow)

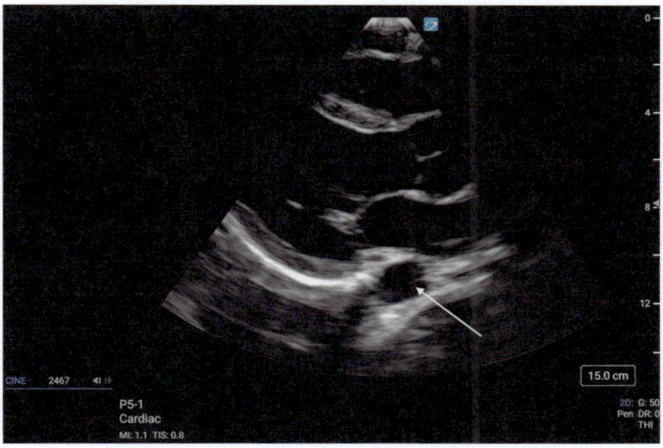

Fig. 9.9 Descending aorta: The descending aorta (arrow) can be seen posterior to the heart in a parasternal long view

  - Measure the maximal outer-to-outer diameter of the aorta in:
    - Proximal (just below diaphragm).
    - Mid (at renal arteries).
    - Distal (above iliac bifurcation).
  - Keep the transducer perpendicular to the long axis of the aorta and follow the aorta down through the bifurcation at approximately the level of the umbilicus.
    - Figure 9.10—Transducer placement for imaging the aorta in a transverse plane
- Sagittal imaging of the abdominal aorta
  - Place the transducer over the epigastrium with the transducer marker pointed cephalad.
  - Figure 9.11—Transducer placement for imaging the aorta in a sagittal plane.

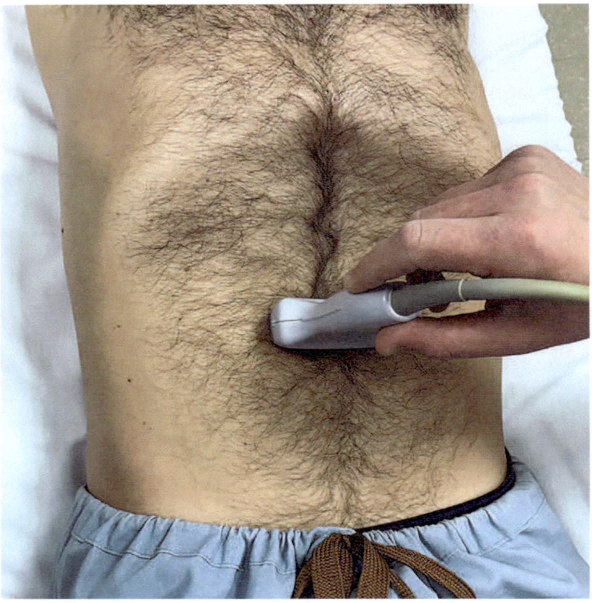

Fig. 9.10 Transducer placement for aorta in transverse plane: Beginning just below the xiphoid process, scan the aorta from proximal to the distal bifurcation in a transverse orientation

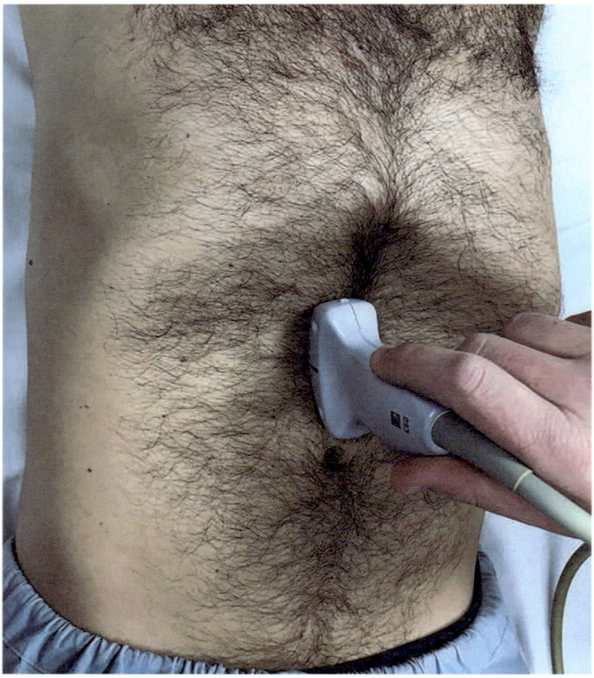

Fig. 9.11 Transducer placement for aorta in sagittal plane: Orient the transducer with the marker pointed cephalad to obtain a sagittal view of the aorta. Slide the transducer inferior or superior to visualize the entire aorta

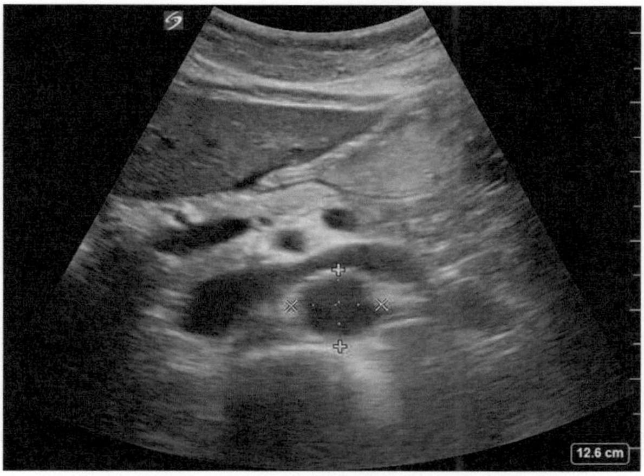

Fig. 9.12 Normal Aorta Measurement Proximal: Proximal measurement of the aorta measuring outer wall to outer wall

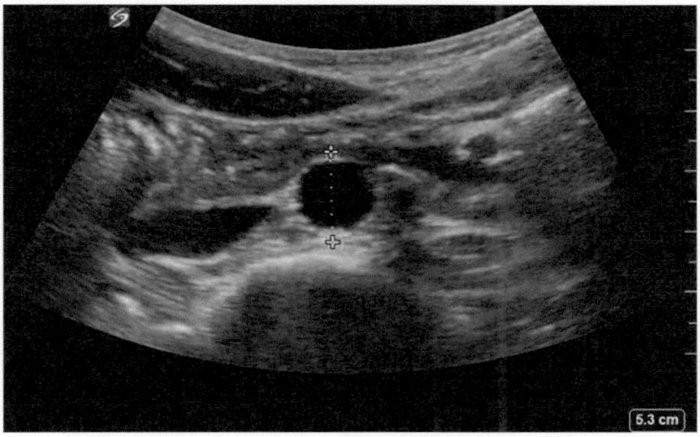

Fig. 9.13 Normal Aorta Measurement Distal: Distal measurement of aorta from outer wall to outer wall

- The abdominal aortic diameter should be measured from outer wall to outer wall in cross-sectional and anterior-posterior planes.
  - Figure 9.12—Normal aorta measurement proximal
  - Figure 9.13—Normal aorta measurement distal

Abdominal Aortic Pathology

(a) Abdominal Aortic Aneurysm
- Defined as an aortic diameter of greater than 3.0 cm [1–3].
- Will most commonly be located infrarenal [1].
- Can be fusiform (most common) or saccular (less common).
  - Fusiform aneurysms are demonstrated by a uniform concentric dilation of the circumference of the aorta [1] and are best measured as the distance between the outer walls of the aorta perpendicular to its long axis.
    - Figure 9.14—Fusiform aneurysm in a sagittal plane
    - Video 9.7—Fusiform aneurysm in a sagittal plane

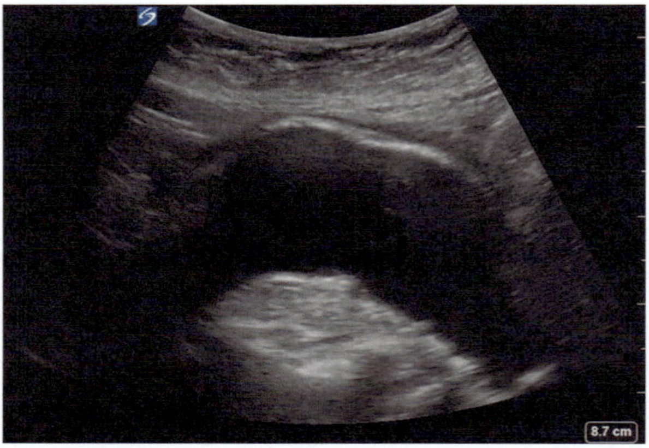

Fig. 9.14 Fusiform aneurysm: Uniform concentric dilation of a fusiform aneurysm in a sagittal plane

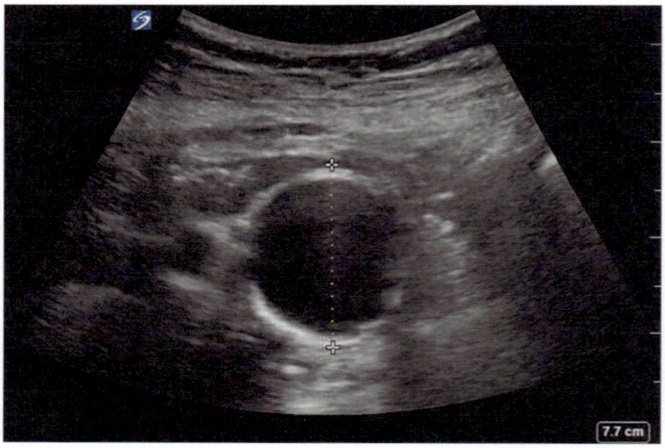

Fig. 9.15 Abdominal aortic aneurysm: Transverse view of a fusiform aneurysm measuring greater than 3.0 cm

    - Figure 9.15—Fusiform aneurysm in transverse
    - Video 9.8—AAA (fusiform) in transverse plane
  - Saccular aneurysms are characterized by a localized outpouching of a portion of the aortic wall [1]. Note that there is no diameter threshold for saccular aneurysms, and if found to be present will require repair due to high risk of rupture
    - Figure 9.16—Saccular aneurysm
- Mural thrombus can often be seen within the periphery of a AAA, with a central lumen for blood flow.
  - Care must be taken to measure the outer wall-to-outer wall diameter of a AAA, including the thrombus if present, to avoid falsely measure the central lumen only.
    - Figure 9.17—AAA with thrombus
    - Video 9.9—AAA with thrombus

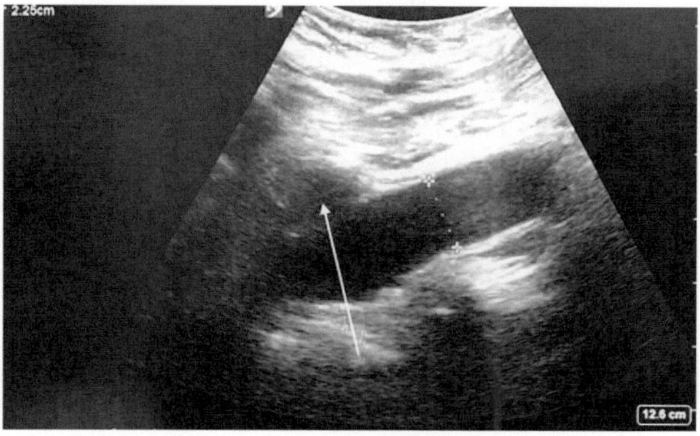

Fig. 9.16 Saccular aneurysm: Noticed here in sagittal plane is an outpouching of the aorta creating a saccular aneurysm

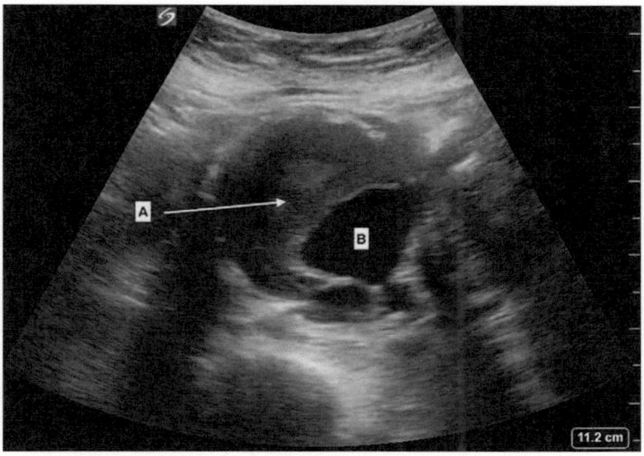

Fig. 9.17 AAA with thrombus: Large dilated aorta, with internal thrombus (A). Note the small area of continued flow (B)

(b) Thoracic Aortic Dissection

- Aortic dissection occurs when the inner wall of the artery tears allowing blood to flow between layers of the wall of the aorta creating a false lumen [8].
- Stanford criteria are frequently utilized to classify aortic dissections based on whether the ascending aorta is involved, thereby dictating a specific management pathway:
  - Stanford Type A involves the ascending aorta and aortic arch, and may or may not involve the descending aorta. Can be life-threatening and usually requires emergency surgery or endovascular therapy [6].
  - Stanford Type B involves the descending aorta or the arch distal to the left-subclavian artery, without the involvement of the ascending aorta [6].
- Ascending aortic dissection can be diagnosed if there is a dissection flap, identified as a hyperechoic linear band through the lumen of the aorta, which is visualized when imaging the heart in a parasternal long axis [8].

- Ascending dissection may also be suspected if the aortic root is significantly dilated. Current guidelines suggest surgical intervention when the aortic root diameter reaches 5.0 cm to 5.5 cm depending on the patient's individual risk factors and medical history [7].
  - Figure 9.18 Dilated aortic root
  - Video 9.10—Dilated aortic root
- Aortic arch dissection may be seen with a suprasternal notch view allowing visualization of the aortic arch and potential identification of an intimal flap indicative of a dissection.
  - Figure 9.19 Aortic arch dissection
  - Video 9.11—Aortic arch dissection

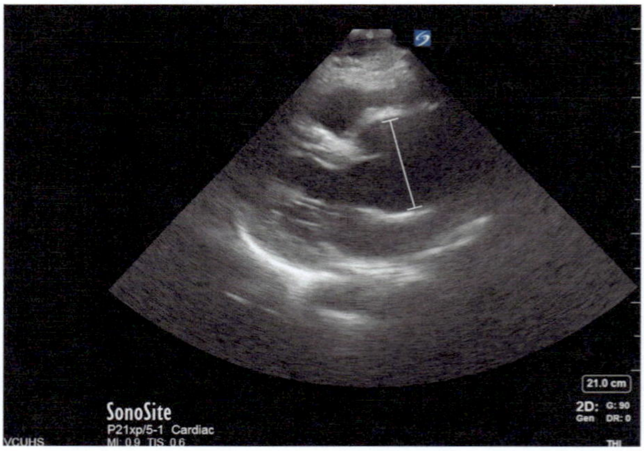

Fig. 9.18 Dilated Aortic Root: Ultrasound image of the proximal aorta demonstrating a dilated aortic root exceeding normal diameter thresholds. This appearance is suggestive of aortic root aneurysm

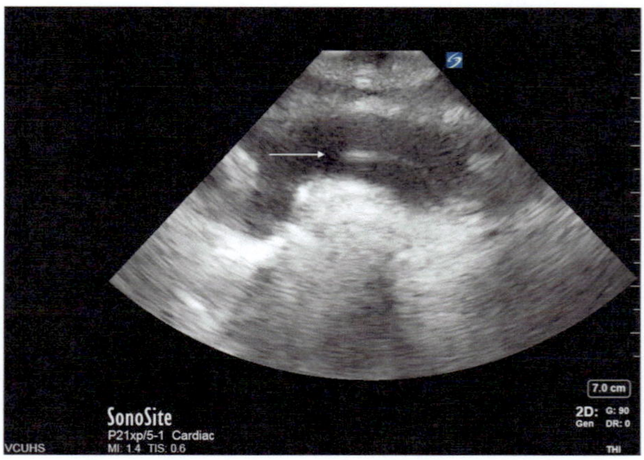

Fig. 9.19 Aortic Arch Dissection: Ultrasound image of the aortic arch revealing an intimal flap separating the true and false lumens, consistent with aortic dissection

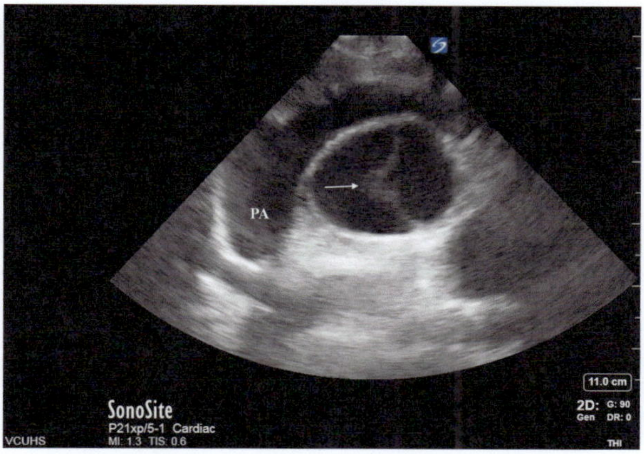

Fig. 9.20 Descending Thoracic Aortic Dissection: Ultrasound image of the descending thoracic aorta showing a clear intimal flap separating the true and false lumens, characteristic of aortic dissection

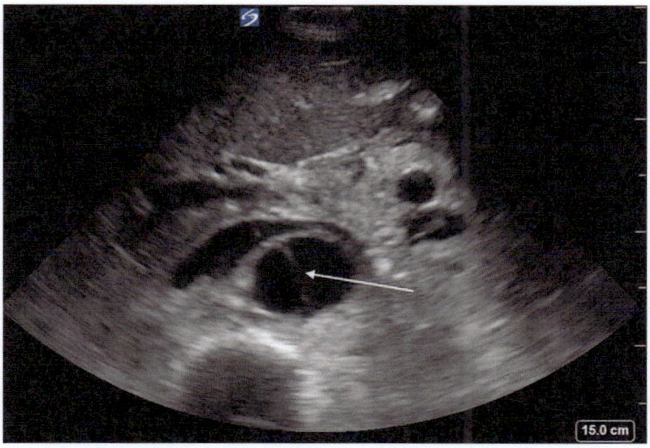

Fig. 9.21 Dissection: Hyperechoic dissection flap (*arrow*) is seeing in the middle of this aorta

- Descending aortic dissection is identified using a parasternal long cardiac window to visualize the aorta posterior to the heart. A dissection flap can be seen as a transverse hyperechoic linear band through the lumen.
  - Figure 9.20 Descending thoracic aortic dissection
  - Video 9.12—Descending thoracic aortic dissection

(c) Abdominal Aortic Dissection

- Dissection flap, if present, will be visualized within the lumen of the aorta:
  - Appears as a hyperechoic linear band through the lumen
  - Figure 9.21—Dissection
  - Video 9.13—Aortic dissection
  - Images should be taken in multiple planes to distinguish true dissection from artifact
  - Figure 9.22—Artifact
  - Video 9.14—Artifact

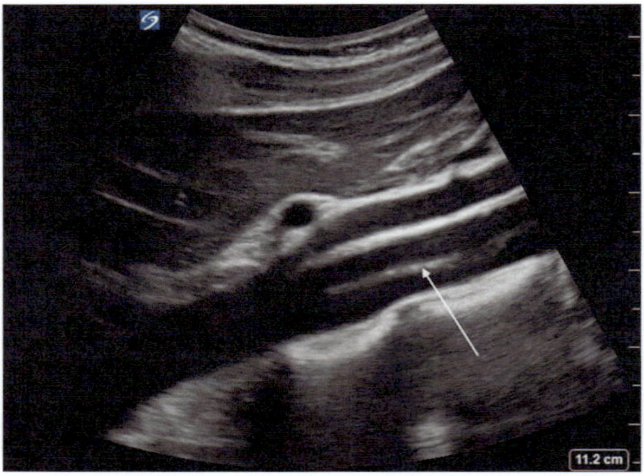

Fig. 9.22 Artifact: This image displays a mirror artifact where the aorta wall is doubled (*arrow*). Note there is no beginning or end to the flap, and it only is where the wall is next to another vessel, thus raising suspicion for artifact. Imaging in multiple planes will help delineate this

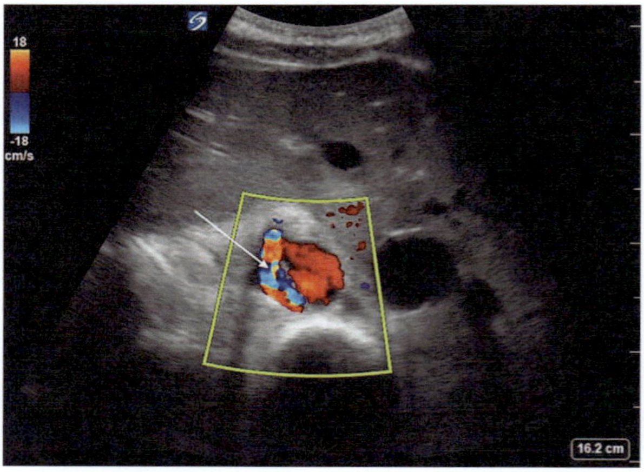

Fig. 9.23 Dissection with color Doppler: Color flow imaging of dissection shows more turbulent flow in the dissected portion of the aorta (*arrow*)

- Color Doppler may show flow only in one portion of the aorta in a transverse orientation, and not the false lumen [1] or with more turbulent flow in the false lumen
  - Figure 9.23—Dissection with color Doppler
  - Video 9.15—Dissection with color Doppler

Key Points

- Ultrasound is a Rapid, First-line Tool for Evaluating Aortic Emergencies:
  - Ultrasound enables emergency physicians to quickly assess for life-threatening aortic pathology such as abdominal aortic aneurysm (AAA) and aortic dissection. It plays a critical role in patients with abdominal pain, hypotension, flank pain, or syncope, where vascular pathology may be the cause.

- Proper Image Acquisition and Measurement Technique Is Essential:
  - Use a curvilinear probe in the supine position.
  - Image the aorta in both transverse and sagittal planes.
  - Always measure outer wall to outer wall, as underestimation may miss a diagnosis of AAA.
  - Ensure measurements are perpendicular to the long axis to avoid false underestimation.
- Abdominal Aortic Aneurysms Are Commonly Infrarenal and ≥3.0 cm:
  - Most AAAs occur below the renal arteries and are classified as aneurysmal when the diameter exceeds 3.0 cm. The fusiform type, with uniform dilation, is most common. Measurements must include the outer walls, not just the lumen, to avoid underestimating size- especially in the presence of mural thrombus.
- Recognizing Aortic Landmarks Ensures Accurate Scanning:
  - Familiarity with aortic anatomy—including the celiac trunk, superior mesenteric artery (SMA), and renal arteries—is essential for complete evaluation. These landmarks help confirm probe positioning and ensure that the entire abdominal aorta is visualized from the diaphragm to the iliac bifurcation.
- Ultrasound is not sensitive for diagnosing aortic rupture
  - Most ruptured AAAs will result in retroperitoneal bleeding which is difficult to visualize with ultrasound

References

1. Reardon RF, Clinton ME, Madore F, Cook T. Chapter 9: Abdominal aortic aneurysm. In: Ma OJ, Mateer JR, Reardon RF, Joing SA, editors. Emergency ultrasound. 3rd ed. China: McGraw-Hill Education; 2014. p. 225–46.
2. Wu S, Blackstock U, Lewiss R, Saul T, Bagley W. Focus on: bedside ultrasound of the abdominal aorta. ACEP News Website. 2010. https://www.acep.org/Clinical%2D%2D-Practice-Management/Focus-On%2D%2DBedside-Ultrasound-of-the-Abdominal-Aorta/. Accessed 17 Apr 2017.
3. SonoSim Ultrasound Training Solution [Video]. Santa Monica: SonoSim Inc.; 2017.
4. Anagnostakos J, Lal BK. Abdominal aortic aneurysms. Prog Cardiovasc Dis. 2021;65:34–43. https://doi.org/10.1016/j.pcad.2021.03.009.
5. Lang RM, et al. Recommendations for cardiac chamber quantification by echocardiography in adults: an update from the American Society of Echocardiography and the European Association of Cardiovascular Imaging. J Am Soc Echocardiogr. 28(1):1-39.e14.
6. Fukui T. Management of acute aortic dissection and thoracic aortic rupture. J Intensive Care. 2018;6:15. https://doi.org/10.1186/s40560-018-0287-7. PMID: 29507729; PMCID: PMC5831732
7. Brewster DC, Cronenwett JL, Hallett JW Jr, Johnston KW, Krupski WC, Matsumura JS. Joint Council of the American Association for Vascular Surgery and Society for Vascular Surgery. Guidelines for the treatment of abdominal aortic aneurysms. Report of a Subcommittee of the Joint Council of the American Association for Vascular Surgery and Society for Vascular Surgery. J Vasc Surg. 2003;37(5):1106–17. https://doi.org/10.1067/mva.2003.363.
8. Gibbons RC, Smith D, Feig R, Mulflur M, Costantino TG. The sonographic protocol for the emergent evaluation of aortic dissections (SPEED protocol): a multicenter, prospective, observational study. Acad Emerg Med. 2024;31(2):112–8. https://doi.org/10.1111/acem.14839. Epub 2023 Dec 19

Biliary Ultrasound

10

Adam Weltler, Angela Lindsay, Michael J. Vitto, Jordan Tozer, and Michael Joyce

Abdominal pain is one of the most common ailments among patients within all facets of medicine. Right upper quadrant pain and its associated pathology, such as cholecystitis and cholelithiasis, can occur in patients seeing their primary care physician, seeking care in the emergency department, and in those admitted to the intensive care unit, general floor, or long-term care facilities. Ultrasound is an efficient, easy, and economical modality for a provider to evaluate the gallbladder and its surrounding structures for disease processes. This chapter will focus on performing the biliary ultrasound, basic gallbladder and biliary system anatomy, image acquisition, and interpretation of pathology.

Clinical Application and Indications

- Evaluate for causes of right upper quadrant pain, specifically cholelithiasis, cholecystitis, and choledocholithiasis.

Supplementary Information The online version contains supplementary material available at https://doi.org/10.1007/978-3-032-27643-8_10.

A. Weltler (✉)
Department of Emergency Medicine, Virginia Commonwealth University, Richmond, VA, USA
e-mail: angela.creditt@vcuhealth.org

A. Lindsay · M. J. Vitto · J. Tozer · M. Joyce
Department of Emergency Medicine, Virginia Commonwealth University Health, Richmond, VA, USA
e-mail: michael.vitto@vcuhealth.org; jordan.tozer@vcuhealth.org; john.joyce@vcuhealth.org

A. Lindsay et al. (eds.), *Clinical Ultrasound*,
https://doi.org/10.1007/978-3-032-27643-8_10

Normal Biliary Anatomy

- The gallbladder is a fluid-filled, hollow structure that lies inferior to the liver within the gallbladder fossa, medial and anterior to the kidney, and lateral to the inferior vena cava (IVC).
- There are three distinct regions of the gallbladder: fundus, body, and neck.
  - Body and fundus contain stored bile and are variable in size depending on the patient's prandial state.
  - Gallbladder neck is contiguous with the cystic duct, which joins the common hepatic duct to form the common bile duct.
  - A normal fully distended gallbladder will be no larger than 8 cm × 4 cm.
    - Average gallbladder measurements include length 6.16 ± 1.09 cm, height 2.75 ± 0.58 cm, and width 2.98 ± 0.59 cm [1].
  - The gallbladder wall is normally less than 3 mm thick [2–4].
  - Patients who are postprandial may have a small and contracted gallbladder measuring greater than 3 mm.
    - Average gallbladder wall thickness is 2.29 ± 0.525 [3].
- Common Bile Duct (CBD) travels anterior to the main portal vein and often to the right of the hepatic artery [2] forming the portal triad.

Imaging Overview

(a) Transducer Selection
  - Curvilinear transducer
  - Phased array transducer

(b) Patient Position
  - Patient should be lying in a supine position.
  - A left lateral decubitus position may bring the gallbladder out from beneath the rib cage and closer to the skin, allowing easier visualization.
  - Imaging on deep inspiration with a breath hold can also help bring the gallbladder out from beneath the rib cage, allowing easier visualization.
  - Alternatively, using a phased array probe, the gallbladder can be visualized through the intercostal spaces using the liver as an acoustic window.

(c) Standard Exam Views
  - Image the gallbladder in long axis
    - Begin with the transducer placed below the rib margin at approximately the midclavicular line with the marker pointed cephalad.
    - With the transducer, follow the rib margin laterally until you find the gallbladder, which is typically located between the nipple line and the anterior axillary line.
    - Once you locate the gallbladder, orient the transducer to mirror the long axis of the gallbladder to obtain a long-axis view.

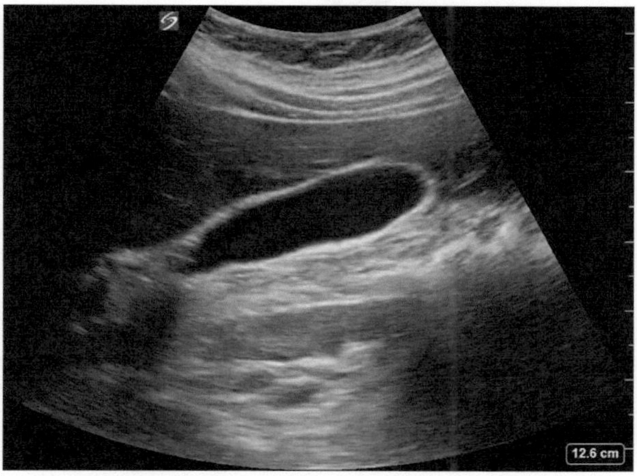

Fig. 10.1 Gallbladder in long axis: Gallbladder imaged in long axis

- Scan through the gallbladder by fanning the transducer from left to right.
  - Figure 10.1—Gallbladder in long axis
  - Video 10.1—Gallbladder in long axis

- Image the gallbladder in short axis
  - Rotate the transducer approximately 90° counterclockwise to obtain a short-axis view. The marker should be pointing toward the patient's right for this view.
  - Scan through the gallbladder in short axis by fanning from fundus to neck.
    - Figure 10.2—Gallbladder in short axis
    - Video 10.2—Gallbladder in short axis
- Measure the anterior gallbladder wall when in short-axis view.
  - Avoid measuring the gallbladder wall at the lateral or posterior positions. Ultrasound artifacts (edge artifact, shadowing, and posterior acoustic enhancement) will preclude accurate measurement in those locations.
  - If unable to obtain a clear image of the anterior wall in short axis, measure the gallbladder wall that abuts against the liver in long axis.
  - Figure 10.3—Anterior wall measurement in short axis
  - Figure 10.4—Wall measurement in long axis
- Image the common bile duct
  - Place the transducer inferior to costal margin at the midclavicular line with the transducer perpendicular to the costal margin and the marker pointed cephalad.
  - Locate the gallbladder, then rotate the transducer to the patients right and follow the main lobar fissure to find the portal vein.
  - Locate the portal vein, which is a thick hyperechoic-walled vein posterior to the neck of the gallbladder. Rotate the transducer so the portal vein is visualized longitudinally.
    - Figure 10.5—Portal vein

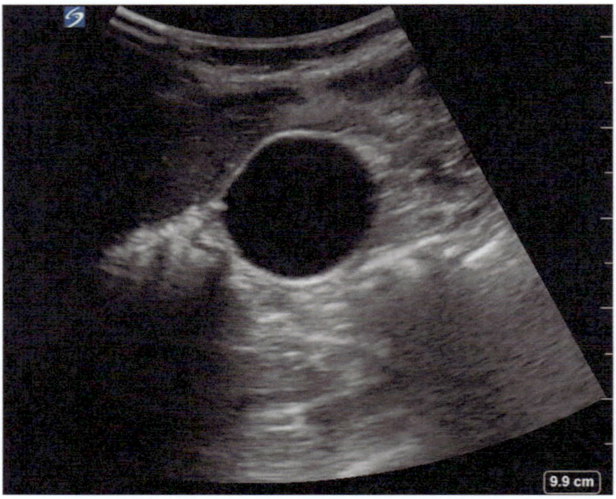

Fig. 10.2 Gallbladder in short axis: Gallbladder imaged in short axis

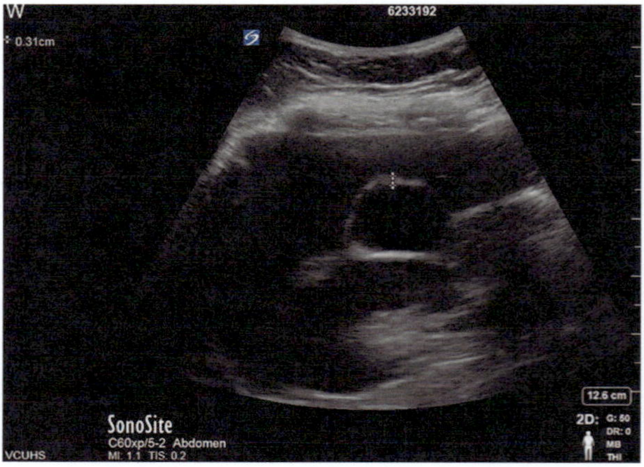

Fig. 10.3 Gallbladder wall measurement in short axis: The gallbladder wall should ideally be measured at the thickest location of the anterior wall when in short axis

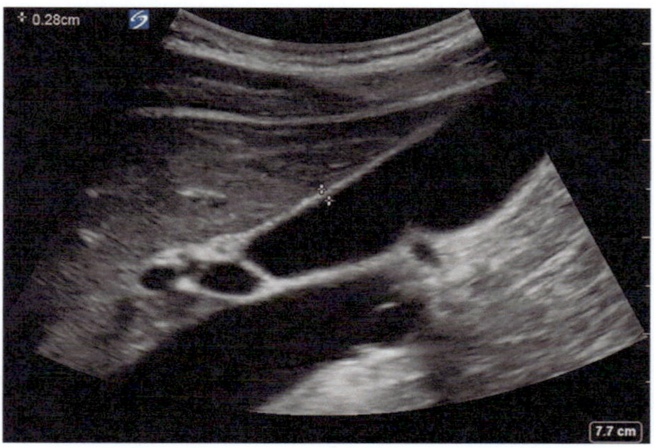

Fig. 10.4 Wall measurement in long axis: If unable to obtain an anterior wall measurement, measure the gallbladder wall that abuts against the liver in long axis at the thickest location

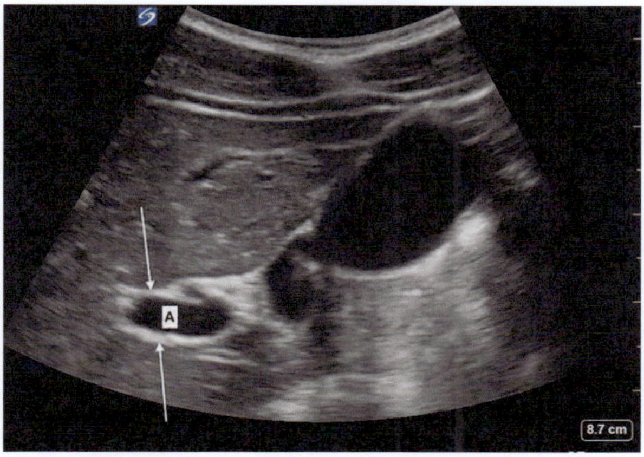

Fig. 10.5 Portal vein: The portal vein (A) has a thick hyperechoic wall (*arrows*), which makes it easy to identify within the liver

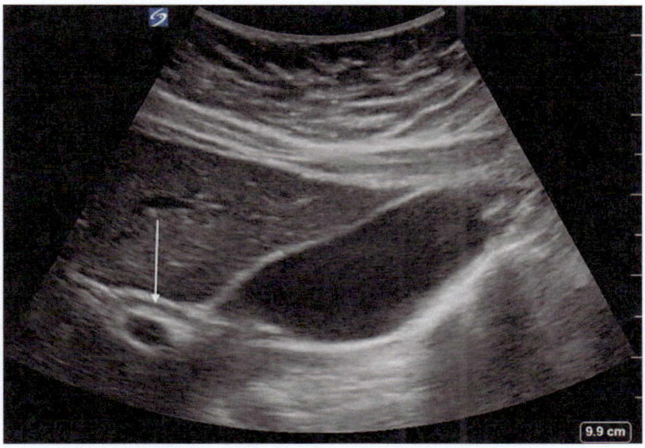

Fig. 10.6 CBD: Common bile duct (*arrow*) lies anterior to the portal vein

- CBD will be found anterior to and parallel to the portal vein, appearing as if they share a wall.
  - Figure 10.6—CBD
  - Video 10.3—Common bile duct
- A normal CBD can be difficult to differentiate from the hepatic artery.
  - Use color flow Doppler to assist in confirmation of the CBD. Both the portal vein and hepatic artery will demonstrate color Doppler, indicating flow, whereas the CBD should not.
  - Figure 10.7—Portal triad with color Doppler
  - Video 10.4—Portal triad with color Doppler
- In cross-section, the portal triad appears as three hypoechoic circles, commonly referred to as "Mickey Mouse sign" [2]
  - The larger portal vein is located at the base.
  - The smaller hepatic artery will be more medial at approximately the 2 o'clock position relative to the portal vein.

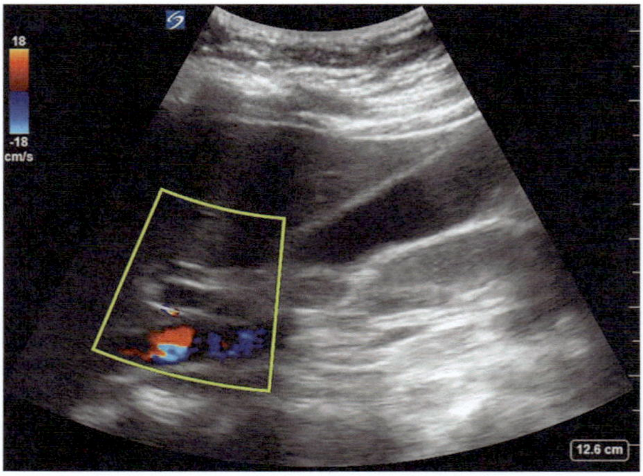

Fig. 10.7 Portal triad with color Doppler: Color Doppler can assist in locating the CBD. The portal vein and hepatic artery will both demonstrate color flow, whereas the common bile duct will not

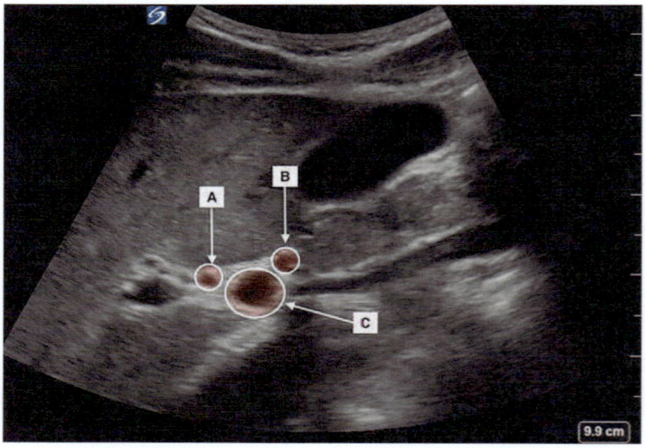

Fig. 10.8 Mickey Mouse sign: In cross section, the portal triad will appear as three hypoechoic circles, referred to as the Mickey Mouse sign: common bile duct (A), hepatic artery (B) and the portal vein (C)

    - CBD will be more lateral at approximately the 10 o'clock position relative to the portal vein.
    - Figure 10.8—Mickey Mouse sign
- Measure the common bile duct diameter from inner wall to inner wall.
    - Normal common bile duct diameter is less than 7 mm [2].
    - Figure 10.9—Normal CBD measurement
    - In patients who are status post cholecystectomy, CBD diameter should be less than 10 mm [5].

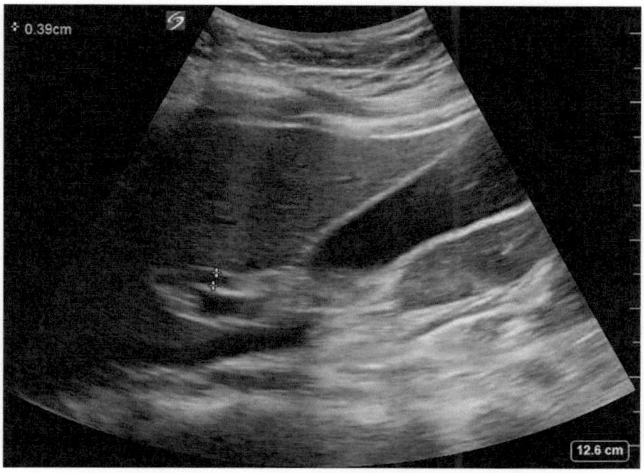

Fig. 10.9 Normal CBD measurement: Measure the common bile duct should be measured from inner wall to inner wall as pictured here

Gallbladder Pathology

(a) Cholelithiasis
- Cholelithiasis is the presence of stones within the gallbladder.
- Stones appear as hyperechoic, round or oval-shaped structures within the gallbladder and exhibit almost complete posterior acoustic shadowing.
- Posterior acoustic shadowing may not be seen with stones less than 2 mm [2].
  - Figure 10.10—Large gallstone
  - Video 10.5—Large gallstone
  - Figure 10.11—Multiple small gallstones
  - Video 10.6—Multiple small gallstones
- Gallstones are usually mobile, such that rolling the patient will cause the stones to move within the gallbladder.
- Wall echo shadow (WES) sign is a specific sign that indicates a contracted gallbladder filled with multiple stones [2] or a single large stone [6].
  - Sometimes referred to as "double arc shadow" sign [6, 7].
  - It is often difficult to appreciate, as the shadowing from multiple stones is often confused with bowel gas shadowing [7, 8].
    - Gallstones will produce clean shadowing, whereas bowel gas will produce irregular shadowing [8].
  - This finding will also preclude visualization of the gallbladder anatomy.
  - Figure 10.12—Wall echo shadow sign in short axis
  - Figure 10.13—Wall echo shadow sign in long axis
  - Video 10.7—Wall echo shadow sign

Fig. 10.10 Large Gallstone: Large gallstone with posterior acoustic shadowing

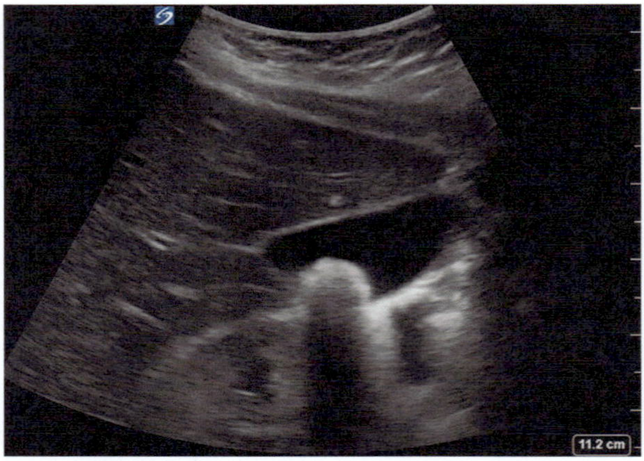

Fig. 10.11 Multiple gallstones: Multiple small gallstones with posterior acoustic shadowing

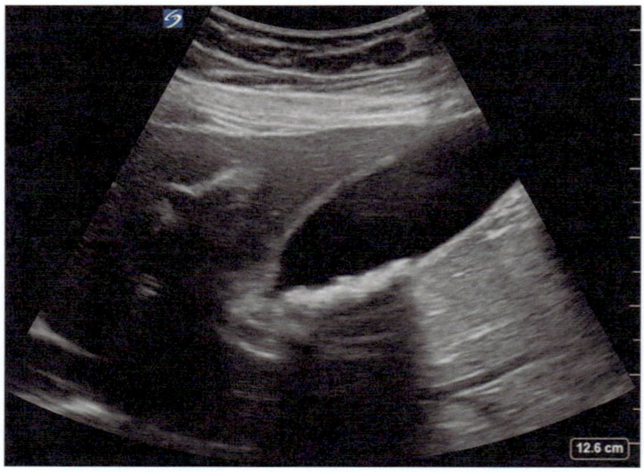

Fig. 10.12 Wall echo shadow sign in short axis: Wall echo sign (*arrow*) is seen when the gallbladder is contracted around many small stones or a single large stone

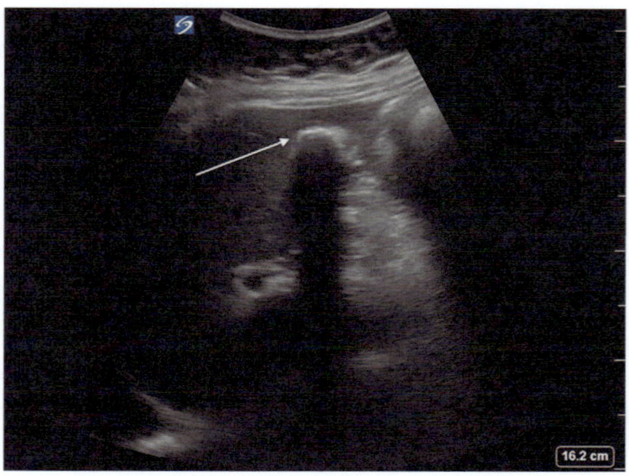

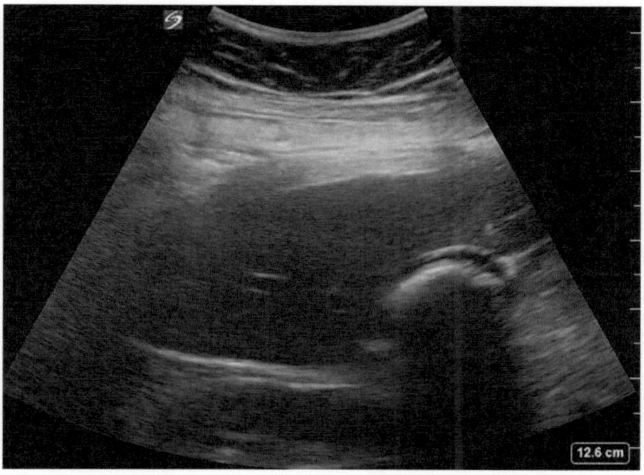

Fig. 10.13 Wall echo shadow sign in long axis: A long axis view depicting WES sign with a gallbladder that is completely full of stones, leaving no to very little cavity visible

(b) Biliary Sludge
- Sludge is particulate solids that have precipitated from bile but have not formed into stones.
- Sludge will appear as hyperechoic fluid layering within the gallbladder in a gravity-dependent fashion.
- Sludge will move when the patient is rotated.
- Figure 10.14—Sludge
- Video 10.8—Biliary sludge

(c) Acute Cholecystitis
- Inflammation of the gallbladder.
- Findings on ultrasound consistent with acute cholecystitis include thickened gallbladder wall, pericholecystic fluid, and sonographic Murphy's sign [2].
  - Video 10.9—Acute cholecystitis
- Thickened gallbladder wall
  - Will measure greater than 3 mm on the anterior wall [2–4].
  - Figure 10.15—Thickened wall in short axis
  - Figure 10.16—Thickened wall in long axis
- Pericholecystic fluid
  - Fluid surrounding the gallbladder that develops secondary to inflammation.
  - Will appear as a hypoechoic stripe between the liver and gallbladder.
  - Figure 10.17—Pericholecystic fluid
  - Video 10.10—Pericholecystic fluid
- Sonographic Murphy's sign
  - Defined as reproduction of the patient's pain while compressing the gallbladder with the transducer under direct visualization.
  - Combined with visualized stones, has a positive predictive value for acute cholecystitis >90% [9].

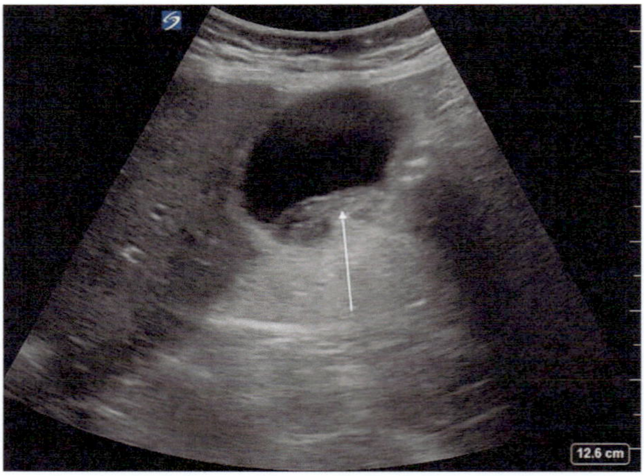

Fig. 10.14 Sludge: Sludge appears as hyperechoic fluid layering in the dependent portions of the gallbladder, without posterior shadowing

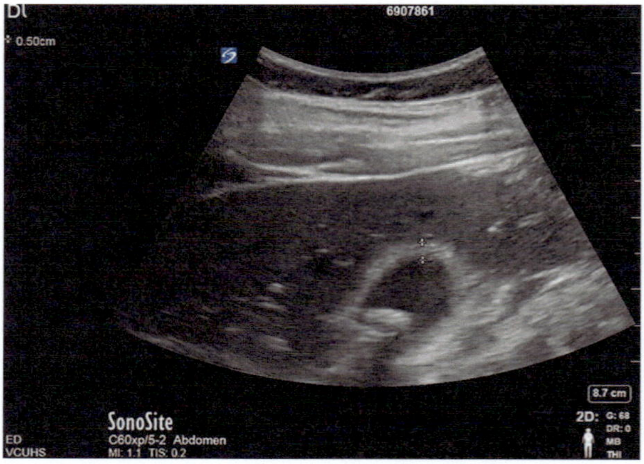

Fig. 10.15 Thickened wall in short axis: Anterior gallbladder wall is measuring 5 mm, consistent with a thickened wall and concerning for acute cholecystitis

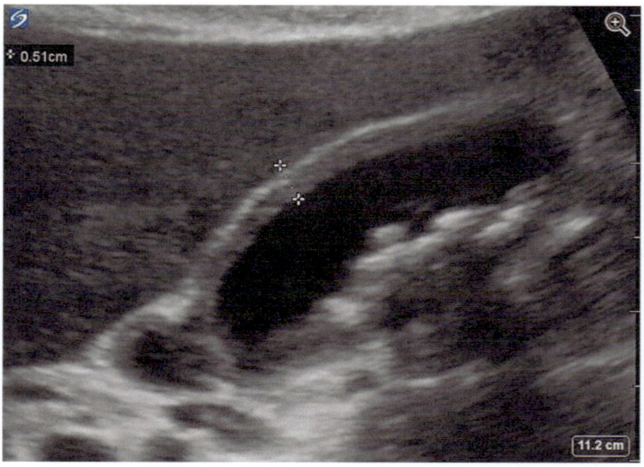

Fig. 10.16 Thickened wall in long axis: In long axis, the gallbladder wall is 5.1 mm consistent with thickened wall and concerning for acute cholecystitis

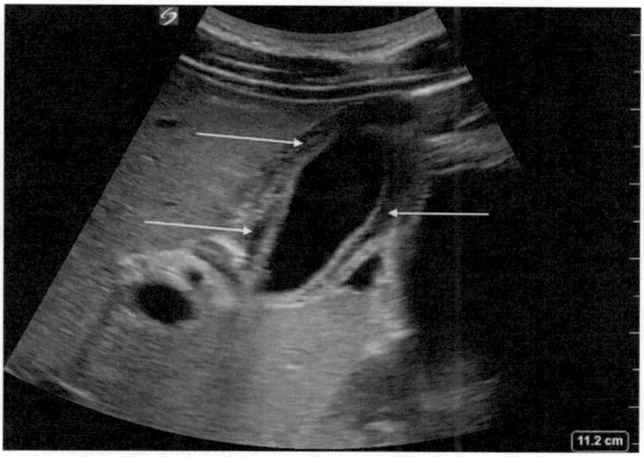

Fig. 10.17 Pericholecystic fluid: Pericholecystic fluid (*arrows*) is seen between the gallbladder and liver due to inflammation and likely acute cholecystitis

(d) Chronic Cholecystitis
- The gallbladder will appear contracted with thickened gallbladder walls due to fibrosis [2] from recurrent acute cholecystitis.
- Consider other causes of wall thickening such as postprandial contracture, pancreatitis, CHF, renal failure, and ascites.

(e) Adenomyomatosis
- Benign mucosal hyperplasia of gallbladder wall, either focal or diffuse.
- Echogenic foci with comet tail artifact (Rokitansky–Aschoff sinuses).

(f) Acalculous Cholecystitis
- Similar to acute cholecystitis due to cholelithiasis, however, the gallbladder will be devoid of stones.
- Typically seen as echogenic sludge within a dilated gallbladder that has a thickened wall.
- Most commonly occurs with reduced gallbladder function such as in trauma, postoperative, burn, sepsis, and patients who are immobilized or on TPN [10]
- Figure 10.18—Acalculous cholecystitis
- Video 10.11—Acalculous cholecystitis

(g) Emphysematous Cholecystitis
- Rare form of cholecystitis in which necrosis of the gallbladder occurs due to gas-forming bacteria resulting in air within the gallbladder wall [2].
- Will appear as small brightly echogenic areas along the anterior wall with reverberation artifact [11] or "dirty" shadowing from the gallbladder wall
- More often associated with acalculous cholecystitis.
- Will often progress to gangrenous cholecystitis and perforation if untreated.

(h) Gallbladder Polyps
- Non-shadowing, nonmobile outgrowths of the gallbladder wall.
- Often incidental in nature
  - Rarely become malignant.
  - May cause obstruction if they are very large and located near the neck.
  - Figure 10.19—Gallbladder polyp

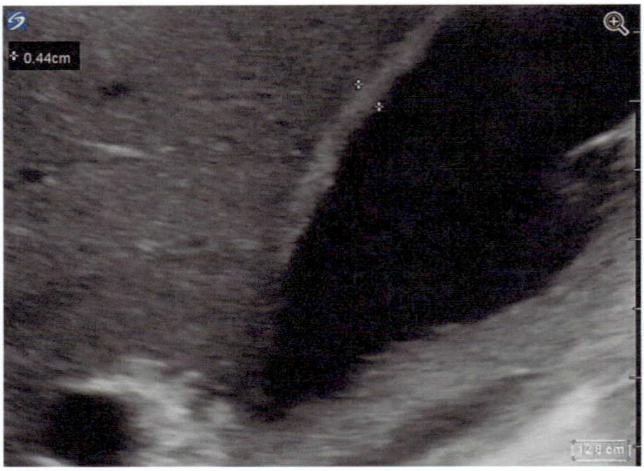

Fig. 10.18 Acalculous cholecystitis: Thickened gallbladder wall in the absence of gallstones

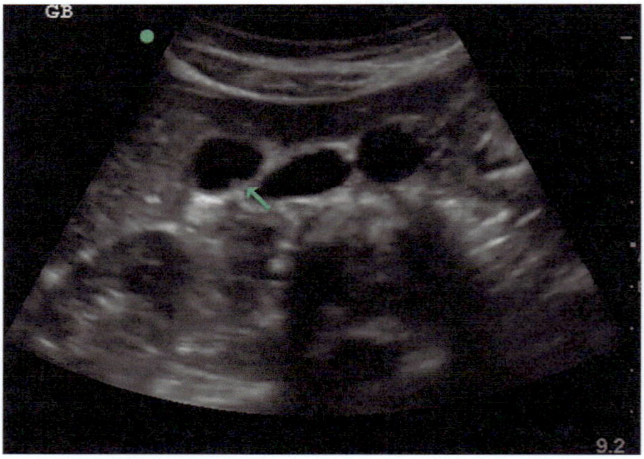

Fig. 10.19 Gallbladder polyp: Outgrowth from the gallbladder wall that has no posterior acoustic shadowing and is not mobile with patient movements

Common Bile Duct Pathology

- Common Bile Duct Dilation
  - Considered dilated once it becomes greater than 7 mm in normal patients or 10 mm in post-cholecystectomy patients [2, 5].
  - Normal size can increase with age.
  - Most common cause is obstruction, which can occur with an impacted stone, obstructing mass of the CBD or pancreas, or stricture of the CBD.
  - Non-obstructing causes of CBD dilation include cirrhosis and rarely, medications.
  - Figure 10.20—Dilated CBD

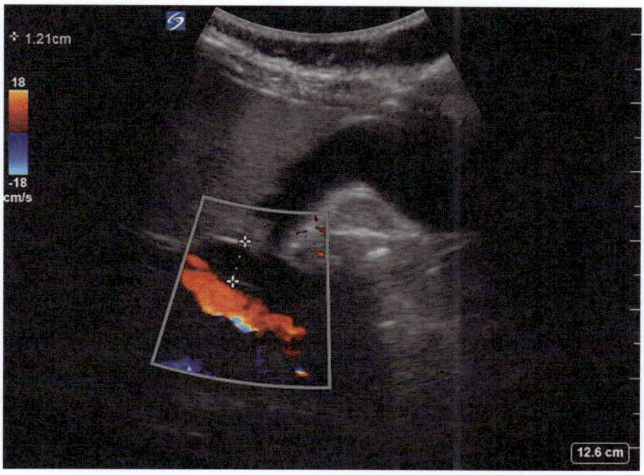

Fig. 10.20 Dilated CBD: Common bile duct in this patient is measuring 12.1 mm indicating a dilated duct, which is most commonly due to obstruction

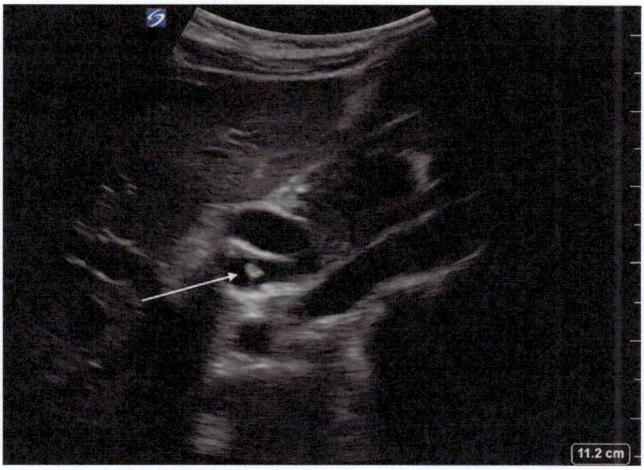

Fig. 10.21 Choledocholithiasis: A gallstone located within the common bile duct (*arrow*)

- Choledocholithiasis
  - Gallstone within the common bile duct.
  - Dilation of the CBD is usually the only ultrasound finding that a patient may have choledocholithiasis. This is because the distal CBD is rarely visualized secondary to overlying bowel gas.
  - Figure 10.21—Choledocholithiasis
  - Video 10.12—Choledocholithiasis

Key Points

- Patients who are recently postprandial may have a small and contracted gallbladder. A contracted gallbladder will give the appearance of a thickened wall.
- Gallbladder wall thickening can be seen in conditions that are unrelated to the gallbladder including pancreatitis, cirrhosis, congestive heart failure, renal failure, and ascites [2].
- Posterior acoustic shadowing may not be seen with stones less than 2 mm.

References

1. Adeyekun AA, Ukadike IO. Sonographic evaluation of gallbladder dimensions in healthy adults in Benin City, Nigeria. West Afr J Radiol. 2013;20(1):4–8. http://www.wajradiology.org/article.asp?issn=1115-3474;year=2013;volume=20;issue=1;spage=4;epage=8;aulast=Adeyekun. Accessed 24 Apr 2017
2. Lewiss RE, Theodoro DL. Chapter 10: Hepatobiliary. In: Ma OJ, Mateer JR, Reardon RF, Joing SA, editors. Emergency ultrasound. 3rd ed. China: McGraw-Hill Education; 2014. p. 247–72.
3. Mohammed S, Tahir A, Ahidjo A, Mistapha Z, Franza O, Okoye I, Shugaba A. Sonographic gallbladder wall thickness in normal adult populations in Nigeria. S Afr J Radiol. 2010;14(4):84. https://www.ajol.info/index.php/sajr/article/viewFile/70566/59167. Accessed 24 Apr 2017
4. Blackstock U, Wu S, Lewiss R, Saul T, Bagley W. Focus on: bedside biliary ultrasound. ACEP News Website. November 2010. https://www.acep.org/Content.aspx?id=64648. Accessed 24 Apr 2017.
5. Sharma S, Goyal S, Goyal RA. Prospective study to determine the effect of cholecystectomy on common bile duct diameter in Indian population. Int J Clin Exp Physiol. 2015;2(1):61–5. http://www.ijcep.org/article.asp?issn=2348-8832;year=2015;volume=2;issue=1;spage=61;epage=65;aulast=Sharma. Accessed 24 Apr 2017
6. Datta A, Garg N, Lema PC. The significance of the wall echo shadow triad on ultrasonography: a case series. Crit Ultrasound J. 2010;2(3):107–8. http://link.springer.com/article/10.1007/s13089-010-0038-z. Accessed 24 Apr 2017
7. Raptopoulos V, D'Orsi C, Smith E, Reuter K, Moss L, Kleinman P. Dynamic cholecystosonography of the contracted gallbladder: the double-arc-shadow sign. Am J Roentgenol. 1982;138(2):–275, 8. http://www.ajronline.org/doi/pdf/10.2214/ajr.138.2.275. Accessed 24 Apr 2017
8. Brown BS, Hoffmann B, Noble VE. Chapter 45: Emergency biliary ultrasonography. In: Adams JG, Barton ED, Collings J, DB PMC, Gisondi MA, Nadel ES, editors. Emergency medicine: clinical essentials. 2nd ed. Philadelphia: Saunders, an imprint of Elsevier Inc.; 2013. p. 370–81.
9. Hassan T. Ultrasonographic frequency of acute cholecystitis in the patients presenting with right hypochondriac pain. Arch Gen Intern Med. 2023;7(4):186.
10. Huffman JL, Schenker S. Acute acalculous cholecysrtitis: a review. Clin Gastroenterol Hepatol. 2010;8(1):15–22. http://www.cghjournal.org/article/S1542-3565(09)00880-5/pdf. Accessed 24 Apr 2017
11. Smith EA, Dillman JR, Elsayes KM, Menias CO, Bude RO. Cross-sectional imaging of acute and chronic gallbladder inflammatory disease. Am J Roentgenol. 2009;192(1):188–96. http://www.ajronline.org/doi/full/10.2214/AJR.07.3803. Accessed 15 June 2017

11 Renal and Bladder Ultrasound

Chelsea Bunce, Lindsay Taylor, Michael J. Vitto,
Angela Lindsay, and Michael Joyce

Point-of-care evaluation of the urinary system is focused on assessing the kidneys and bladder. Commonly, renal ultrasound is used to evaluate for hydronephrosis and/or evidence of renal stones in patients who present with signs and symptoms of nephrolithiasis. It is also frequently used to image the bladder and obtain measurements for calculating bladder volume in patients who report urinary retention and allows providers to evaluate for causes of gross hematuria or troubleshoot issues with indwelling Foley catheters. At times, incidental findings are noted, such as a bladder or renal mass, that will necessitate further workup, making it important to learn how to recognize these structures. This chapter will review the basic genitourinary anatomy, image acquisition, normal ultrasound anatomy, and interpretation of pathology.

Supplementary Information The online version contains supplementary material available at https://doi.org/10.1007/978-3-032-27643-8_11.

C. Bunce
Department of Emergency Medicine, Virginia Commonwealth University Medical Center, Richmond, VA, USA

L. Taylor (✉) · M. J. Vitto · A. Lindsay · M. Joyce
Department of Emergency Medicine, Virginia Commonwealth University Health, Richmond, VA, USA
e-mail: Lindsay.Taylor@vcuhealth.org; Michael.Vitto@vcuhealth.org; Angie.Creditt@vcuhealth.org; John.Joyce@vcuhealth.org

A. Lindsay et al. (eds.), *Clinical Ultrasound*,
https://doi.org/10.1007/978-3-032-27643-8_11

Clinical Application and Indications

- Evaluate for the cause of abdominal pain, flank pain, pelvic pain, hematuria, and urinary retention:
  - Common pathologies include renal stones, ureteral stones, renal mass, hydronephrosis, hydroureter, enlarged prostate, bladder mass, and malfunctioning urinary catheter.
- Calculate bladder volume

Genitourinary Anatomy

- Kidney
  - Paired retroperitoneal structures:
    - Right kidney is found inferior to the liver
    - Left kidney is found inferior to the spleen
  - The renal capsule surrounds the kidney with adjacent perinephric fat.
  - Just deep to the capsule will be the renal parenchyma that consists of the cortex, medulla, and medullary pyramids:
    - Medullary pyramids empty urine into minor calyces, which form major calyces. Major calyces then unite to form the renal pelvis.
  - Within the hilum is the renal vasculature and renal pelvis, which connect to the ureter.
  - Ureters course posteriorly within the abdomen toward the bladder.
- Bladder
  - The bladder is a highly distensible structure.
  - Surrounding the bladder is the bladder wall composed largely of the detrusor muscle [1].
  - Ureters from the right and left kidney drain into the bladder at the trigone.

Image Acquisition

1. Transducer Selection
   (a) Curvilinear
   (b) Phased array
2. Patient Position
   (a) The patient should be lying supine.
   (b) Occasionally, a right lateral decubitus position may be needed to bring the left kidney closer to the skin surface.
3. Standard Exam Views
   (a) Right kidney:
      - Position the transducer at the right anterior axillary line just inferior to the costal margin with the transducer marker pointed cephalad.
      - The liver will be used as an acoustic window to image the right kidney.

- Visualize the kidney in long axis:
  - Figure 11.1—Right kidney
  - Video 11.1—Right kidney
  - The echogenic renal capsule appears bright white.
  - Internal to this is the renal parenchyma containing the outer renal cortex, which should be isoechoic relative to the liver parenchyma with the hypoechoic medullary pyramids throughout [1].
  - Buried within the hyperechoic fat of the renal pelvis is the central collecting system, which consists of the minor and major calyces [2].
- Rotate the transducer 90° counterclockwise and view the kidney in short axis:
  - Figure 11.2—Right kidney in short axis
  - Video 11.2—Right kidney in short axis
- Alternatively, the right kidney can also be imaged with the transducer placed anteriorly just beneath the costal margin and the marker pointed cephalad.

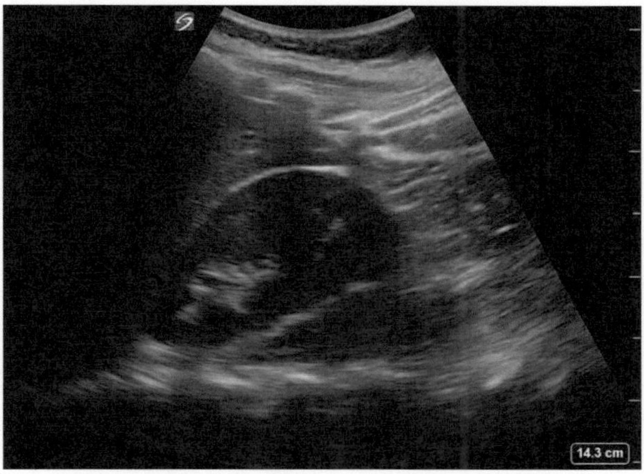

Fig. 11.1 Right kidney: The right kidney is visualized next to the liver in long axis

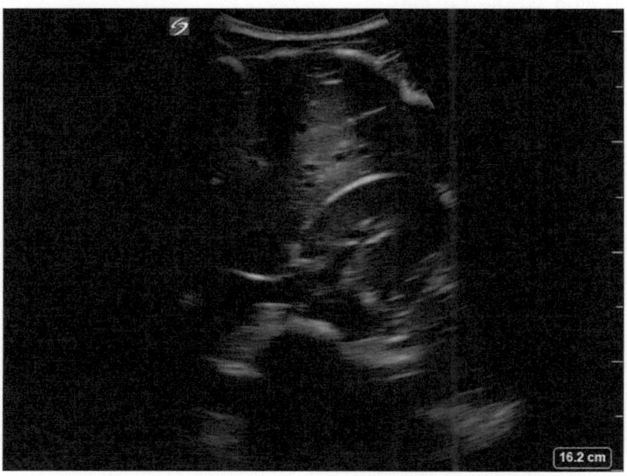

Fig. 11.2 Right kidney in short axis: In short axis, the kidney will appear more rounded

(b) Left kidney:
  - Position the transducer at the left posterior to midaxillary line inferior to the costal margin with the transducer marker pointed cephalad.
  - The spleen will be used as an acoustic window to image the left kidney.
  - The left kidney is typically located more superior than the right; therefore, the transducer may need to be placed higher up, occasionally as high as the tenth or eleventh intercostal space:
    - Figure 11.3—Left kidney in long axis
    - Video 11.3—Left kidney in long axis
  - Rotate the transducer 90° counterclockwise and visualize the left kidney in short axis:
    - Figure 11.4—Left kidney in short axis
    - Video 11.4—Left kidney in short axis

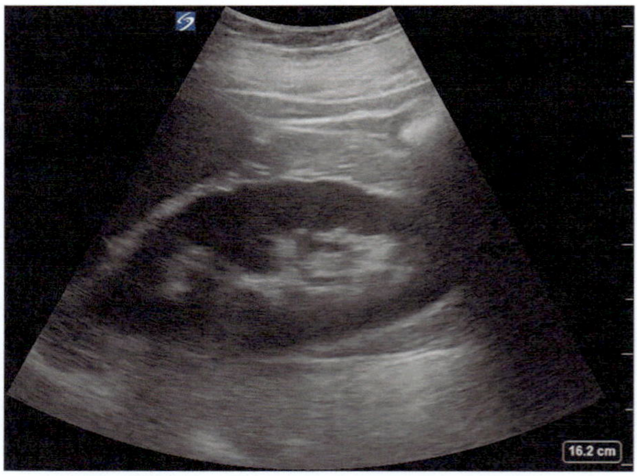

Fig. 11.3 Left kidney: The left kidney is visualized next to the spleen in long axis

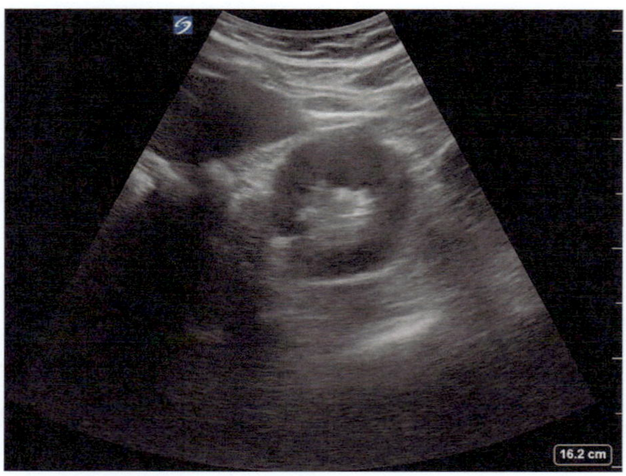

Fig. 11.4 Left kidney in short axis: The left kidney in short axis next to the spleen

(c) Bladder:

- The transducer should be placed superior to the pubic bone, angled inferiorly, with the transducer marker pointed toward the patient's right to obtain a cross-sectional view:
  - Figure 11.5—Bladder in transverse
  - Video 11.5—Bladder in transverse
- Rotate the transducer 90° with the marker pointed cephalad to obtain a longitudinal/sagittal view:
  - Figure 11.6—Bladder in sagittal
  - Video 11.6—Bladder in sagittal
- The bladder appears as an anechoic fluid collection surrounded by a thin hyperechoic line representing the bladder wall.
- In females, the uterus will be posterior and superior to the bladder:
  - Figure 11.7—Uterus posterior to the bladder

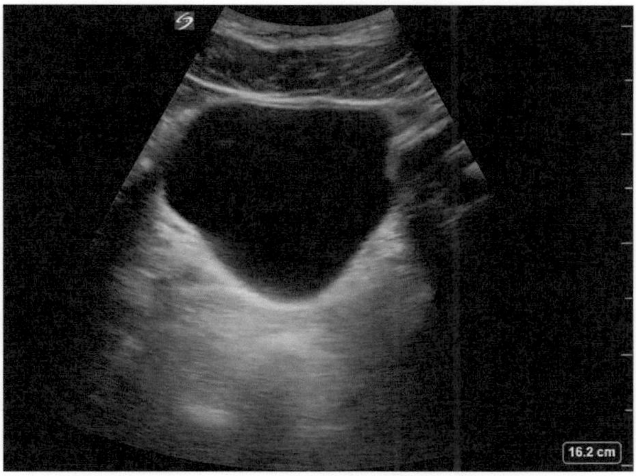

Fig. 11.5 Bladder in transverse: Cross-sectional view of the bladder

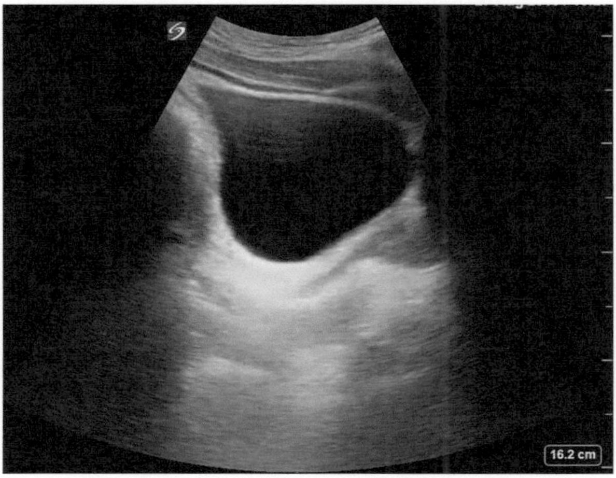

Fig. 11.6 Bladder in sagittal: Sagittal view of the bladder. Note the posterior acoustic enhancement that is normal for fluid-filled structures

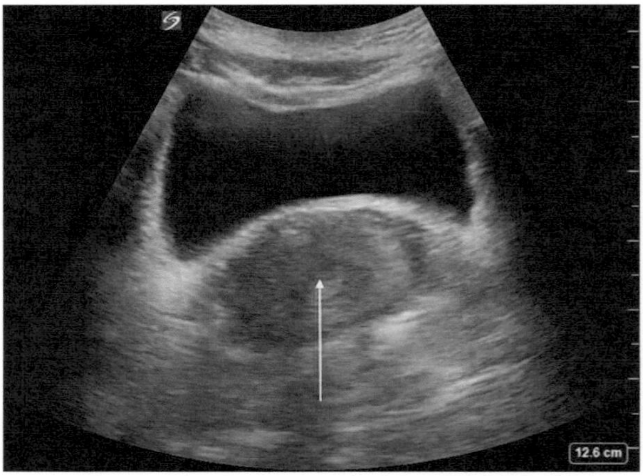

Fig. 11.7 Uterus posterior to bladder: In females, the uterus is located directly posterior to the bladder (*arrow*)

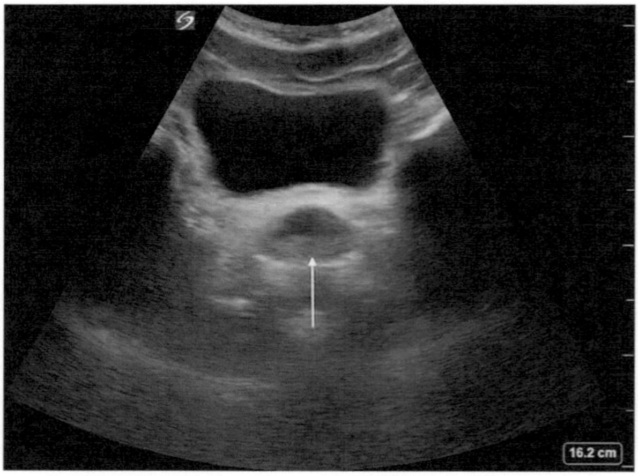

Fig. 11.8 Prostate posterior to bladder: In males, the prostate is located posterior to the bladder (*arrow*)

- In males, the prostate, a hypoechoic round mass, will be posterior to the bladder:
  - Figure 11.8—Prostate posterior to the bladder
- Normal bladder wall thickness is 5 mm when empty and 3 mm when full [3]:
  - Figure 11.9—Normal bladder wall thickness
- In a cross-sectional view, visualize ureteral flow jets representing urine entering the bladder:
  - Video 11.7—Ureteral flow jets
  - Color or Power Doppler can be a useful adjunct to image this process
  - Figure 11.10—Ureteral flow jets with color Doppler
  - Video 11.8—Ureteral flow jets with color Doppler

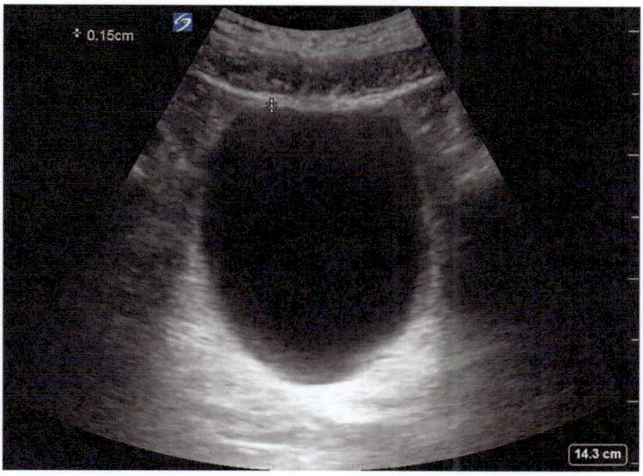

Fig. 11.9 Normal bladder wall thickness: Bladder wall thickness measured at 0.15 cm. Normal bladder wall thickness is less than 5 mm when empty and less than 3 mm when full

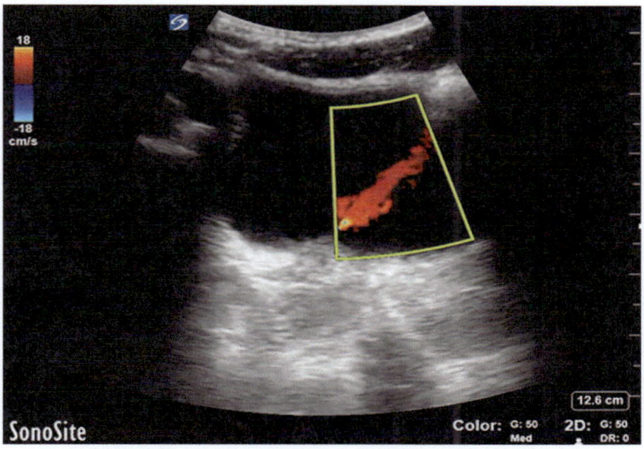

Fig. 11.10 Ureteral flow jets with color Doppler: In a transverse plane, ureteral flow jets representing urine entering the bladder can be seen. Color Doppler can enhance the detection of ureteral flow jets

- Measuring bladder volume:
  - Bladder volume is estimated by measuring height, width, and depth:
    - Most ultrasound machines have bladder volume calculators.
    - Alternatively, the formula length (L) times width (W) times height (H) times 0.75 ($L \times W \times H \times 0.75$) can be used [4].
  - Width and depth measurements are taken while in the transverse/cross-sectional window:
    - Figure 11.11—Bladder volume measurement in transverse
  - Height is measured in the longitudinal/sagittal view with a measurement caudal to cephalad:
    - Figure 11.12—Bladder volume measurement in sagittal
  - A normal post-void residual volume is less than 50 mL[2].

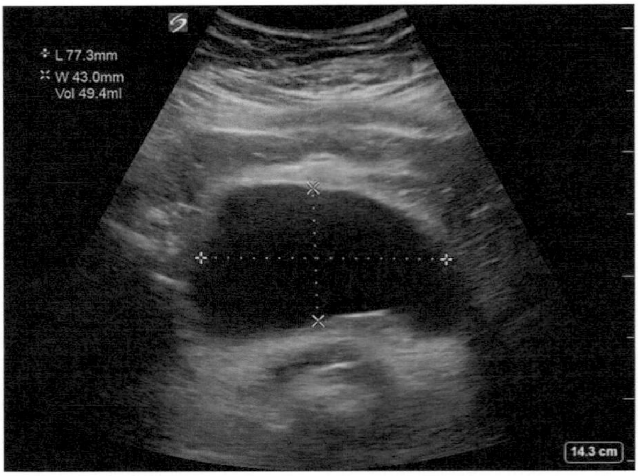

Fig. 11.11 Bladder volume measurement in transverse: In a transverse plane, measure across the bladder to obtain length (*L*) and from anterior to posterior to obtain width (*W*)

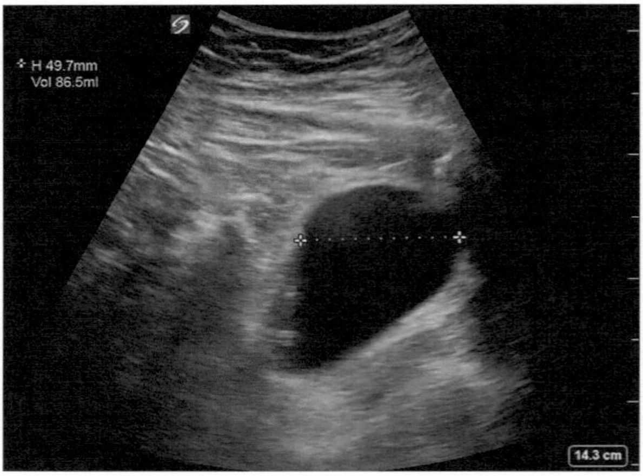

Fig. 11.12 Bladder volume measurement in sagittal: In sagittal orientation, measure superior to inferior to obtain the height (*H*) measurement

Renal Pathology

(a) Hydronephrosis

- Dilation of the renal collecting system due to intrinsic or extrinsic obstruction:
  - Common etiologies include large ureteral stone, enlarged prostate, bladder mass, and extrinsic compression of the collecting system.
- Appears as an anechoic fluid collection within the renal sinus.
- Hydronephrosis can be mild, moderate, or severe:
  - Mild: Dilation of renal pelvis and anechoic areas within the hyperechoic renal sinus [1]:
    - Figure 11.13—Mild hydronephrosis
    - Video 11.9—Mild hydronephrosis

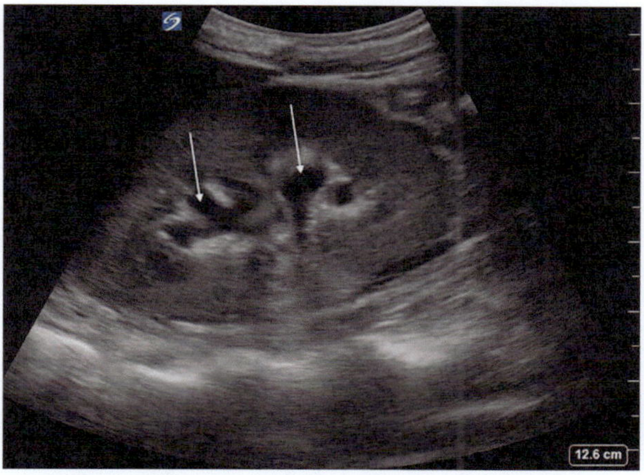

Fig. 11.13 Mild hydronephrosis: Mild dilation of the collecting system (*arrows*)

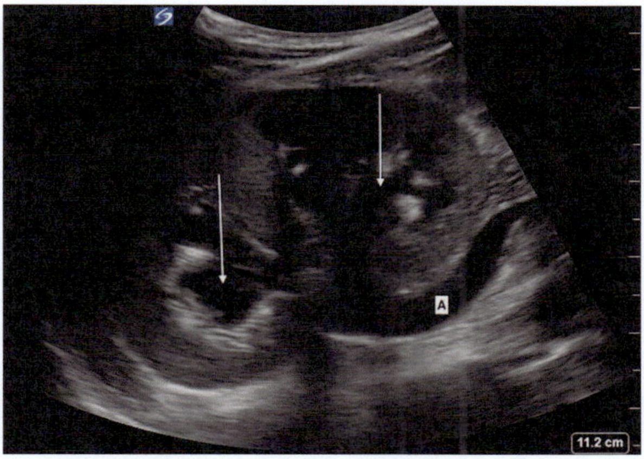

Fig. 11.14 Moderate hydronephrosis: Moderate dilation of the collecting system (*arrows*) with associated hydroureter (A)

- Moderate: Separation of minor and major calyces [1]:
  - Figure 11.14—Moderate hydronephrosis
  - Video 11.10—Moderate hydronephrosis
- Severe: Notable for thinning of the renal cortex [4] and significant dilation of the renal pelvis and minor and major calyces [1]:
  - Figure 11.15—Severe hydronephrosis
  - Video 11.11—Severe hydronephrosis

- Considerations when evaluating for hydronephrosis:
  - Right-sided hydronephrosis is common in pregnancy.
  - Bilateral mild hydronephrosis can occur in a well-hydrated patient without pathology and in patients with a full bladder [1].
  - Have the patient void and then reimage their kidneys for comparison.
  - A dehydrated patient may not demonstrate signs of hydronephrosis.
  - A large abdominal aortic aneurysm (AAA) can compress the ureter and cause hydronephrosis.

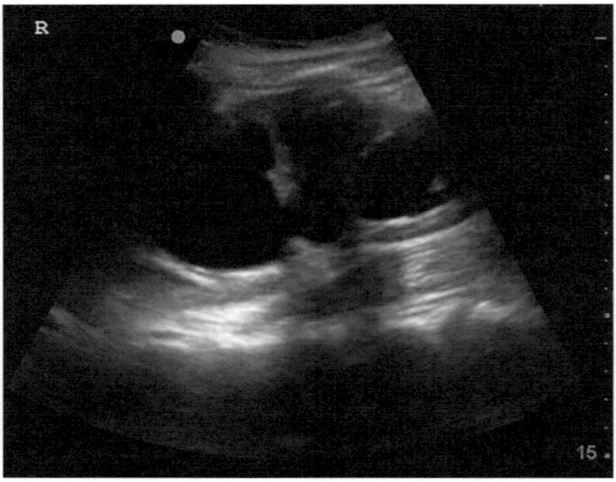

Fig. 11.15 Severe hydronephrosis: Significant dilation of the renal pelvis and collecting system with thinning of the renal cortex

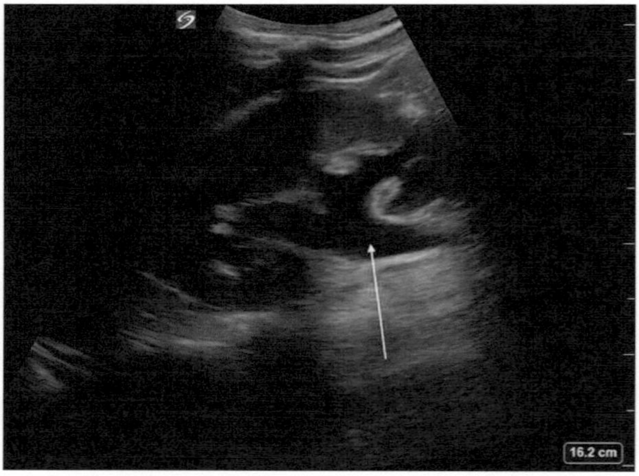

Fig. 11.16 Hydroureter: The ureter is seen exiting the renal collecting system and is dilated (*arrow*)

(b) Hydroureter
  - Dilated ureter
  - Can be seen with severe hydronephrosis
  - Figure 11.16—Hydroureter
  - Video 11.12—Hydroureter
  - Figure 11.17—Hydroureter with color Doppler

(c) Nephrolithiasis
  - Stones within the kidney.
  - They appear brightly echogenic and are usually found within the renal pelvis or parenchyma.
  - Demonstrate posterior acoustic shadowing, similar to a gallstone.
  - Rarely, stones can be visualized in the urinary tract, more commonly at the ureteropelvic or ureterovesicular junctions [4].
  - Figure 11.18—Stone within the renal pelvis.
  - Figure 11.19—Parenchymal stone
  - Video 11.13—Renal stone

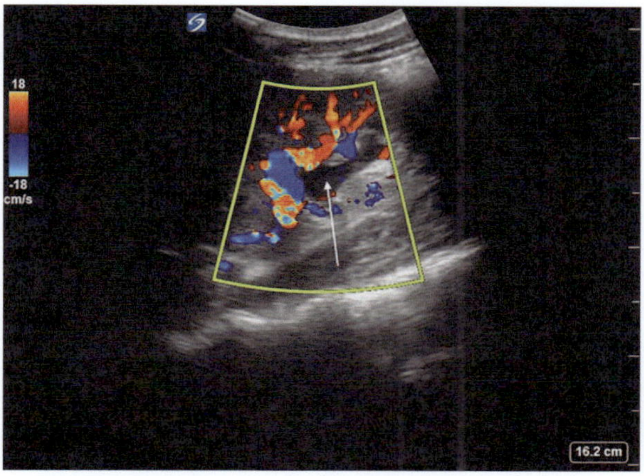

Fig. 11.17 Hydroureter with color Doppler: Place color Doppler over the ureter to help verify the ureter is what is being imaged and that the structure is not renal vasculature. The ureter (*arrow*) will not exhibit color flow

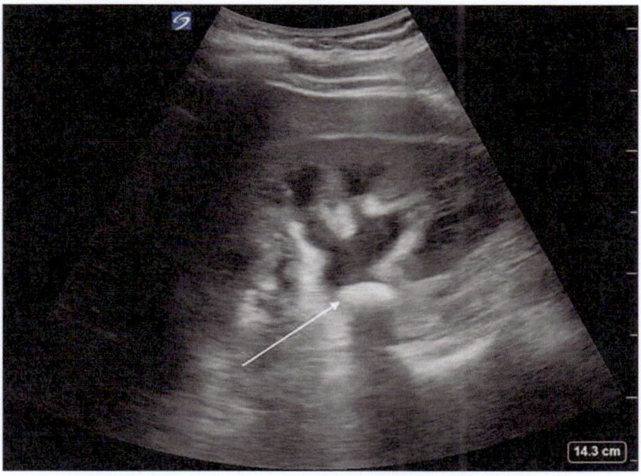

Fig. 11.18 Stone within the renal pelvis: Large renal stone within the renal collecting system, with posterior shadowing. Also, note the moderate hydronephrosis and hydroureter

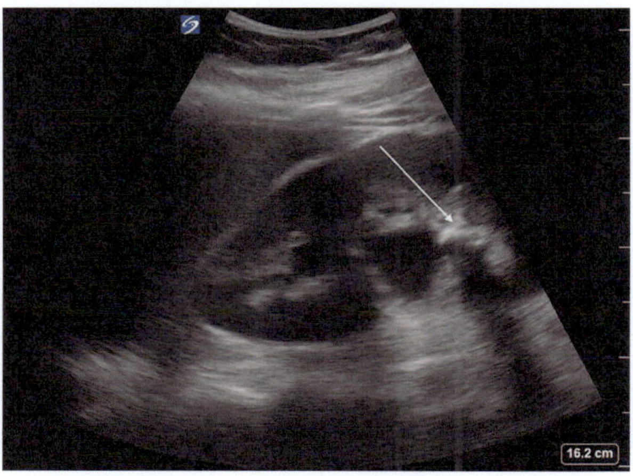

Fig. 11.19 Parenchymal stone: A stone (*arrow*) within the parenchyma of the kidney will not cause dilation of the collecting system

(d) Renal Cyst
- Abnormal cystic structure that appears within the renal parenchyma and distorts the typical architecture of the normal kidney:
  - Seen more frequently in elderly patients.
- On ultrasound appears as an anechoic fluid collection.
- Will have a smooth, thin wall, round or oval shape, and posterior enhancement without any internal echoes or solid components [4]:
  - Figure 11.20—Simple renal cyst
  - Video 11.14—Simple renal cyst
- Polycystic kidney disease will have numerous variable-sized cysts, typically bilateral:
  - Figure 11.21—Polycystic kidney disease
  - Video 11.15—Polycystic kidney disease

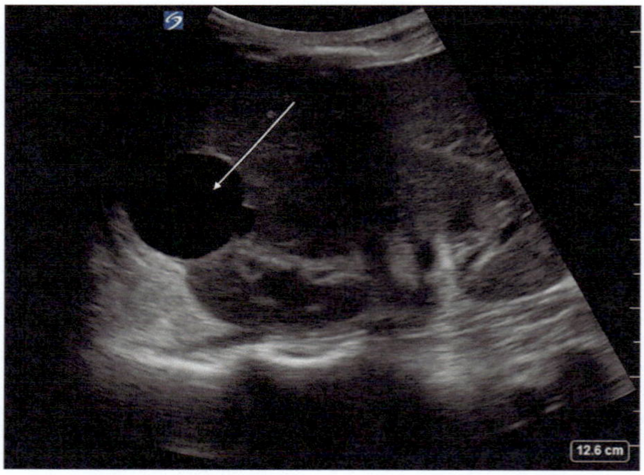

Fig. 11.20 Simple renal cyst: A large renal cyst (*arrow*) with a smooth, thin outer wall and simple, anechoic fluid

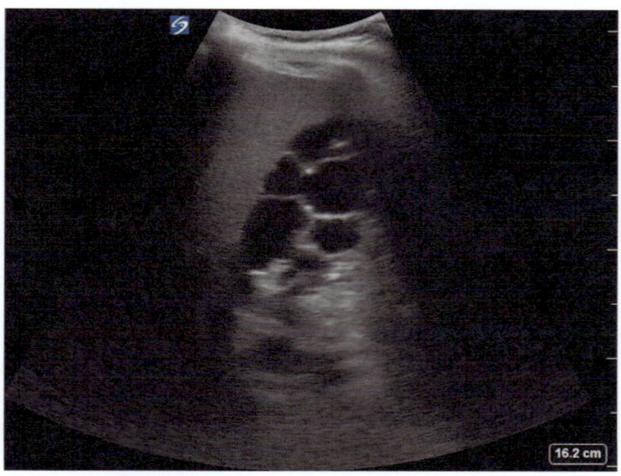

Fig. 11.21 Polycystic kidney disease: Multiple cysts of variable sizes distorting the normal architecture of the kidney

(e) Renal Mass
   - Benign or malignant growth within the kidney parenchyma.
   - Renal cell carcinoma tumors appear heterogeneous on ultrasound and may be hyperechoic, hypoechoic, or isoechoic to the renal parenchyma [4].
   - Can also have a cystic appearance [4].

Bladder Pathology

- Bladder Mass
  - Benign and malignant masses can appear as an irregular growth projecting from the bladder wall into the lumen of the bladder or as a focal area of bladder wall thickening [4]:
    - Figure 11.22—Bladder mass
    - Video 11.16—Bladder mass
  - In patients with gross hematuria, it is important to consider that a bladder mass can be a hematoma:
    - In this situation, it would be appropriate to consider bladder irrigation and then reimage the bladder for resolution or change in the appearance of the mass.
    - Figure 11.23—Bladder hematoma
    - Video 11.17—Bladder hematoma
- Thickened Bladder Wall
  - A bladder wall is considered thickened if it is greater than 5 mm when non-distended and greater than 3 mm when distended [1]:
    - Artifacts can contribute to a thickened bladder wall when non-distended.

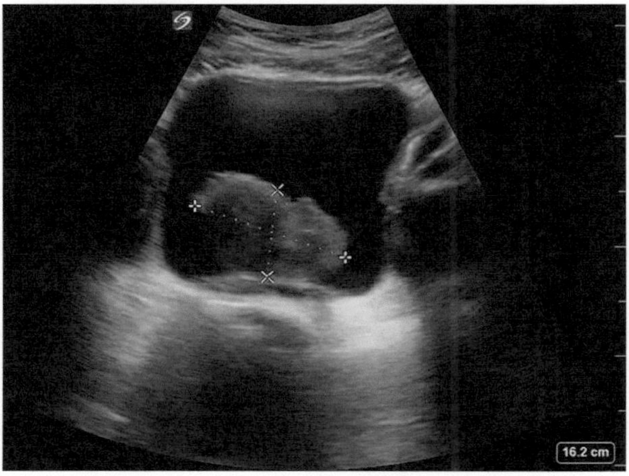

Fig. 11.22 Bladder mass: A bladder mass will appear as large irregular growth originating from the bladder wall

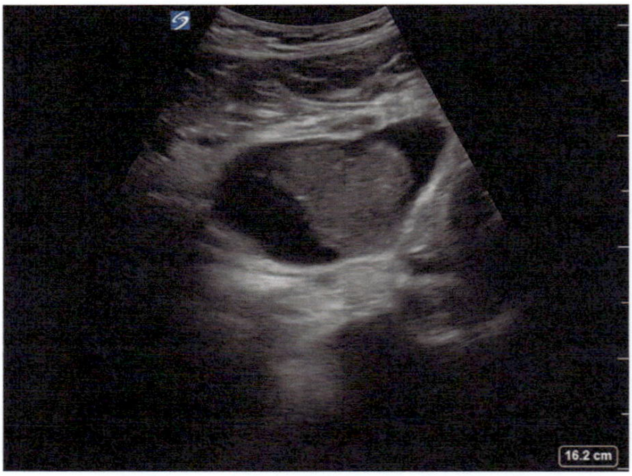

Fig. 11.23 Bladder hematoma: Bladder hematoma, as seen here, can be easily confused with a bladder mass

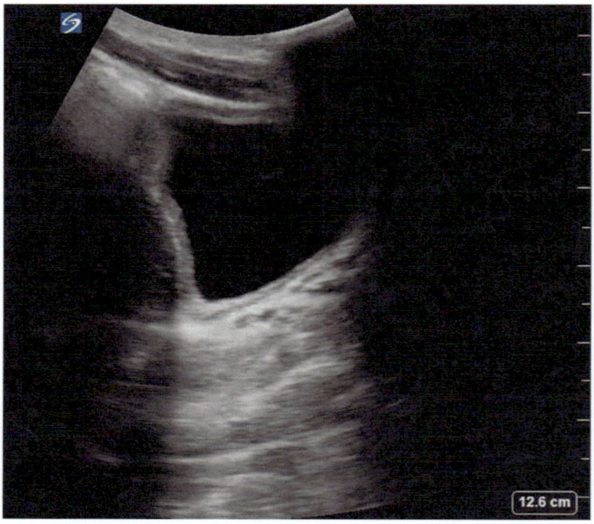

Fig. 11.24 Thickened bladder wall: Thickened bladder wall throughout the entire bladder

   - Generalized bladder wall thickening can have multiple etiologies including cystitis from radiation, recurrent urinary tract infection, and neurogenic bladder:
     - Figure 11.24—Thickened bladder wall
   - Focal wall thickening can be due to hematoma, benign or malignant tumor, polyp, and less commonly cystitis.
- Enlarged Prostate
   - A normal prostate measures up to 5 cm in diameter [4].
   - A prostate that measures greater than 5 cm is abnormal.
   - Prostate enlargement can extend into the bladder and be mistaken for a bladder mass. Therefore, it is important to obtain views of any abnormality in multiple planes.

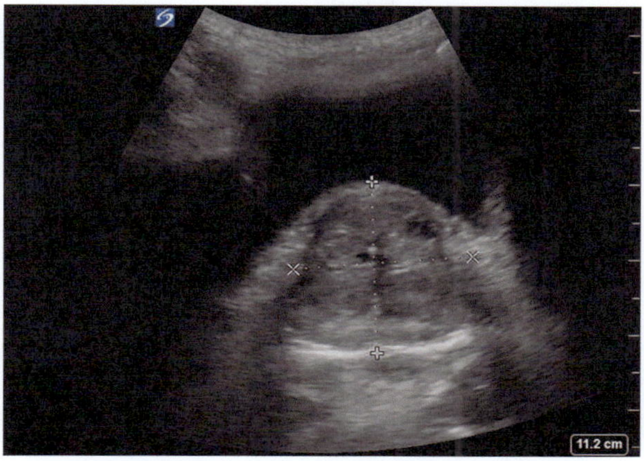

Fig. 11.25 Enlarged prostate due to BPH: Symmetrically enlarged prostate posterior to the bladder in a transverse plane. With these characteristics, this enlargement is likely due to BPH

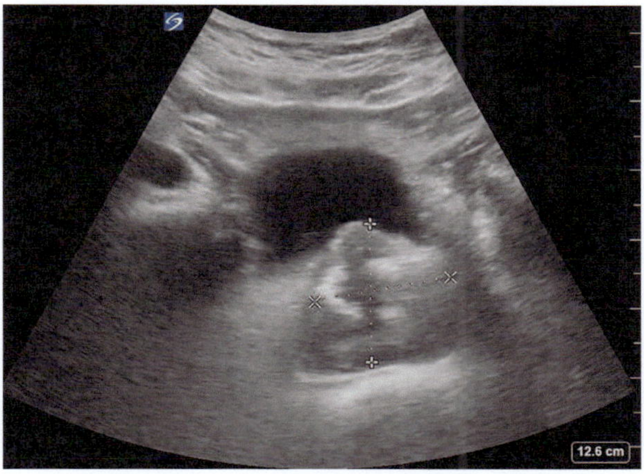

Fig. 11.26 Enlarged prostate due to prostate cancer: Enlarged prostate with abnormal and irregular shape indicates that this is more likely to be due to prostate cancer

– Benign prostatic hyperplasia (BPH) and prostate cancer can appear similar on ultrasound; further studies will be needed to determine the cause of prostate enlargement:
  - Figure 11.25—Enlarged prostate due to BPH
  - Figure 11.26—Enlarged prostate due to prostate cancer
  - Video 11.18—Enlarged prostate

Key Points
- When evaluating hydronephrosis, consider the various obstructive causes vs. normal physiology from being well hydrated.
- AAA should be considered in the differential diagnosis in any patient who presents with flank pain, signs or symptoms of renal colic, and is over the age of 50.
- If uncertain about a possible abnormality, compare with the other kidney.
- Benign renal cysts should be anechoic. If a cyst appears to be complex with internal echoes, septations, etc., consider malignancy.

References

1. SonoSim Ultrasound Training Solution [Video]. Santa MonicaCA: SonoSim Inc.; 2017.
2. Southgate SJ, Herbst MK. Ultrasound of the urinary tract [Internet]. Treasure Island: StatPearls Publishing; 2024. [updated 2023 Jan 16; cited 2025 July 25]. Available from: https://www.ncbi.nlm.nih.gov/books/NBK535381/
3. Patel U. Chapter 2: Imaging modalities used for assessment of the bladder. In: Patel U, editor. Imaging and urodynamics of the lower urinary tract. 2nd ed. London: Springer; 2010. p. 9–21.
4. Seif D, Swadron S. Chapter 12: Renal. In: Ma OJ, Mateer JR, Reardon RF, Joing SA, editors. Emergency ultrasound. 3rd ed. China: McGraw-Hill Education; 2014. p. 319–52.

Abdominal Ultrasound

12

Angela Lindsay and Michael J. Vitto

Ultrasound is an efficient way to evaluate for acute pathology in patients who present to the Emergency Department, or other clinical area, with abdominal pain. Given the potentially emergent nature of various abdominal conditions, bedside ultrasound can expedite patients' diagnosis and treatment. Furthermore, many cases of appendicitis and intussusception occur in younger patients, making the utility of ultrasound particularly advantageous to prevent unnecessary radiation. This chapter will review indications for performing an abdominal ultrasound, basic abdominal anatomy, image acquisition, normal ultrasound anatomy, and interpretation of pathology.

Clinical Application and Indications

- Acute abdominal pain with concern for appendicitis, bowel obstruction, ileus, and intussusception
- Unexplained shock or sepsis
- Evaluate for ascites
- Evaluate for free air in the abdomen

Supplementary Information The online version contains supplementary material available at https://doi.org/10.1007/978-3-032-27643-8_12.

A. Lindsay (✉) · M. J. Vitto
Department of Emergency Medicine, Virginia Commonwealth University Health, Richmond, VA, USA
e-mail: angela.creditt@vcuhealth.org; michael.vitto@vcuhealth.org

A. Lindsay et al. (eds.), *Clinical Ultrasound*,
https://doi.org/10.1007/978-3-032-27643-8_12

Normal Abdominal Anatomy

- Abdominal Wall
  - Abdominal wall layers include (from superficial to deep) the skin, subcutaneous tissue, superficial fascia, external oblique muscle, internal oblique muscle, transversus abdominis muscle, transversalis fascia, preperitoneal adipose, and, finally, the peritoneum [1].
    - Nerves, blood vessels, and lymphatics are present throughout each layer.
- Appendix
  - A blind-ended, tubular pouch, arising from the cecum, typically located in the right lower quadrant.
    - Position can be variable such as in pregnancy, displacing the appendix more laterally and superiorly.
- Small Bowel
  - Composed of the duodenum, jejunum, and ileum.
    - Jejunum is often located in the left upper quadrant (LUQ) and mid abdomen; ileum is located in the right mid to lower abdomen [2].
  - Tube-like structure that contains plicae circulares, often with peristalsis
  - Small bowel wall thickness is typically less than 2 mm [3].
- Large Bowel
  - Includes the cecum (and appendix), ascending, transverse, descending, and sigmoid colon, rectum, and anus.
    - Ascending colon courses in the right flank anterior to the kidney, transverse colon runs inferior to the stomach, and descending colon can be found in the left flank anterior to the kidney [2].
    - Sigmoid colon may be difficult to identify by ultrasound [2].
    - Rectum is visualized posterior to the uterus or prostate [2].
  - Contains longitudinal bands called taeniae coli and haustra.
  - Large bowel wall thickness is typically less than 2 mm [3].

Image Acquisition

(a) Transducer Selection
- Curvilinear
- Phased array
- Linear array transducer
  - Can be used on smaller or thinner patients, including pediatric patients, or when evaluating the appendix.

(b) Patient Position and Procedure
- The patient should be supine with the head of the bed flat and their knees flexed to allow abdominal muscles to relax.

(c) Standard Exam Views
- Appendix
  - Have the patient point to the site of maximal pain and begin with a low-frequency transducer at this site in a transverse plane with the marker pointed toward the patient's right.
    - Scan both inferior and superior and try to identify the appendix
    - Terminal ileum will cross over the psoas muscle where it connects with the cecum [2].
    - Appendix will typically be visualized anterior to the iliac vessels originating from the cecum.
    - The appendix is a compressible tubular structure with a blind end and an outer diameter measuring approximately 4 cm [2].
    - Rotate the transducer 90° with the marker pointed toward the patient's head to obtain views in a sagittal plane.
  - Alternatively, place the transducer at the hepatic flexure and trace the ascending colon down to the cecum.
  - Use graded compression by exerting gentle pressure over the areas of interest with the ultrasound transducer in effort to displace bowel gas to better visualize intra-abdominal structures.
  - A normal appendix will exhibit peristalsis and compressibility [4].
- Small and Large Bowel
  - Begin with the transducer in a transverse plane with the marker pointed toward the patient's right.
  - Scan through and obtain images from the patient's epigastrium, bilateral colic gutters, and suprapubic region. Oblique views may be needed to identify bowel in the appropriate plane.
  - Consider a "lawn mower" pattern path to ensure the bowel is fully examined [2].
  - Apply gentle downward pressure every few centimeters to assess for bowel compression.

Abdominal Pathology

(a) Appendicitis

- Inflammation of the appendix.
- Typically identified on ultrasound as an aperistaltic, noncompressible, blind-ended tubular structure with an outer diameter of greater than 6 mm [4].
  - Figure 12.1—Appendicitis
  - Video 12.1—Appendicitis
  - Figure 12.2—Appendicitis with measured diameter
- The following may also indicate acute appendicitis:
  - Target sign appearance

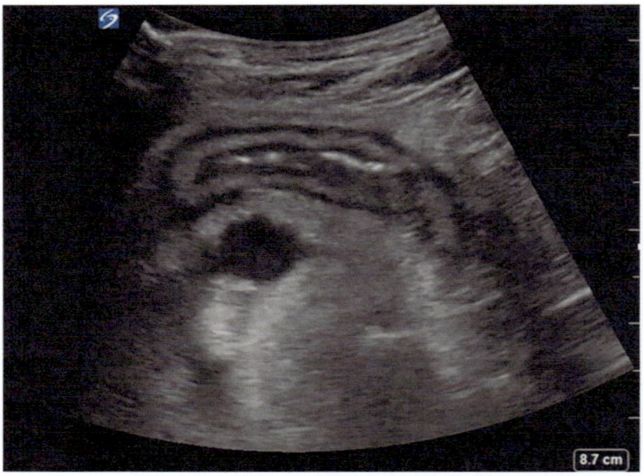

Fig. 12.1 Appendicitis. Acute appendicitis can be identified as an aperistaltic, noncompressible, blind-ended tubular structure

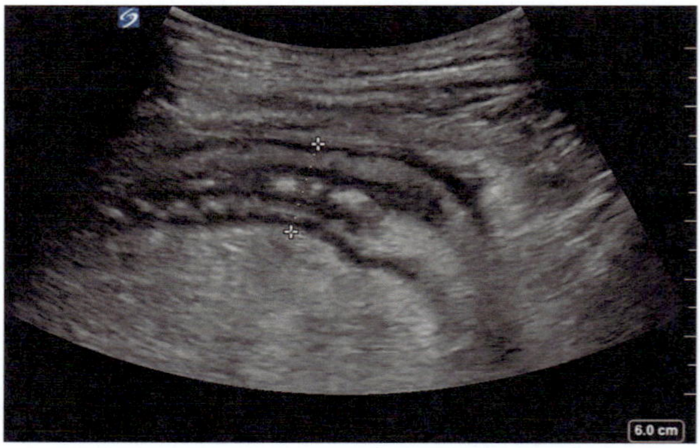

Fig. 12.2 Appendicitis. A diameter greater than 6 mm is indicative of acute appendicitis

    - Figure 12.3—Target sign
    - Video 12.2—Target sign
  - Appendicolith with posterior acoustic shadowing [5]
    - Figure 12.4—Appendicolith
    - Video 12.3—Appendicolith
  - Periappendiceal fluid collection [5]
    - Figure 12.5—Appendicitis with surrounding fluid
    - Video 12.4—Appendicitis with surrounding fluid
  - Wall thickness greater than 3 mm [6].
  - Increased periappendiceal echogenicity due to fat stranding [7].
  - Color Doppler can be used to demonstrate increased vascularity in the setting of acute appendicitis, often termed "ring of fire" [4].
- Perforation may be identified by a fluid collection, hypoechoic mass, or thickening of adjacent bowel wall; complex abscess fluid collections may also be present.

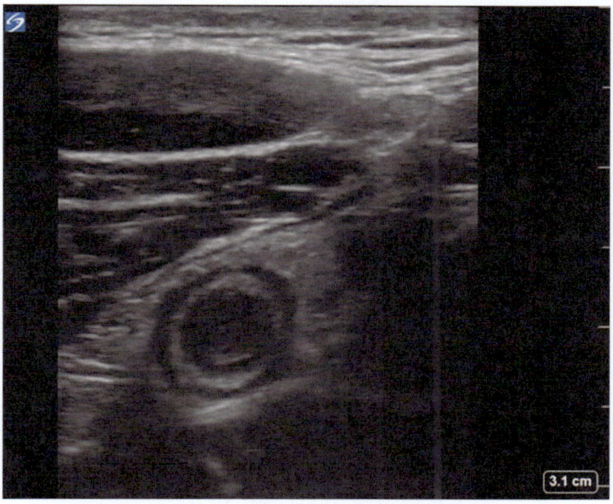

Fig. 12.3 Target sign. In short axis, acute appendicitis will often look similar to a target thereby earning the classic finding of "target sign"

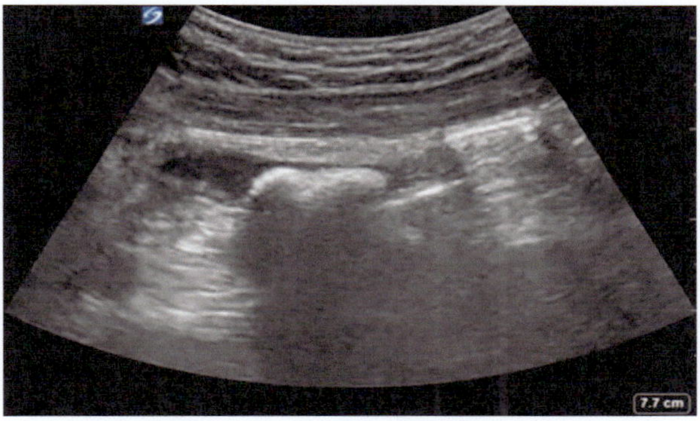

Fig. 12.4 Appendicolith. Within the inflamed appendix may be a fecalith, which is visualized as a hyperechoic rounded structure with posterior acoustic shadowing

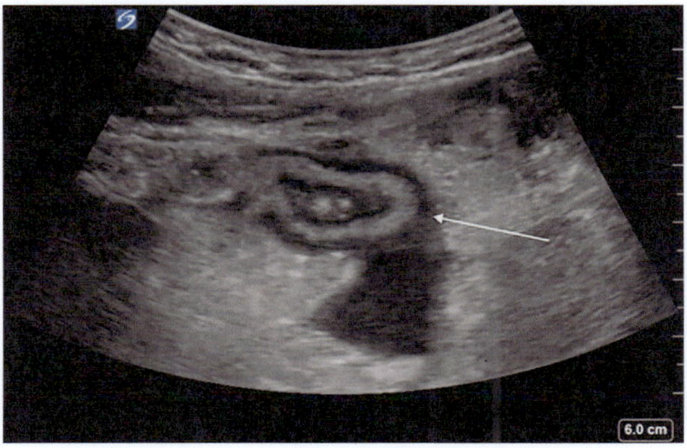

Fig. 12.5 Appendicitis. Another ultrasonographic finding of acute appendicitis is periappendiceal fluid (arrow)

(b) Small Bowel Obstruction
- Mechanical blockage of food and liquid passing through the small intestine. As material accumulates in the lumen of the small bowel, it will become distended, and the wall may thicken due to edema [2]
- Look for dilated, noncompressible small bowel proximal to a collapsed, compressible bowel.
  - Small bowel will be greater than 2.5 cm in diameter, but more often greater than 3.0 cm [2].
- Typically, there will be fluid and echogenic material within the lumen of the bowel moving to-and-fro in a whirling pattern.
  - Figure 12.6—Small bowel obstruction
  - Video 12.5—Small bowel obstruction
- Piano key or keyboard sign can be seen due to prominent plicae circulares silhouetted against small bowel contents.
  - Figure 12.7—Keyboard sign
  - Video 12.6—Keyboard sign
  - "Tanga sign", a triangular pocket of free intraperitoneal fluid between dilated loops of fluid-filled small bowel, may also be seen [8].

(c) Large Bowel Obstruction
- Mechanical blockage of stool passing through the large intestine.
- Dilated colon proximal to the obstruction, typically seen in the periphery of the abdomen, often filled with dense spot echoes [2].
- A dilated colon will often cause the haustra to become more widely spaced [2].

(d) Intussusception
- Telescoping of one section of bowel into another, usually at the ileocecal junction

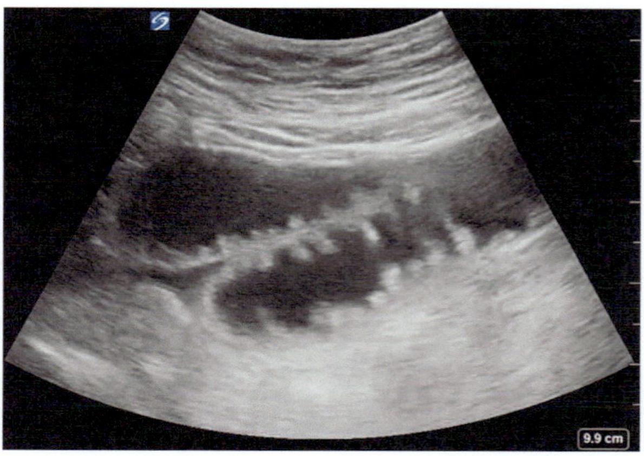

Fig. 12.6 Small bowel obstruction. Small bowel obstruction can be identified by dilated, noncompressible small bowel that is greater than 2.5 cm in diameter. There will typically be echogenic material within the lumen of the bowel exhibits and to-and-fro whirling pattern

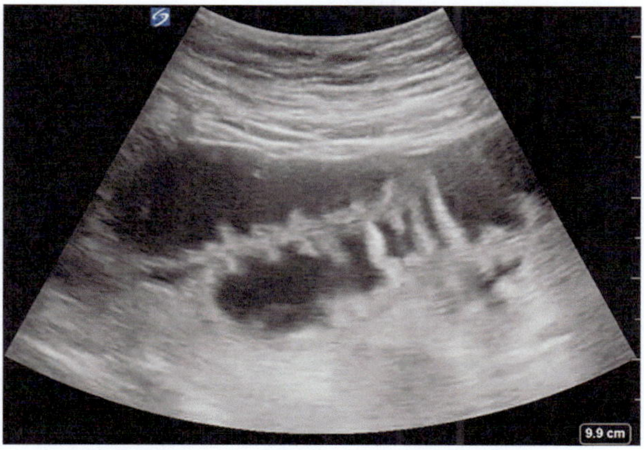

Fig. 12.7 Keyboard sign. Keyboard sign can be seen with small bowel obstruction due to prominent plicae circulares, representing piano keys, silhouetted against small bowel contents

    - Common cause of obstruction in children, but it is rare in adults
    - Causative lesion can be identified in more than 80% of adults, most commonly a polypoid tumor of the small bowel [2].
  - In a transverse plane, there will be concentric alternating hypoechoic and hyperechoic rings representing layers of bowel with adjacent free fluid and inner fecal matter [4] known as "doughnut" or "target sign."
    - Figure 12.8—Intussusception
    - In a longitudinal view, intussusception may appear as "pseudo-kidney sign" [8]

(e) Ascites
  - Free intraperitoneal fluid caused by varying pathology, most commonly due to cirrhosis.
  - Simple fluid collects in dependent portions of the abdomen
    - Figure 12.9—Ascites
    - Video 12.7—Ascites
  - Free fluid is often first identified in the right paracolic gutter or right upper quadrant of the abdomen.
  - See Chap. 18 for procedural guidance on obtaining a sample of peritoneal fluid.

(f) Pneumoperitoneum and Perforated Viscus
  - Free intraperitoneal air, often accompanied by free fluid, is usually due to a perforated viscus [2].
  - It is easiest to detect pneumoperitoneum in the right upper quadrant [9] over the ventral surface of the liver.
  - Free air will appear as a sharp echogenic line (accentuation of the peritoneal stripe) [3] with posterior reverberation artifacts [9].
  - Reverberation artifacts can also be seen throughout the abdomen in areas where air has collected.
    - Figure 12.10—Free intraperitoneal air
    - Video 12.8—Free intraperitoneal air

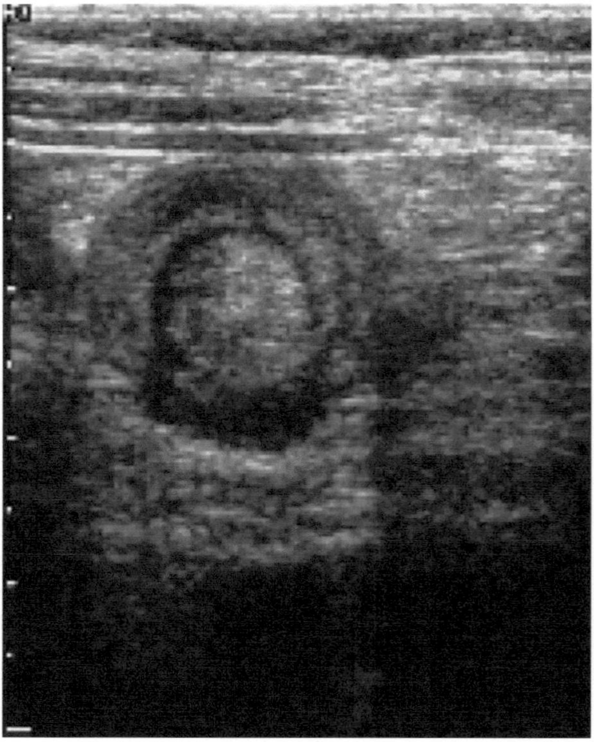

Fig. 12.8 Intussusception. Intussusception is characterized by telescoping of one section of bowel into another. In a transverse plane, there will be concentric alternating hypoechoic and hyperechoic rings representing layers of bowel with adjacent free fluid and inner fecal matter

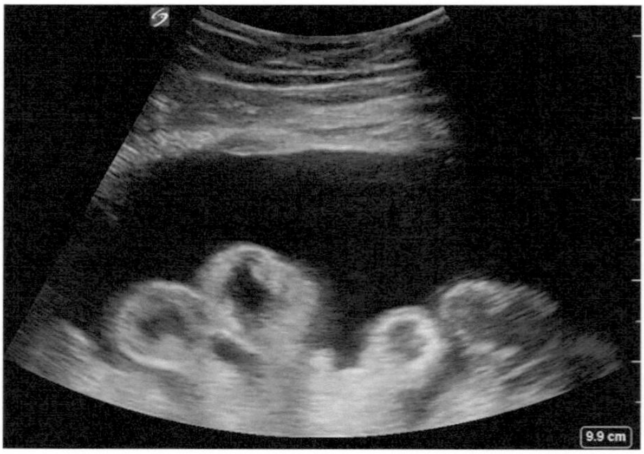

Fig. 12.9 Ascites. Ascites is identified by anechoic free intraperitoneal fluid within the abdomen often appearing as if the bowel is floating within the fluid

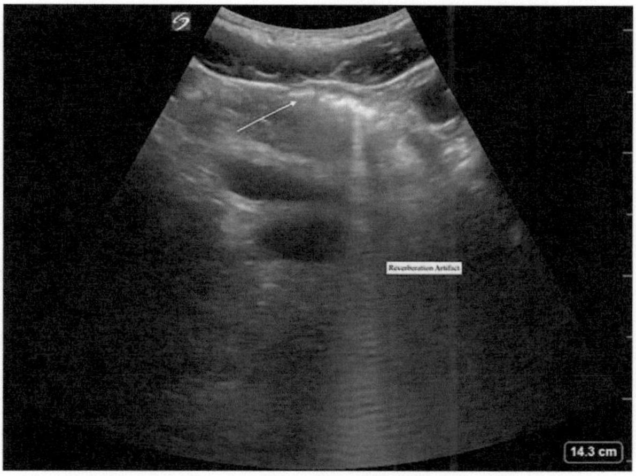

Fig. 12.10 Free intraperitoneal air. Free intraperitoneal air will appear as an echogenic line (arrow) with reverberation artifact as seen in this image of a patient with perforated gastric ulcer

- B-lines and dirty air shadowing may be present.
- Free air and fluid may be identified adjacent to loops of bowel as free fluid with internal grey echoes [2]. This combination may also be seen in the dependent areas of the abdomen, such as the pelvis.
- Fluid contains echogenic spots representing feculent or purulent fluid [2].

Key Points

- When scanning the abdomen, use an organized approach to ensure you scan each area. Visualize the abdomen as a lawn and pass over each area like you would with a lawn mower. Limitations in abdominal bedside ultrasound occur in patients who are morbidly obese, pregnant, or who have a significant amount of bowel gas. Artifact or distortion of typical landmarks may create difficulty in obtaining optimal images.
- A normal appendix is seen less than 15% of the time [4] due to its small size and non-inflamed pathology.
  - Inability to visualize a normal appendix does not rule out the presence of appendicitis.
- Bowel wall thickening greater than 4 mm can be suggestive of colitis [4].
  - Figure 12.11—Thickened bowel wall
  - Video 12.9—Thickened bowel wall

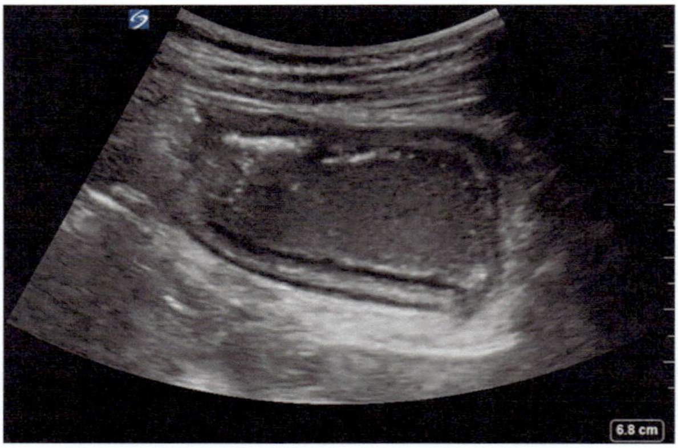

Fig. 12.11 Thickened bowel wall. Bowel wall thickening greater than 4 mm is suggestive of colitis, as seen in this image of a patient with pancolitis

References

1. Gray JE, Mizell JS. Anatomy of the abdominal wall. UpToDate website. https://www.uptodate.com/contents/anatomy-of-the-abdominal-wall. Updated November 5, 2015. Accessed 17 Apr 2017.
2. Oakley E, Jang T, Ma O. Gastrointestinal and abdominal wall. In: Ma O, Mateer JR, Reardon RF, Byars DV, Knapp BJ, Laudenbach AP, editors. Ma and Mateer's emergency ultrasound, 4e. McGraw-Hill Education; 2021. https://accessemergencymedicine.mhmedical.com/content.aspx?bookid=2966&sectionid=249993246. Accessed 26 Mar 2024.
3. Gilja OH, Nylund K. Point-of-care ultrasound of the gastrointestinal tract. J Med Ultrasound. 2023;31(1):1–7. https://doi.org/10.4103/jmu.jmu_5_23.
4. SonoSim Ultrasound Training Solution [Video]. Santa Monica: SonoSim Inc.; 2017.
5. Chao A, Gharahbaghian L. Tips and tricks: ultrasound in the diagnosis of acute appendicitis. American College of Emergency Physicians; 2015. Website. https://www.acep.org/Content.aspx?id=101803. Accessed 15 Apr 2017.
6. Paspulati RM. Chapter 23: Ultrasonography of bowel disorders. In: Dogra V, Rubens D, editors. Ultrasound secrets. Philadelphia: Elsevier Health Sciences; 2004. p. 207–11.
7. Old JL, Dusing RW, Yap W, Dirks J. Imaging for suspected appendicitis. Am Fam Phys. 2005;71(1):71–8. http://www.aafp.org/afp/2005/0101/p71.html. Accessed 15 Apr 2017
8. Li JJ, Boivin Z, Bhalodkar S, Liu R. Point of care abdominal ultrasound. Semin Ultrasound CT MR. 2024;45(1):11–21. https://doi.org/10.1053/j.sult.2023.12.003.
9. Hefny AF, Abu-Zidan FM. Sonographic diagnosis of intraperitoneal free air. J Emerg Trauma Shock. 2011;4(4):511–3. https://www.ncbi.nlm.nih.gov/pmc/articles/PMC3214511/. Accessed 17 Apr 2016.

Gynecologic Ultrasound

13

Jordan Tozer, Angela Lindsay, and Michael J. Vitto

In outpatient clinics and, more specifically, within the emergency department, women frequently present for evaluation of pelvic complaints. Fortunately, with increasing knowledge and the advancement of ultrasound, a more thorough assessment can be completed without exposing patients to unnecessary radiation. Transvaginal ultrasound allows providers to obtain valuable information about pelvic organs to aid in the diagnostic discovery of a patient's complaint such as acute pelvic pain or abnormal vaginal bleeding. To this point, in most cases, gynecologic problems are best imaged using ultrasound. This chapter will focus on performing a gynecologic ultrasound, basic pelvic anatomy, image acquisition using a transvaginal approach, and interpretation of pathology.

Clinical Application and Indications

- Lower abdominal or pelvic pain in a female
- Evaluate for ovarian cyst, ovarian torsion, or tubo-ovarian abscess
- Evaluate for uterine pathology such as fibroids and intrauterine device location

Supplementary Information The online version contains supplementary material available at https://doi.org/10.1007/978-3-032-27643-8_13.

J. Tozer · A. Lindsay (✉) · M. J. Vitto
Department of Emergency Medicine, Virginia Commonwealth University Health, Richmond, VA, USA
e-mail: jordan.tozer@vcuhealth.org; Angela.creditt@vcuhealth.org; Michael.vitto@vcuhealth.org

A. Lindsay et al. (eds.), *Clinical Ultrasound*,
https://doi.org/10.1007/978-3-032-27643-8_13

Normal Gynecologic Anatomy

- The uterus and paired ovaries are centrally located in the pelvis between the more anterior bladder and more posterior rectum.
- The uterus is a muscular organ comprised of outer myometrium and inner endometrium.
  - It is typically anteverted, meaning the fundus or superior most part of the uterus points anteriorly above the bladder.
  - Alternatively, the uterus can be retroverted, meaning the fundus points posteriorly away from the bladder.
  - The endometrium varies in thickness in a cyclical fashion that mirrors the menstrual cycle, sloughing off at each menstruation before developing again in anticipation of embryo implantation.
  - In women of reproductive age, the average uterus will measure 7 cm × 4 cm × 5 cm [1].
- The adnexa are bilateral structures that include the ovaries, fallopian tubes, and ligaments.
  - Each ovary is ovoid in shape.
  - Ovarian size is variable based on patient age and timing of the reproductive cycle.
    - Ovarian size is typically measured by volume with a calculated formula of length × width × height × 0.523 [2].
    - Normal ovarian volume in premenopausal women is less than 20 cm [3] and less than 10 cm [3] in postmenopausal women [2].
  - Ovarian location can vary from patient to patient due to the free-floating nature of their connection to the uterus.
  - The paired fallopian tubes project from the more fundal and lateral portion of the uterus and end in fingerlike fimbria that lie adjacent to the ovary.

Image Acquisition

(a) Transducer Selection

- Endocavitary transducer, also known as transvaginal transducer
  - By convention, the "marker dot" rests on top of the transducer, and the "trigger" of the transducer therefore points away from the marker dot.
    - Figure 13.1—Endocavitary transducer
    - Figure 13.2—Transducer position for sagittal images
    - Figure 13.3—Transducer position for coronal images
- Curvilinear transducers can also be used for transabdominal imaging; however, transvaginal ultrasound provides better image resolution, quality, and therefore diagnostic capability.

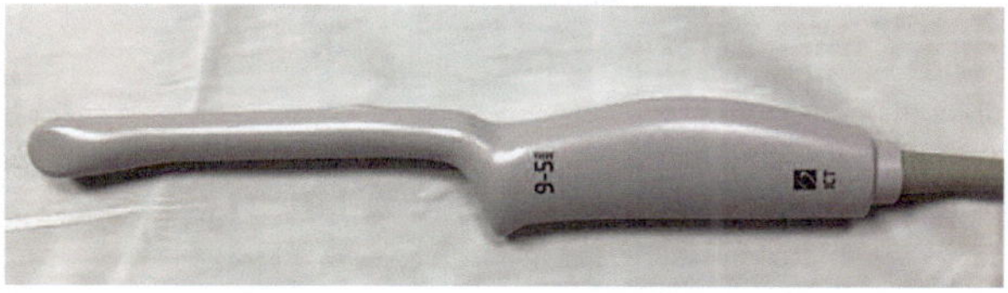

Fig. 13.1 Endocavitary transducer also known as transvaginal transducer

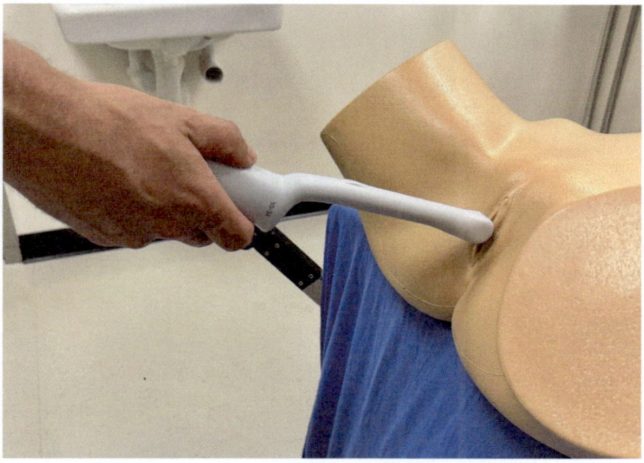

Fig. 13.2 Transducer position for sagittal images. To obtain sagittal views of the uterus, the "trigger" or transducer marker should be pointed toward the floor

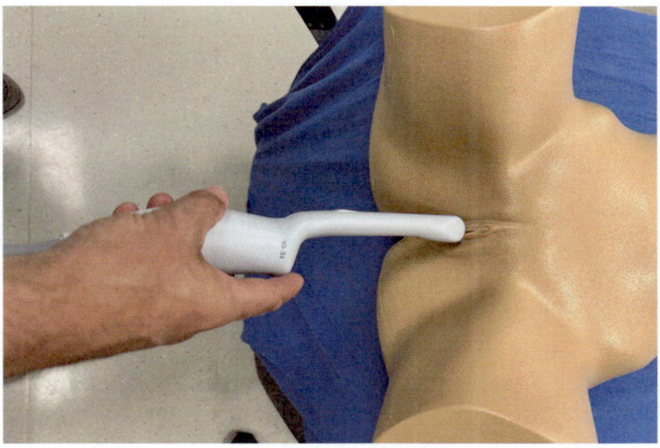

Fig. 13.3 Transducer position for transverse images. To obtain transverse views of the uterus and ovaries, the "trigger" or transducer marker is pointed toward the patient's left

(b) Patient Position

- For a transvaginal approach, patients should be placed in the lithotomy position, ideally on a pelvic-specific stretcher with footrests.
- The patient should be covered during all portions of the procedure, except during transducer insertion when direct visualization is required.
- Ensure the patient has an empty bladder; a full bladder can cause discomfort as well as distort the anatomy and make visualizing the ovaries more difficult.

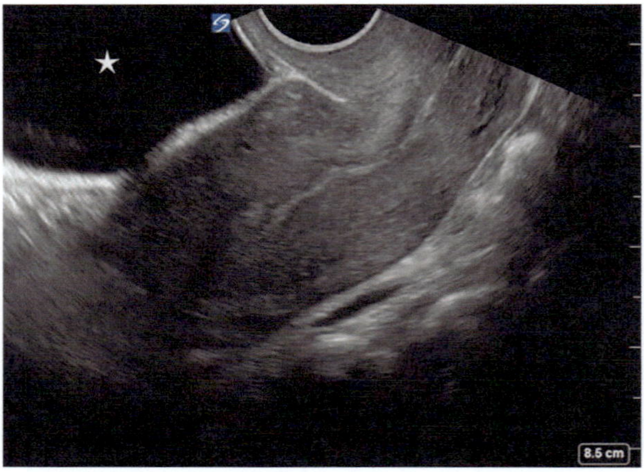

Fig. 13.4 Bladder in sagittal view. In a sagittal plane using an endovaginal approach, the bladder (star) will be seen anterior to the uterus or on the left of the image. The uterine stripe is seen traversing the center of the uterus

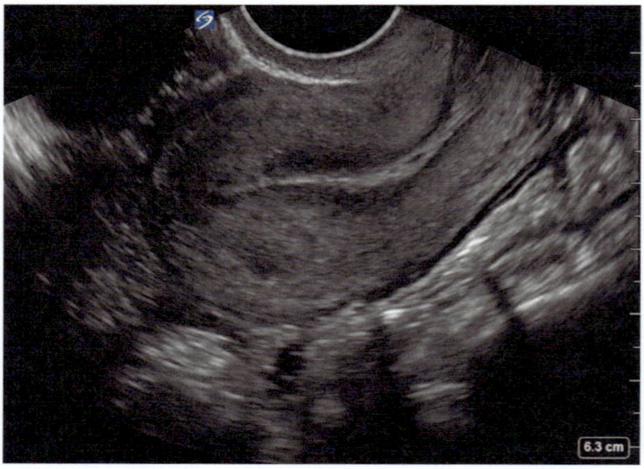

Fig. 13.5 Long axis of uterus. The uterus is imaged in a sagittal plane from cervix (on the right of the image) to fundus (left of the image) with the echogenic uterine stripe in the midline

(c) Standard Exam Views
- Sagittal view
  - Insert the transducer into the vagina with the trigger pointed toward the floor and the transducer footprint in a vertical orientation.
  - In this view, the bladder will be seen on the left side of the image and can be visualized more completely by lowering the scanning hand to point the transducer head toward the ceiling.
    - Figure 13.4—Bladder in sagittal view
  - The uterus lies in the mid position and should be fully evaluated by fanning from the patient's right to left.
  - Identify the long axis of the uterus by finding the endometrial stripe, a hyperechoic line within the uterus, extending from the fundus to the cervix.
    - Figure 13.5—Long axis of uterus
    - Video 13.1—Long axis of uterus

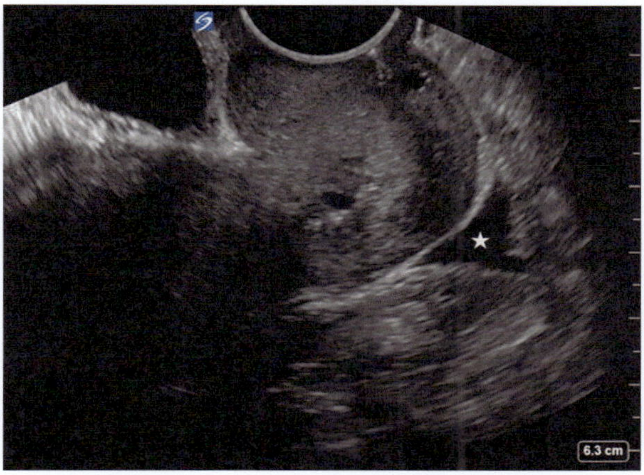

Fig. 13.6 Pouch of Douglas. Posterior to the uterus and anterior to the rectum is the posterior cul-de-sac or pouch of Douglas. A small amount of free fluid is visualized here within the pouch of Douglas (star), which can be normal in reproductive-aged females

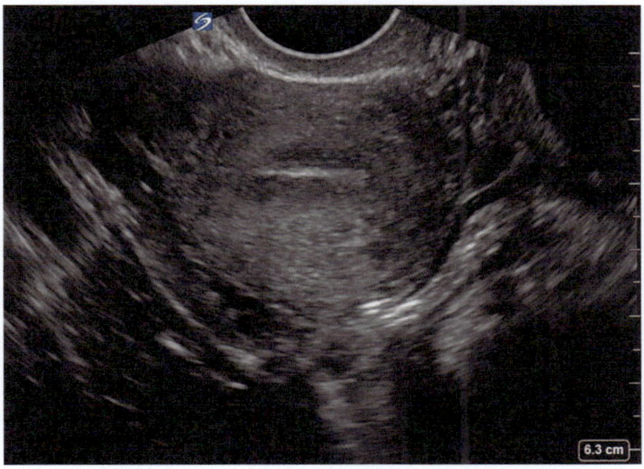

Fig. 13.7 Uterus in transverse. In a transverse plane, the uterus is seen in short axis with the echogenic uterine stripe visualized as a small horizontal line within the center of the uterus

  - Posterior cul-de-sac, also known as rectouterine pouch or pouch of Douglas, can be seen by raising the scanning hand anteriorly to point the transducer head toward the floor.
    - Figure 13.6—Pouch of Douglas
    - Video 13.2—Pouch of Douglas
- Transverse View
  - Return to a midline sagittal view centered on the endometrial stripe and rotate the transducer 90° counterclockwise, so that the transducer trigger is pointed toward the patient's left.
    - Figure 13.7—Uterus in transverse
    - Video 13.3—Uterus in transverse
  - View the uterus completely by fanning the transducer anterior to posterior
    - Lowering the scanning hand will image toward the fundus.
    - Raising the scanning hand will image toward the cervix.

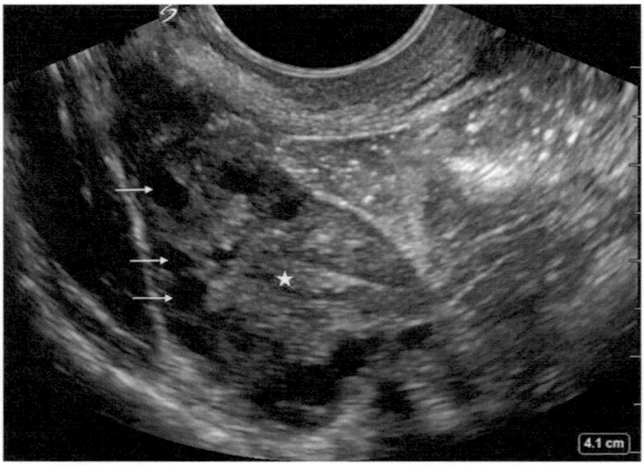

Fig. 13.8 Normal ovary. Multiple small cysts (arrows) in the cortex surround the medulla (star) in this normal ovary, giving the appearance of what is often referred to as a "chocolate chip cookie"

- Adnexa should be imaged initially in the transverse plane by directing the transducer toward the adnexa in question.
  - Moving the scanning hand toward the patient's left will move the transducer head toward the patient's right, and therefore image the right adnexa and vice versa.
- Once the transducer head is directed toward the adnexa of choice, fan the transducer up and down to search for the ovaries, adjusting the depth and gain as necessary.
- Ovaries are hyperechoic structures with hypoechoic follicles that are located lateral to the uterus and medial and anterior to the iliac vessels, often said to have a "chocolate chip cookie" appearance.
- Ovarian position can be variable however, and they can be difficult to locate on some patients.
  - Figure 13.8—Normal ovary
  - Video 13.4—Normal ovary
- Fallopian tubes may not be easily visualized in a healthy patient

Gynecologic Pathology

- Simple Cyst
  - A simple ovarian cyst is a collection of fluid surrounded by a membrane within or on the surface of an ovary.
  - Simple cysts are anechoic with smooth walls, posterior acoustic enhancement, and no internal echoes.
    - Referred to as a physiologic cyst when the diameter measures less than 2.5 cm and a follicular cyst when it is greater than 2.5 cm [1].
    - Figure 13.9—Simple physiologic cyst
    - Figure 13.10—Simple follicular ovarian cyst
    - Video 13.5—Simple ovarian cysts

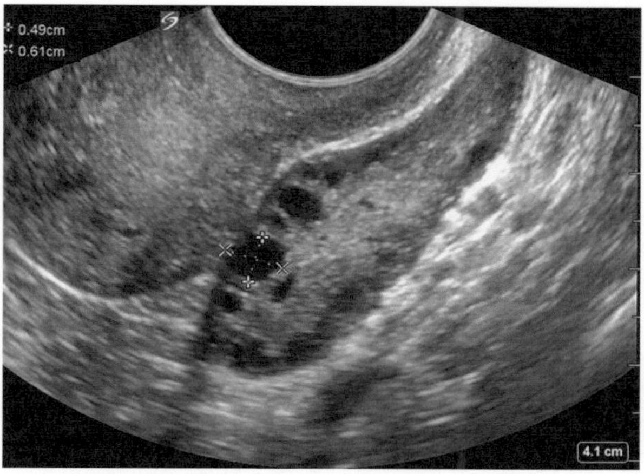

Fig. 13.9 Simple physiologic ovarian cyst. When the diameter of a simple ovarian cyst measures less than 2.5 cm, it is referred to as a physiologic cyst

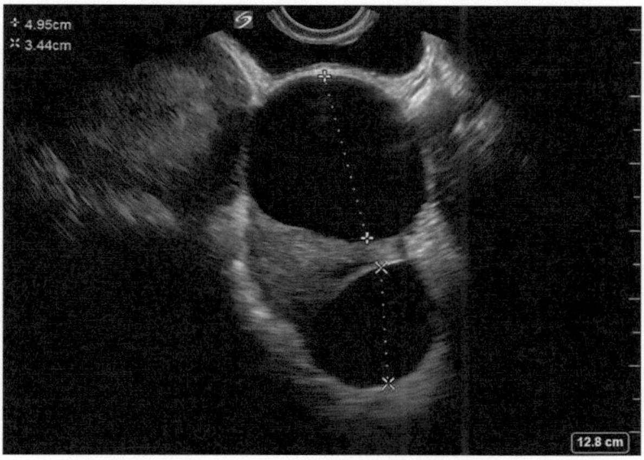

Fig. 13.10 Simple ovarian cyst. When the diameter of a simple ovarian cyst measures greater than 2.5 cm, it is referred to as a simple follicular cyst

- Polycystic Ovarian Syndrome
  - Syndrome that occurs due to imbalance of reproductive hormones with a multifactorial etiology.
  - Will appear as multiple small, usually less than one centimeter, simple cysts along the periphery of the ovary, sometimes referred to as "beads on a string" [1].
    - Figure 13.11—Polycystic ovarian syndrome
- Complex Cyst
  - A complex ovarian cyst contains both fluid and solid components, often with mixed echogenicity within the cyst itself.
    - Figure 13.12—Complex ovarian cyst
    - Video 13.6—Complex ovarian cyst

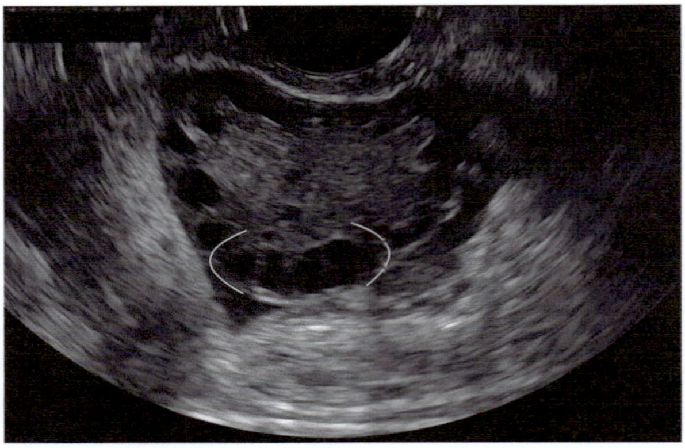

Fig. 13.11 Polycystic ovarian syndrome. Polycystic ovarian syndrome often appears as "beads on a string" (between parentheses) with multiple small simple cysts lining the periphery of the ovary

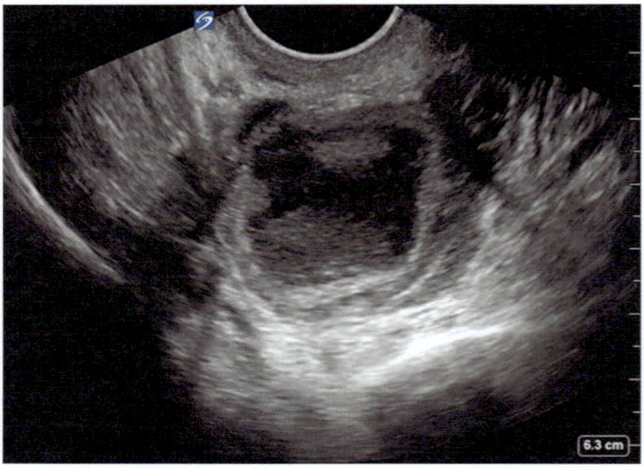

Fig. 13.12 Complex ovarian cyst. Complex ovarian cysts will have varying echogenicities within the cyst itself, often representing hemorrhage or other complex fluid

- Complex cysts can be benign or malignant
  - Benign complex cysts include hemorrhagic, endometriomas, and dermoid cysts.
  - Complex cyst can also represent a tubo-ovarian abscess (TOA) in the right clinical setting.
  - It is not always possible to determine the cause of complex cysts with ultrasound alone.
- Hemorrhagic cysts contain hyperechoic internal echoes. They also may contain fluid levels, exhibit a fishnet appearance, or appear as a clot.

- Ovarian Torsion
  - Occurs when the ovary rotates around its pedicle causing occlusion of the blood supply to the ovary.
  - Large ovarian cysts are the most common risk factor for torsion, with cysts greater than 5 cm and larger being classically associated with this condition [3].

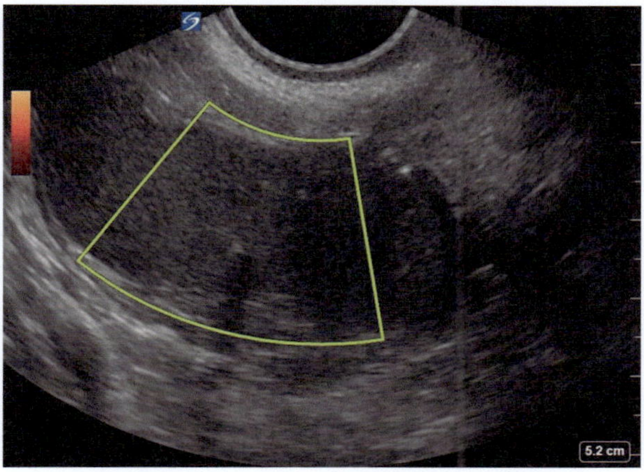

Fig. 13.13 Ovarian torsion. Note the enlarged ovary with loss of architecture and absence of color flow with power Doppler (orange color bar) in this image of ovarian torsion

- An ovary with prolonged torsion is typically enlarged [1] and heterogeneous due to edema.
  - Figure 13.13—Ovarian torsion
  - Video 13.7—Ovarian torsion
- A torsed ovary may demonstrate both hyperechoic and hypoechoic areas if hemorrhage and necrosis are present [3].
- Peripherally arranged follicles can be present [1, 3–5].
- Free fluid is often found within the pouch of Douglas or around the ovary [5]
- Evaluate the ovary for blood flow using color Doppler.
  - Venous occlusion will occur first, prior to arterial occlusion; therefore. the presence of flow using color Doppler does not rule out ovarian torsion
  - Complete absence of blood flow is typically a late finding
  - Compare flow to the contralateral side to evaluate for decreased flow of the ovary in question.
  - Figure 13.14—Ovary with color Doppler.
  - Figure 13.15—Ovarian torsion with color Doppler.
  - Video 13.8—Ovary with color Doppler.
  - Video 13.9—Ovarian torsion with color Doppler.
- Evaluate the ovary for blood flow using power Doppler, and adjust the color gain to the appropriate sensitivity to detect a small amount of flow
  - Figure 13.16—Ovary with power Doppler
- Finally, apply spectral Doppler to the vessels that were identified with color or power Doppler to evaluate the arterial waveform
- Ovarian lesions with irregular walls, nodules, solid echogenic elements, or thick septations are concerning for malignancy.
- Diagnosis of ovarian torsion is difficult, and it is important to remember that the ovaries receive dual blood supply so you can detect blood flow via color Doppler in a torsed ovary.
- The presence of arterial flow, venous flow, or both does not rule out ovarian torsion.

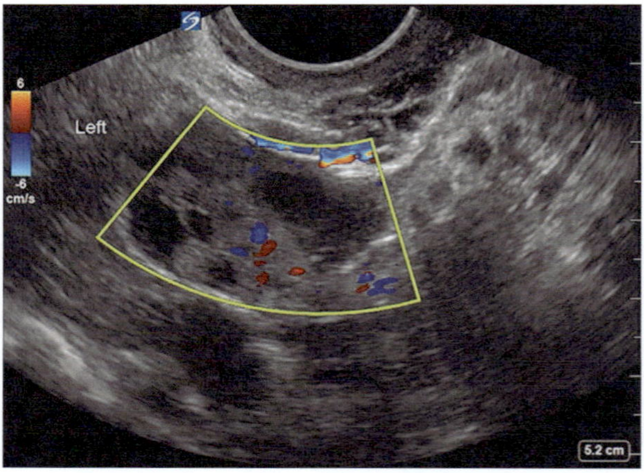

Fig. 13.14 Ovary with color Doppler. Normal appearing ovary with normal flow on color Doppler

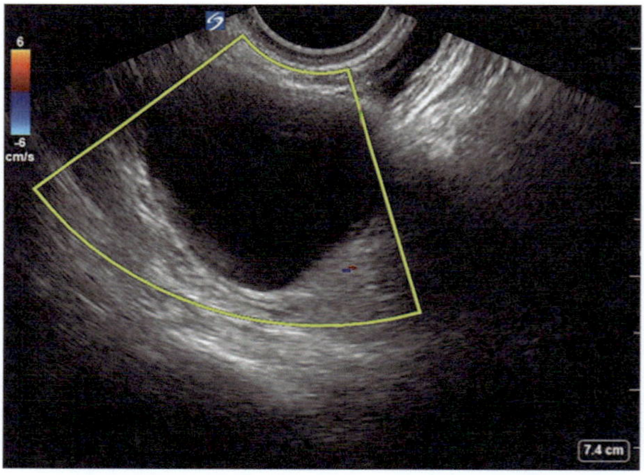

Fig. 13.15 Ovarian Torsion with color Doppler. Large ovarian cyst with reduced flow using color Doppler. In ovarian torsion, blood flow may be reduced or in advanced cases completely absent. Importantly, the presence of flow using color Doppler does not rule out ovarian torsion

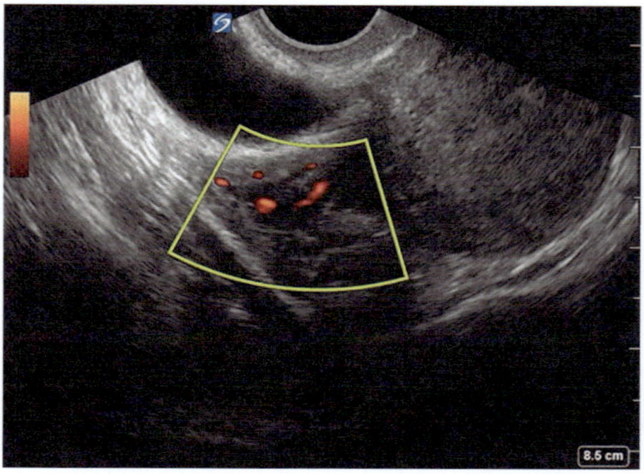

Fig. 13.16 Ovary with power Doppler. Power Doppler is the preferred method for evaluating ovarian flow because it is more sensitive to low-flow states

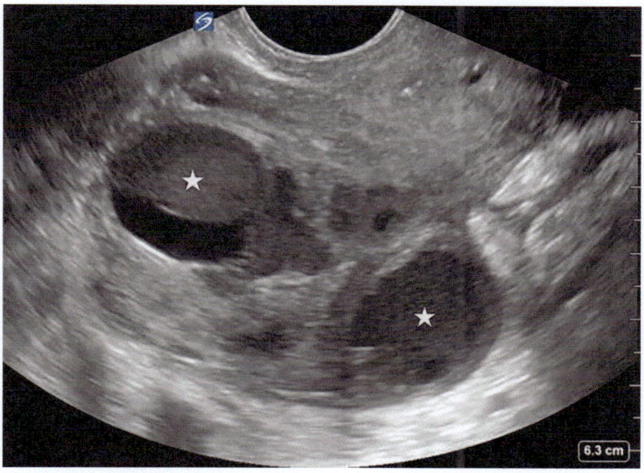

Fig. 13.17 TOA. A tubo-ovarian abscess (star) will appear as a peri-uterine or adnexal mass containing complex fluid

- Tubo-Ovarian Abscess
  - Consider TOA in a nonpregnant female with clinical signs or symptoms of pelvic inflammatory disease and a complex adnexal mass found on ultrasound [6].
  - TOA will appear as a peri-uterine or adnexal mass with echogenic fluid within the pelvis.
    - Figure 13.17—TOA
    - Video 13.10—TOA
  - "Cogwheel sign" may also be visualized on cross-sectional imaging, which appears due to prominent folds within the fallopian tube projecting inward with central anechoic fluid [7].
- Confirmation of Intrauterine Device Placement
  - Obtain a sagittal and transverse view of the uterus.
  - Evaluate for a highly echogenic structure within the endometrium, which will typically have posterior acoustic shadowing.
    - Figure 13.18—IUD
    - Video 13.11—IUD Placement
  - If unable to identify an IUD in the correct place, consider displacement of the device or device migration causing perforation of the uterus.
- Uterine Fibroids
  - Abnormal growth of the myometrium causing a benign smooth muscle tumor
  - Visualized as hyperechoic, hypoechoic, or isoechoic masses within the myometrium [1].
  - Figure 13.19—Uterine fibroid
  - Video 13.12—Uterine fibroid
  - Figure 13.20—Uterine fibroid

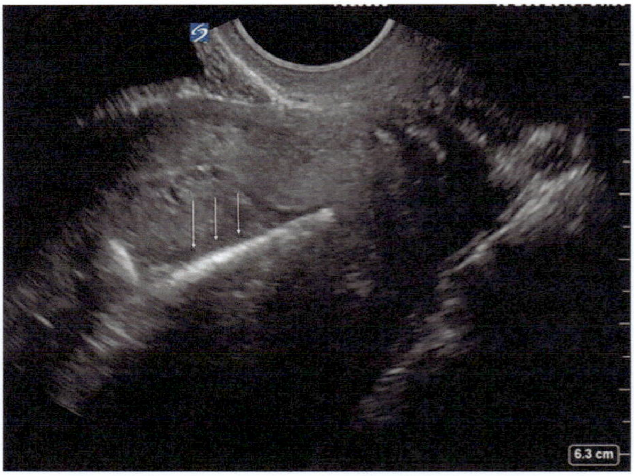

Fig. 13.18 IUD. An IUD will appear as a brightly echogenic structure (arrows) with posterior acoustic shadowing

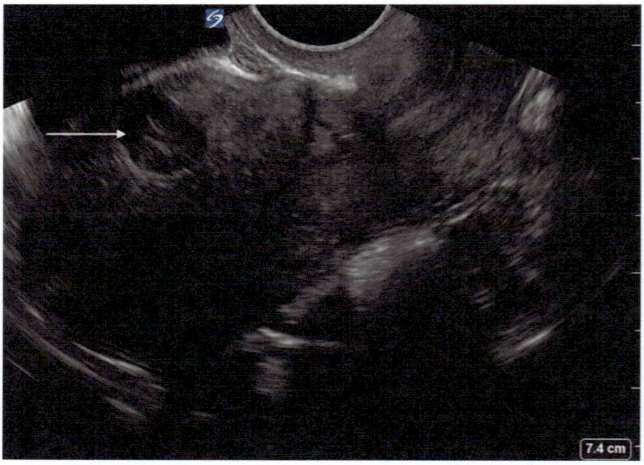

Fig. 13.19 Uterine fibroid. Small uterine fibroid located in myometrium (arrow). Fibroids can have varying size, shape, echogenicity, and number but almost uniformly represented as benign smooth muscle tumors within the myometrium

Key Points

- Transvaginal ultrasound can be confusing as orientation quickly changes with slight movements of the transducer. If orientation is lost, return to the midline sagittal view (trigger down), then readjust to obtain an image of the uterine stripe at midline.
- Make sure that depth is set correctly to include the entirety of the uterine fundus.
- Ovaries can be difficult to find and may not be located in similar positions on each side of the same patient.
- The presence of blood flow in an ovary does not rule out ovarian torsion.

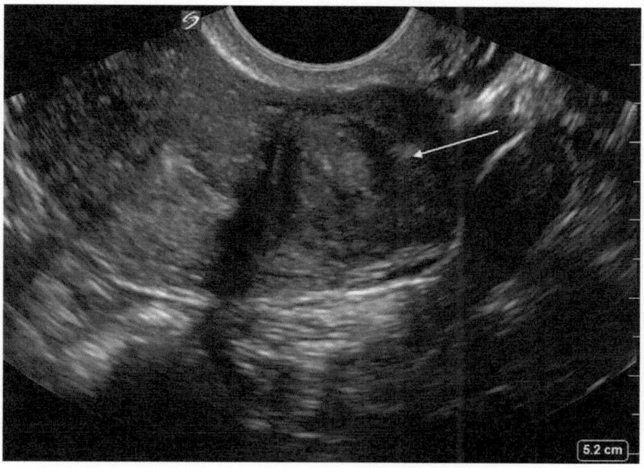

Fig. 13.20 Uterine fibroid. Large uterine fibroid (arrow) appears similar to the uterine architecture representing the varying appearance of fibroids

References

1. Fox JC, Lambert MJ. Chapter 16: Gynecologic concepts. In: Ma OJ, Mateer JR, Reardon RF, Joing SA, editors. Emergency ultrasound. 3rd ed. New York: McGraw-Hill Education; 2014. p. 455–78.
2. Pavlik EJ, DePriest PD, Gallion HH, Ueland FR, Reedy MB, Kryscio RJ, van Nagell Jr JR. Ovarian volume related to age. Gynecol Oncol. 2000;77(3):410–2. http://www.sciencedirect.com/science/article/pii/S0090825800957834?via%3Dihub. Accessed 23 Apr 2017
3. Damigos E, Johns J, Ross J. An update on the diagnosis and management of ovarian torsion. Obstet Gynaecol. 2012;14(4):229–36. http://onlinelibrary.wiley.com/doi/10.1111/j.1744-4667.2012.00131.x/pdf. Accessed 18 Apr 2017
4. Chang HC, Bhatt S, Dogra VS. Pearls and pitfalls in diagnosis of ovarian torsion. RadioGraphics. 2008;28(5):1355–68. http://pubs.rsna.org/doi/pdf/10.1148/rg.285075130. Accessed 18 Apr 2017
5. Mashiach R, Melamed N, Gilad N, Ben-Shitrit G, Meizner I. Sonographic diagnosis of ovarian torsion, accuracy and predictive factors. Am Inst Ultrasound Med. 2011;30:1205–10. http://edus.ucsf.edu/sites/edus.ucsf.edu/files/wysiwyg/1205.full.pdf. Accessed 18 Apr 2017
6. Adhikari S, Blaivas M, Lyon M. Role of bedside transvaginal ultrasound in the diagnosis of tuboovarian abscess in the emergency department. J Emerg Med. 2008;34:4429–33. http://www.sciencedirect.com/science/article/pii/S0736467907007627. Accessed 18 Apr 2017
7. Lambert MJ, Villa M. Gynecologic ultrasound in emergency medicine. Emerg Med Clin North Am. 2004;22(3):683–96. http://www.sciencedirect.com/science/article/pii/S073386270400046X. Accessed 18 Apr 2017

Obstetric Ultrasound

14

Jordan Tozer and Angela Lindsay

There are many pathologic conditions that can affect the pregnant patient, some more concerning than others. Perhaps the most severe is ectopic pregnancy due to its associated morbidity and mortality if undiagnosed. Ultrasound is the standard imaging modality for the diagnosis of intrauterine pregnancy and evaluation of pregnancy-related complaints. A novice sonographer will need to understand how to accurately identify intrauterine pregnancy, determine gestational age and heart rate using specified measurements, and diagnose ectopic pregnancy. This chapter will focus on performing an obstetric ultrasound, basic pelvic anatomy, image acquisition using transvaginal and transabdominal techniques, and interpretation of pathology.

Clinical Application and Indications

- Evaluate for intrauterine pregnancy.
- Evaluate for the cause of vaginal bleeding, abdominopelvic pain, syncope, or shock in the setting of pregnancy.

Supplementary Information The online version contains supplementary material available at https://doi.org/10.1007/978-3-032-27643-8_14.

J. Tozer · A. Lindsay (✉)
Department of Emergency Medicine, Virginia Commonwealth University Health, Richmond, VA, USA
e-mail: jordan.tozer@vcuhealth.org; Angela.creditt@vcuhealth.org

A. Lindsay et al. (eds.), *Clinical Ultrasound*,
https://doi.org/10.1007/978-3-032-27643-8_14

Normal Gynecologic Anatomy

- The uterus and paired ovaries are centrally located in the pelvis between the more anterior bladder and posterior rectum.
- The uterus is a muscular organ comprised of outer myometrium and inner endometrium:
  - It is typically anteverted, meaning the fundus or most superior part of the uterus points anteriorly above the bladder.
  - Less commonly, the uterus can be retroverted, meaning the fundus points posteriorly away from the bladder.
  - The endometrium varies in thickness in a cyclical fashion that mirrors the menstrual cycle, sloughing off at each menstruation before developing again in anticipation of embryo implantation.
- The adnexa are bilateral structures that include the ovaries, fallopian tubes, and ligaments.
  - Each ovary is ovoid in shape.
  - Ovarian size is typically measured by volume with a calculated formula of length × width × height × 0.523 [1].
    - In premenopausal women, the normal ovarian volume is less than 20 cm [2] and less than 10 cm [2] in postmenopausal women [1].
  - The paired fallopian tubes project from the more fundal and lateral portion of the uterus and end in fingerlike fimbria that lie adjacent to the ovary.

Image Acquisition

(a) Transducer Selection
- Curvilinear transducer.
  - Can be used later in the first trimester of pregnancy to visualize the developing fetus, obtain fetal heart rate and dating measurements from a transabdominal perspective.
  - Use with caution in early pregnancy or if suspicion for ectopic is high.
- Linear transducer
  - Provides higher-resolution imaging from a transabdominal perspective.
  - May be used to visualize intrauterine pregnancy in patients with thin body habitus and an anteverted uterus.
- Endocavitary transducer
  - Also known as transvaginal transducer.
  - Provides higher-resolution imaging of pelvic organs.
  - Preferred for imaging in early pregnancy.
  - Not affected by bowel gas or obesity.

(b) Patient Position
- Transabdominal
  - Patients should lay supine with their knees bent to relax abdominal wall muscles.
  - Try to ensure the patient has a full bladder as this will provide a better acoustic window for imaging pelvic organs.
- Transvaginal
  - Patients should be placed in the lithotomy position, ideally on a pelvic-specific stretcher with footrests.
  - The patient should be covered during all portions of the procedure, except during transducer insertion when direct visualization is required.
  - Ensure the patient has an empty bladder for optimal imaging of the pelvic organs; a full bladder can cause discomfort and distort the anatomy, making visualization of the ovaries more difficult.

(c) Transabdominal Ultrasound Standard Exam Views
- Transverse view.
  - Place the transducer above the pubic bone with the marker pointed toward the patient's right.
  - Fan up and down to obtain transverse images of the uterus from fundus to cervix.
  - Figure 14.1—Transabdominal transverse gravid uterus.
  - Video 14.1—Transabdominal transverse gravid uterus.
  - Move the transducer slightly to the left and right of the uterus to visualize each adnexa.
- Sagittal view
  - Rotate the transducer 90° so that the marker is pointed cephalad.
  - Fan left and right to visualize the uterus in a sagittal or long-axis orientation.

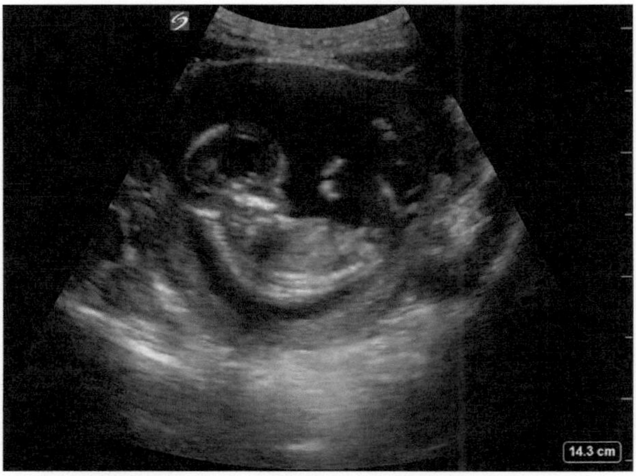

Fig. 14.1 Transabdominal transverse gravid uterus. Using a transabdominal approach, the gravid uterus in visualized here in a transverse plane. The fetus, in this case, is lying in a sagittal plane

- Visualize the endometrial stripe and follow it from fundus to cervix.
- Figure 14.2—Transabdominal uterus in sagittal
- Video 14.2—Transabdominal uterus in sagittal

- In both transverse and sagittal planes, evaluate the rectouterine pouch (pouch of Douglas) for free intraperitoneal fluid.

(d) Transvaginal Ultrasound Standard Exam Views

- Sagittal view
  - Insert the transducer into the vagina with the handle, or trigger, pointed toward the floor.
  - In this view, the bladder will be visualized on the left side of the image and can be seen more completely by lowering the scanning hand to point the transducer head toward the ceiling.
    - Figure 14.3—Bladder with uterus in sagittal plane

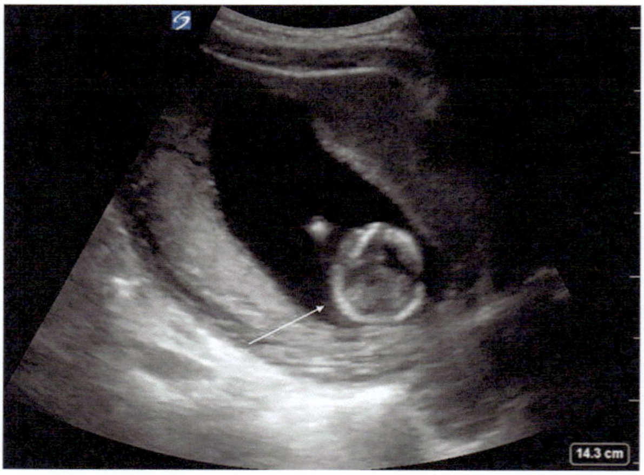

Fig. 14.2 Transabdominal uterus in sagittal. Using a transabdominal approach, the gravid uterus is visualized here in a sagittal view. The fetal head is a hyperechoic structure within hypoechoic fluid (arrow)

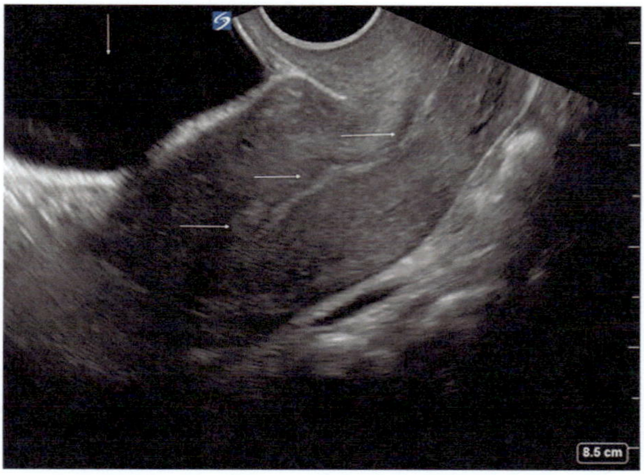

Fig. 14.3 Bladder with uterus in sagittal plane. In this nongravid uterus, the uterine stripe can be seen in the midline of the uterus (horizontal arrows) with the bladder noted to the left (vertical arrow). This uterus is anteverted, the most common uterine position

  - The uterus lies in the mid position and should be fully evaluated by fanning from one side to the other.
  - Identify the long axis of the uterus by finding the endometrial stripe, which is a hyperechoic line within the uterus and extends from the fundus to the cervix.
    - Figure 14.4—Long axis of gravid uterus (sagittal view)
    - Video 14.3—TVUS gravid uterus sagittal
  - The posterior cul-de-sac (also known as rectouterine pouch or pouch of Douglas) can be seen by raising the scanning hand to point the transducer head toward the floor.
    - Figure 14.5—Pouch of Douglas
- Transverse view
  - Rotate the transducer 90° counterclockwise so the transducer handle, or trigger, is pointed toward the patient's left.
    - Figure 14.6—Gravid uterus in transverse
    - Video 14.4—TVUS gravid uterus transverse
  - View the uterus completely by fanning the transducer anterior to posterior.
    - Lowering the scanning hand will image toward the fundus.
    - Raising the scanning hand will image toward the cervix.
  - The adnexa should be imaged initially in the transverse plane by directing the transducer toward the adnexa in question.
    - Moving the scanning hand toward the patient's left will move the transducer head toward the patient's right and image the right adnexa, and vice versa.
  - Once the transducer head is directed toward the adnexa of choice, fan the transducer anterior to posterior to search for the ovaries.
  - The ovaries are hyperechoic structures with hypoechoic follicles that are usually located lateral to the uterus and medial and anterior to the iliac vessels.
    - Figure 14.7—Normal ovary

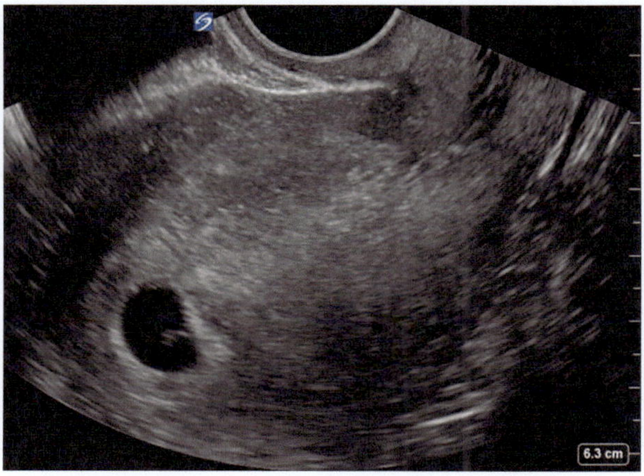

Fig. 14.4 Transvaginal gravid uterus, sagittal. Using a transvaginal approach, the gravid uterus is visualized in a sagittal plane. Note the hypoechoic circular structure in the midline of the uterine stripe within the uterine fundus. This represents a gestational sac containing a yolk sac

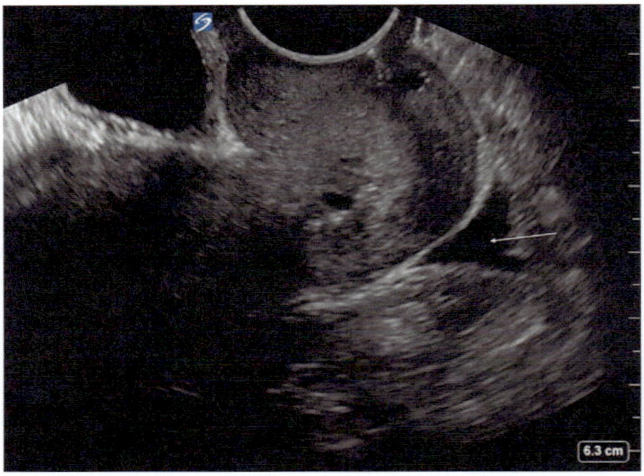

Fig. 14.5 Pouch of Douglas. The pouch of Douglas, also referred to as the cul-de-sac or rectouterine pouch, lies posterior to the uterus and anterior to the rectum (arrow) seen in this sagittal transvaginal view. Trace to small amount of physiologic free fluid is not unusual in women of childbearing age

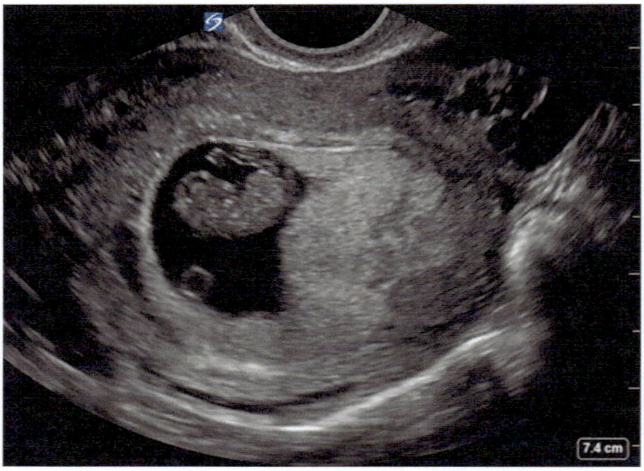

Fig. 14.6 Transvaginal gravid uterus, transverse. Using a transvaginal approach, the gravid uterus is visualized in a transverse plane with a large gestational sac on the left of the image. A yolk sac and developing fetus are clearly visible

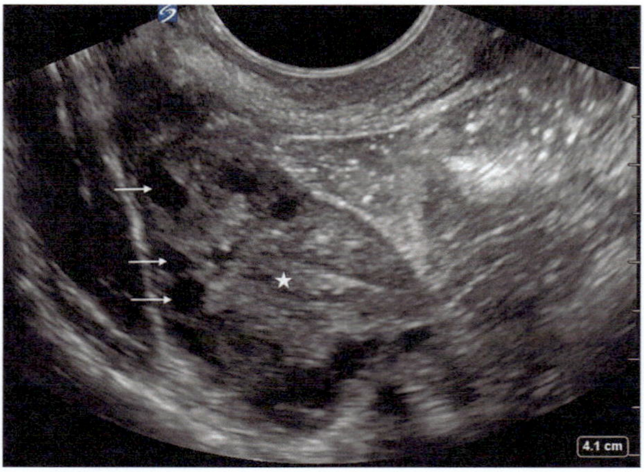

Fig. 14.7 Normal ovary. Multiple small cysts (arrows) in the cortex surround the medulla (star) in this normal ovary, giving the appearance of what is often referred to as a "chocolate chip cookie"

Evaluation for Intrauterine Pregnancy

(a) Gestational Sac
- A gestational sac can be identified at approximately 5 weeks of gestation [3] and in the majority of patients with a bHCG greater than 1000 to 2000 mIU/mL [1–3].
- It will appear as a round or oval hypoechoic fluid collection within the uterine stripe, typically in the fundus.
  - Figure 14.8—Empty gestational sac.
  - Video 14.5—Empty gestational sac.
- Gestational sac can be present in a normal pregnancy prior to development of a yolk sac or fetal pole. However, it can also be seen with an ectopic pregnancy, which is known as pseudogestational sac.
- The presence of a gestational sac without a yolk sac and fetal pole does not confirm intrauterine pregnancy, especially in cases where ectopic pregnancy is suspected.

(b) Double Decidual Sign
- Visualized as alternating hyperechoic rings separated by a thin hypoechoic layer of fluid surrounding a gestational sac.
  - The inner ring is called the decidua capsularis.
  - The outer ring is called the decidua parietalis.
- The presence of a double decidual sign without a yolk sac and fetal pole is suggestive of, but not confirmatory for an intrauterine pregnancy.
  - Figure 14.9—Double decidual sac.
  - Video 14.6—Double decidual sac.

(c) Yolk Sac
- Located within a gestational sac.
- Appears as a small, thin-walled spherical structure with an anechoic center.
  - Figure 14.10—Yolk sac.
  - Video 14.7—Yolk sac.

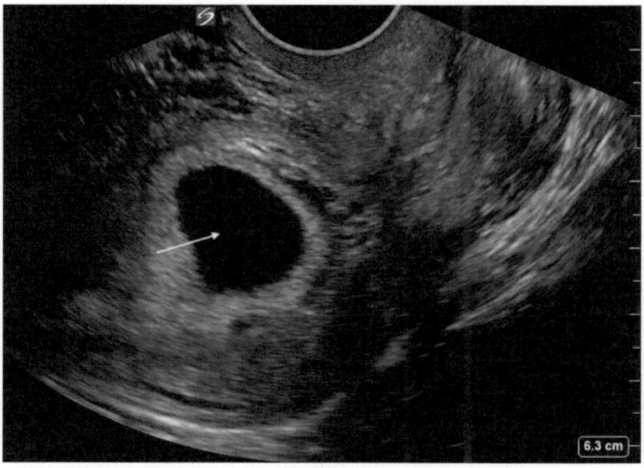

Fig. 14.8 Empty gestational sac. An empty gestational sac (arrow) is visualized here within the uterus. This is the first early sign of a developing pregnancy, but does not in itself confirm an intrauterine pregnancy

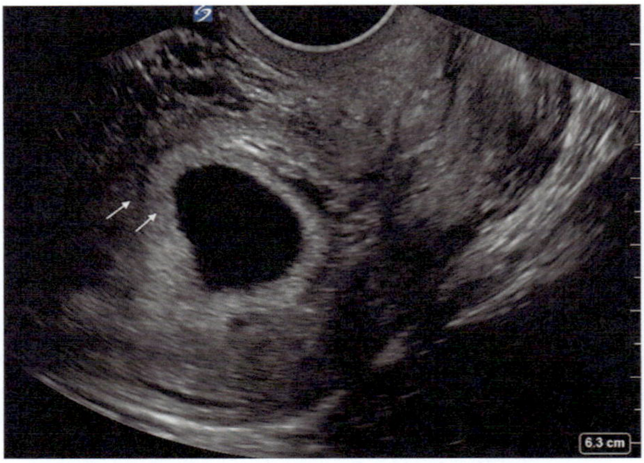

Fig. 14.9 Double decidual sign. Note the alternating hyperechoic rings separated by a thin hypoechoic layer of fluid surrounding a gestational sac

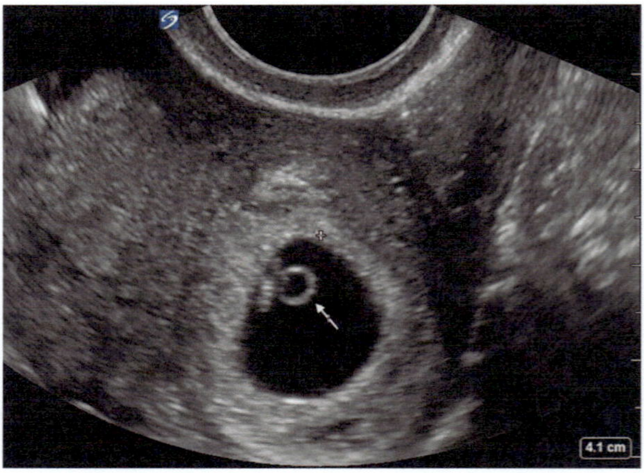

Fig. 14.10 Yolk sac. A yolk sac (arrow) is the first true ultrasonographic confirmation of intrauterine pregnancy

- This is the first confirmatory sign of true intrauterine pregnancy [3].
- Usually appears at approximately 5 to 6 weeks of gestation and disappears by 12 weeks [3].

(d) Fetal Pole

- Located within a gestational sac.
- Visualized as a hyperechoic mass of cells that appear to grow out of the yolk sac.
- Typically present by approximately 6 weeks of gestation [3].
  - Figure 14.11—Fetal pole.
  - Video 14.8—Fetal pole.
- In early pregnancy, distinct fetal parts will not be seen.
- A cardiac flicker may be seen within the fetal pole.
  - Appears as a fluttering motion.
  - Diagnostic for a viable intrauterine pregnancy.
  - Fetal heart rate can be detected at approximately 6 to 6.5 weeks of gestation [2] once the fetal pole is greater than 5 mm [3].

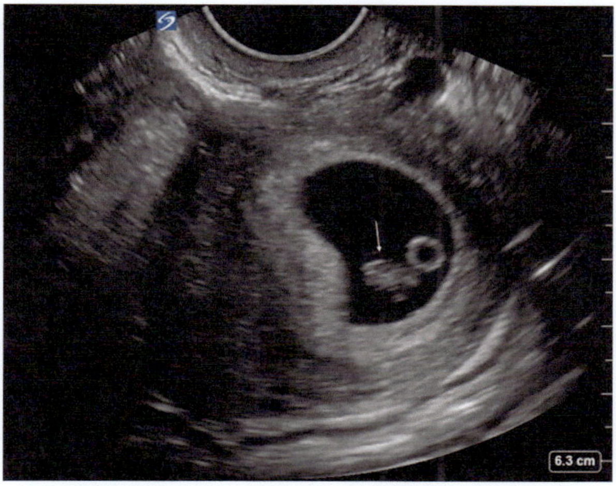

Fig. 14.11 Fetal pole. A fetal pole (arrow) first appears as a thickened area on the yolk sac at approximately 6 weeks of gestational age by transvaginal ultrasound. The circular yolk sac is also visualized

(e) Fetal Heart Rate
- Normal heart rate within the first trimester is 110 to 175 bpm [4].
- Normal heart rate after the first trimester is 120 to 160 bpm [5].
- Use M-mode to calculate fetal heart rate:
  - Place the M-mode vertical line through the cardiac flicker.
  - Plot the fetal heart tracing on the M-mode graph.
  - Use the preprogrammed ultrasound software to calculate the fetal heart rate by measuring one cardiac cycle length [5].
  - Figure 14.12—Fetal heart rate using M-mode.

(f) Gestational Age Measurements
- There are several different measurements that can be done to estimate gestational age. However, the easiest to perform are crown-rump length (CRL) and biparietal diameter (BPD).
- Gestational age measurements are most accurate in the first trimester.
- Crown-rump length
  - This measurement can be obtained at approximately 6 weeks gestation [3].
  - Image the fetus to visualize the spine in a longitudinal plane.
  - Utilize calipers to measure from the top of fetal head to bottom of the buttocks.
    - Figure 14.13—Crown-rump length
  - Software built into the ultrasound machine can then be used to determine gestational age, or the measurement obtained can be compared to standardized CRL-to-gestational age charts.
  - CRL measurement should not include the yolk sac in early first trimester.
- Biparietal diameter
  - This measurement can be obtained toward the end of the first trimester and within the second trimester [3].
  - Obtain a transverse view of the fetal head with the thalami visible and symmetric.

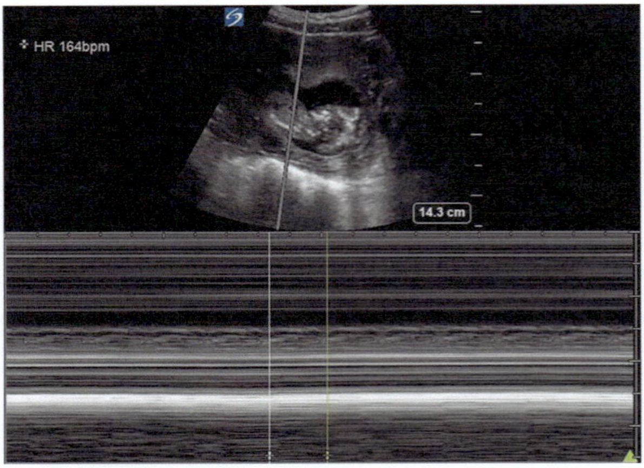

Fig. 14.12 Fetal heart rate using M-mode. Place the M-mode spike over the fetal heart, plot the fetal heart tracing on the M-mode graph, and use the preprogrammed software to calculate a fetal heart rate by measuring between one cardiac cycle length. Here, the fetal heart rate is 164

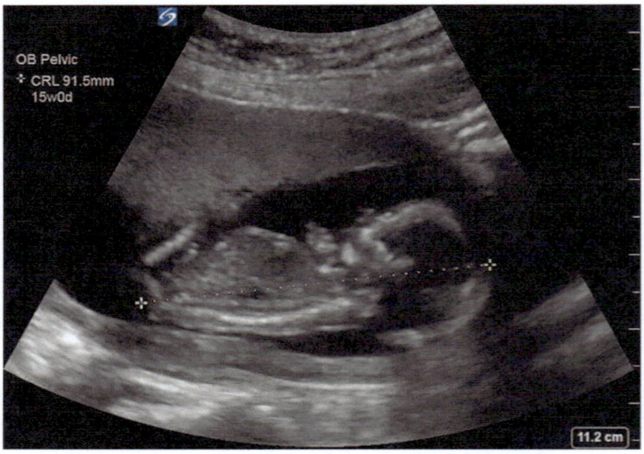

Fig. 14.13 Crown-rump length. To obtain a crown-rump length measurement, use calipers to measure from the top of the fetal head to base of the rump

- Utilize calipers to measure from the outer edge of one bony table to the inner edge of the other [3], across the widest portion of the fetal head.
  - Figure 14.14—Biparietal diameter
- Software built into the ultrasound machine can then be used to determine gestational age, or the measurement obtained can be compared to standardized BPD-to-gestational age charts.

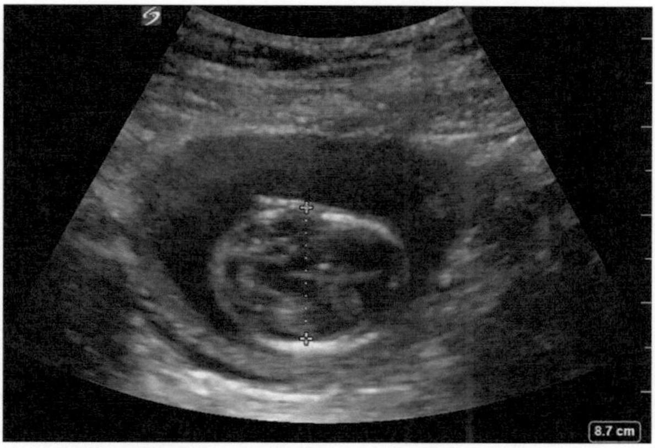

Fig. 14.14 Biparietal diameter. For biparietal diameter, measure from the inner edge of the near skull wall to the outer edge of the far skull wall

Obstetric Pathology

1. Intraperitoneal Pelvic Fluid
   (a) Free fluid is most commonly seen posterior to the uterus in the pouch of Douglas.
   (b) Small amount of fluid may be a normal physiologic finding in women of childbearing age.
      - Figure 14.15—Small amount of free fluid in pouch of Douglas.
      - Video 14.9—Small amount of free fluid in pouch of Douglas.
   (c) Moderate or large amount of fluid is generally considered abnormal and should prompt investigation into potential causes.
      - Figure 14.16—Large amount of free fluid in pelvis.
      - Video 14.10—Large amount of free fluid in pelvis.
      - In the presence of a positive pregnancy test and an empty uterus, an ectopic pregnancy should be suspected.
      - Other causes include ruptured ovarian cyst, trauma, or ascites.
2. Ectopic Pregnancy
   (a) A pregnancy that implants outside the uterus.
      - Figure 14.17—Ectopic pregnancy
   (b) Suspect an ectopic pregnancy in any pregnant patient with vaginal bleeding or abdominal pain in the setting of a positive pregnancy test.
   (c) Suspicion should be raised in a sonographically empty uterus.
   (d) Consider the following:
      - Pseudogestational sac.
        – Difficult to distinguish from a normal gestational sac.
        – Does not contain fetal parts and is centrally located within the endometrial cavity.
      - Pelvic free fluid.
        – The greater the amount of fluid, the higher the likelihood of ectopic pregnancy, including ruptured ectopic pregnancy.

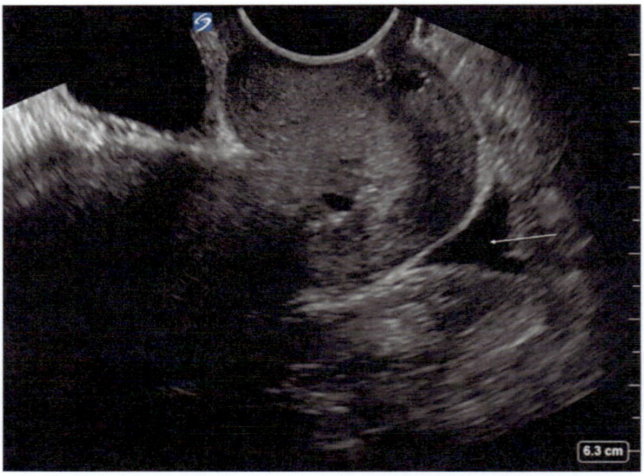

Fig. 14.15 Small amount of free fluid in pouch of Douglas. In a sagittal transvaginal image, the pouch of Douglas will be located posterior to the uterus or on the right side of the screen. Here, a small amount of fluid is seen within the pouch of Douglas (arrow)

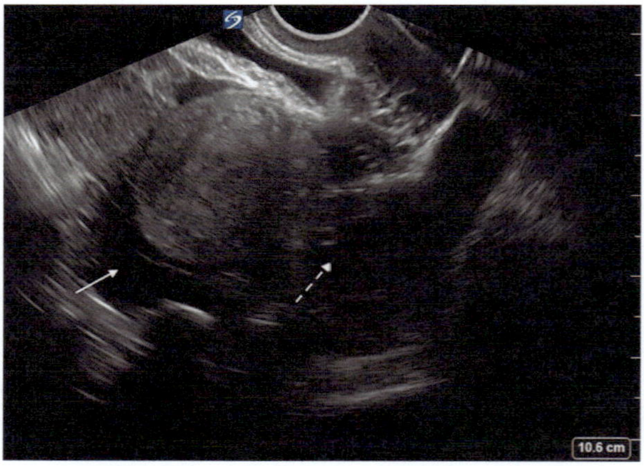

Fig. 14.16 Large amount of free fluid in the pelvis. This sagittal transvaginal view shows a large amount of fluid extending above the fundus (arrow) in this patient with an ectopic pregnancy (dotted arrow)

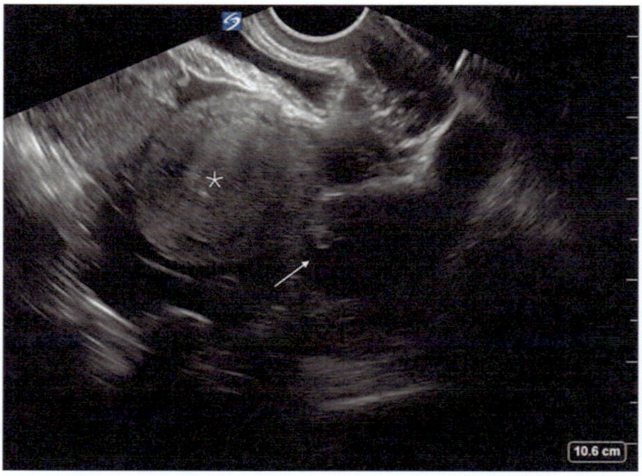

Fig. 14.17 Ectopic pregnancy. An ectopic pregnancy is defined by a gestational sac that implants outside of the uterus. In this sagittal transvaginal image, there is a gestational sac containing a yolk sac (arrow) located posterior to the uterus (star) representing an ectopic pregnancy

  - Small amount of fluid can be normal.
  - With simple, echo-free fluid the risk for ectopic pregnancy is dependent upon the amount present.
    - Trace: Fluid is found posterior to the cervix, confined to the pouch of Douglas.
    - Small: Fluid extends along the lower 1/3 of the posterior wall of the uterus [4].
    - Moderate: Fluid extends between 1/3 and 2/3 the height of the posterior uterus [4].
    - Large: Fluid extends up more than 2/3 the height of the uterus or above the fundus [4].
  - Patients with moderate to large pelvic free fluid have about an 86% chance of having an ectopic pregnancy [3].
  - Patients with free fluid extending up to Morrison's pouch have almost 100% chance of having an ectopic pregnancy [3].
  - Echogenic fluid can represent blood and should raise suspicion for ectopic pregnancy [6].
    - Figure 14.18—Echogenic blood
- Tubal ring sign
  - A concentric hyperechoic structure surrounding a mass or gestational sac within the adnexa [6].
  - When present, there is about a 95% chance the patient has an ectopic pregnancy [3].
- Adnexal mass
  - If visualized, highly suspicious for ectopic pregnancy.
  - The ampulla or isthmic portion of the fallopian tube is the most common extrauterine site of implantation [6].
    - Figure 14.19—Adnexal mass
    - Video 14.11—Adnexal mass
  - Generally, appears as a distinct mass, apart from the ovary.
    - Intraovarian ectopic pregnancies are very rare.
  - Frequently will demonstrate increased flow using power Doppler resembling a "ring of fire" [3, 6].

3. Interstitial Ectopic Pregnancy
   (a) Eccentric location of an intrauterine gestational sac high in the fundus near the highly vascular area at the insertion of the fallopian tubes.
   (b) Uncommon, but carries a higher risk of mortality due to close proximity of uterine artery [7].
   (c) Can be diagnosed by measuring the uterine mantle distance, which is the thickness of the myometrium surrounding the gestational sac.
    - Myometrium that measures less than 5 mm suggests an interstitial ectopic pregnancy [7, 8].
    - Figure 14.20—Interstitial pregnancy.
    - Figure 14.21—Interstitial pregnancy.

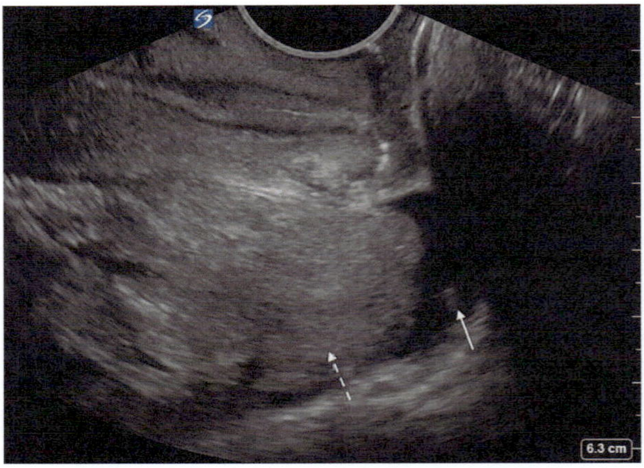

Fig. 14.18 Echogenic blood. Blood within the pelvis can appear anechoic or echogenic, representing clotted blood, which increases the suspicion for ectopic pregnancy. Note both new bleeding (solid arrow) and clotted blood (dotted arrow) posterior to the uterus in this sagittal transvaginal view. The uterus and uterine stripe are seen closest to the transducer or at the top of the image

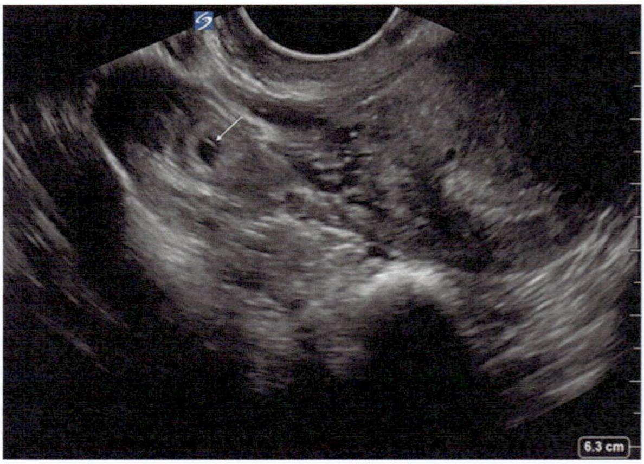

Fig. 14.19 Adnexal mass. This transverse transvaginal image shows a mass outside of the uterus with gestational sac and yolk sac (arrow), located within the adnexa, that represents an ectopic pregnancy

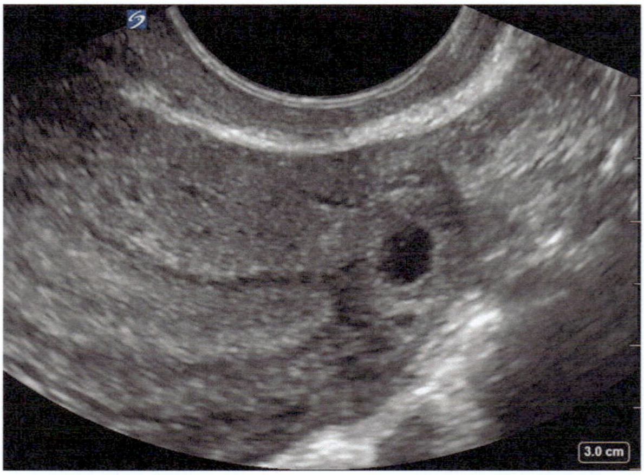

Fig. 14.20 Interstitial pregnancy. Interstitial pregnancy occurs when an intrauterine gestational sac is eccentrically located high in the fundus of the uterus. Note the separation from the uterine stripe

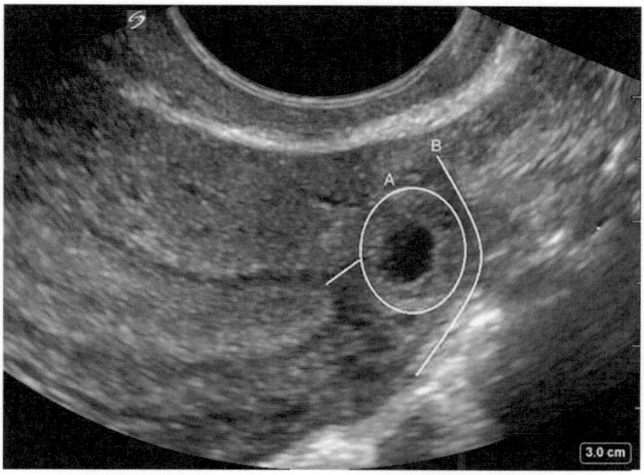

Fig. 14.21 Interstitial pregnancy. To help diagnose an interstitial pregnancy, the uterine mantle should be measured. Uterine mantle is the thickness of the myometrium that surrounds a gestational sac. This measurement can be made by measuring the distance between the gestational sac (**a**) and the outer edge of the uterine wall (**b**)

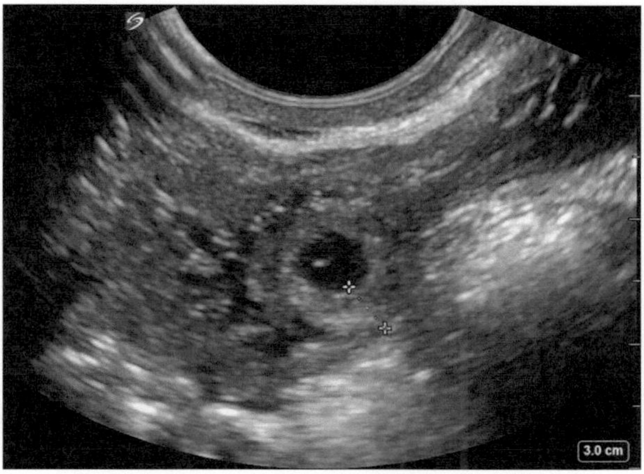

Fig. 14.22 Mantle measurement. A mantle measurement less than 5 mm is highly concerning for interstitial ectopic pregnancy

- Video 14.12—Interstitial pregnancy.
- Figure 14.22—Mantle measurement.

(d) Interstitial line sign.
- Appears as a hyperechoic line connecting the interstitial ectopic mass and the endometrium [7, 8].
- Figure 14.23—Interstitial line sign.

4. Cornual Ectopic Pregnancy

(a) Distinct entity from interstitial ectopic pregnancy, but often used interchangeably.

(b) Occurs when gestational sac and pregnancy develop within one horn (cornua) of a bicornuate or septate uterus [7].

(c) The gestational sac will be surrounded by thin endomyometrium measuring less than 5mm[7], similar to interstitial pregnancy.

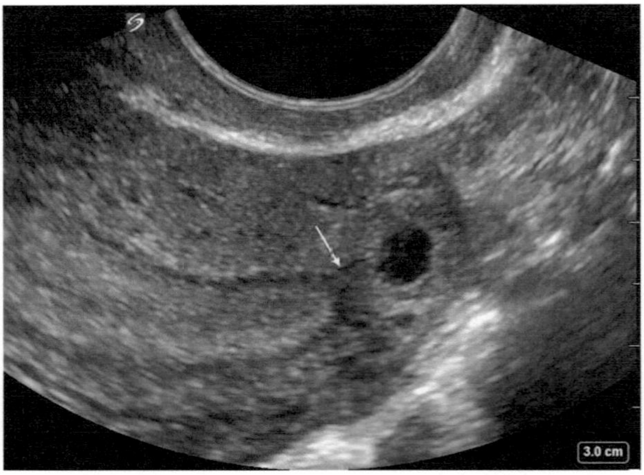

Fig. 14.23 Interstitial line sign. Typically, a hyperechoic line will be seen connecting the interstitial ectopic pregnancy with the endometrial stripe, known as interstitial line sign (arrow)

5. Heterotopic Pregnancy
   (a) Simultaneous intrauterine and extrauterine pregnancies.
   (b) Rare, but occurs more commonly in patients undergoing infertility treatment including medications and in vitro fertilization [6].
6. Fetal Demise
   (a) Findings that may indicate an abnormal pregnancy or fetal demise include:
      - Gestational sac that is distorted or irregular in shape.
      - Empty gestational sac greater than 20 mm [3], known as blighted ovum.
        - Figure 14.24—Blighted ovum (large empty sac).
        - Video 14.13—Blighted ovum.
      - Fetal heart rate less than 70 bpm [4].
      - Fetal pole without cardiac activity at 7 to 8 weeks of gestation.
        - Cardiac activity should be present in embryos with a CRL greater than 5 mm [3].
7. Molar Pregnancy (Hydatidiform mole)
   (a) Most common benign form of gestational trophoblastic disease.
   (b) Complete mole.
      - Usually occupy an enlarged uterine cavity and appear as tissue with variable echogenicity within which are scattered anechoic spaces, often referred to as a "cluster of grapes" [3].
        - Figure 14.25—Molar pregnancy.
        - Video 14.14—Molar pregnancy.
   (c) Incomplete or partial moles:
      - Will appear similar to complete mole [9].
        - Contains tissue with variable echogenicity within uterus.
        - Placenta may be enlarged with diffuse anechoic lesions.
      - Presence of fetal parts on ultrasound is consistent with partial mole [9].
        - Fetus and gestational sac are usually malformed.

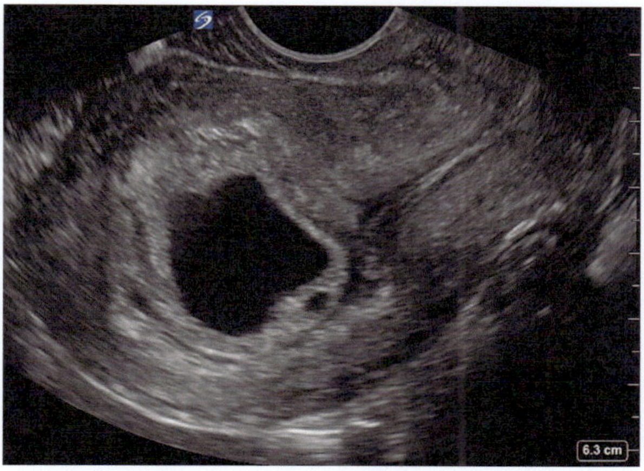

Fig. 14.24 Blighted ovum (large empty sac). An empty, irregular gestational sac greater than 2 cm seen here in this sagittal transvaginal view represents a blighted ovum

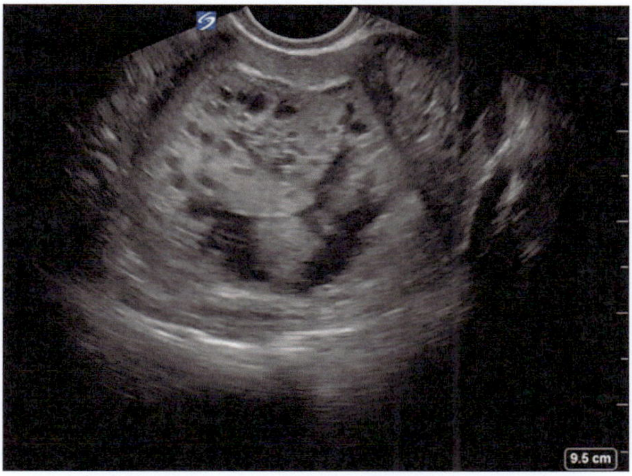

Fig. 14.25 Molar pregnancy. A molar pregnancy will often appear as tissue with variable echogenicity within which are scattered anechoic spaces, commonly referred to as a "cluster of grapes"

Key Points

- Trace to small amounts of free fluid can be normal or "physiologic."
- Moderate to large amounts of free fluid, and especially free fluid present in the RUQ, should raise concern for ruptured ectopic in the correct clinical settings.
- The classic discriminatory zone (bHCG>1500 to find a pregnancy by TVUS) cannot be applied to ectopic pregnancies.
- Ectopic pregnancies can exhibit any bHCG level.
    - Therefore, patients who have signs and symptoms of an ectopic pregnancy should have a transvaginal ultrasound [10].

References

1. Pavlik EJ, PD DP, Gallion HH, Ueland FR, Reedy MB, Kryscio RJ, van Nagell JR Jr. Ovarian volume related to age. Gynecol Oncol. 2000;77(3):410–2. http://www.sciencedirect.com/science/article/pii/S0090825800957834?via%3Dihub. Accessed 23 Apr 2017
2. Murray H, Baakdah H, Bardell T, Tulandi T. Diagnosis and treatment of ectopic pregnancy. Can Med Assoc J. 2005;173(8):905–12. https://www.ncbi.nlm.nih.gov/pmc/articles/PMC1247706/. Accessed 23 Apr 2017
3. Reardon RF, Hess-Keenan J, Roline CE, Caroon LV, Joing SA. Chapter 14: first trimester pregnancy. In: Ma OJ, Mateer JR, Reardon RF, Joing SA, editors. Emergency ultrasound. 3rd ed. New York: McGraw-Hill Education; 2014. p. 381–424.
4. Campos P, Wang RC. Chapter 24: first-trimester pregnancy. In: Soni NJ, Arntfield R, Kory P, editors. Point-of-care ultrasound. Philadelphia: Saunders; 2015. p. 184–98.
5. Byars DV, Knapp BJ. Chapter 15: second and third trimester pregnancy. In: Ma OJ, Mateer JR, Reardon RF, Joing SA, editors. Emergency ultrasound. 3rd ed. New York: McGraw-Hill Education; 2014. p. 425–54.
6. Bhatt S, Ghazale H, Dogra VS. Sonographic evaluation of ectopic pregnancy. Radiograph Clin North Am 2007; 45(3):549–560. http://www.sciencedirect.com/science/article/pii/S0033838907000243. Accessed 22 Apr 2017.
7. Lin EP, Bhatt S, Dogra VS. Diagnostic clues to ectopic pregnancy. Radiographics. 2008;28(6):1661–71. http://pubs.rsna.org/doi/pdf/10.1148/rg.286085506. Accessed 23 Apr 2017
8. Rastogi R, Meena GL, Rastogi N, Rastogi V. Interstitial ectopic pregnancy: a rare and difficult clinicosonographic diagnosis. J Hum Reprod Serv. 2008;1(2):81–2. https://www.ncbi.nlm.nih.gov/pmc/articles/PMC2700669/. Accessed 23 Apr 2017.
9. Shah C, Johnson PT, Durrani H. Partial molar pregnancy. SonoWorld website. https://sonoworld.com/CaseDetails/Partial_molar_pregnancy.aspx?ModuleCategoryId=306. Accessed 24 Apr 2017
10. Robertson J, Koyfman A. Ectopic pregnancy. EmDocs Practice Updates website. http://www.emdocs.net/ectopic-pregnancy/. December 11, 2014. Accessed 23 Apr 2017.

15 Testicular Ultrasound

Michael J. Vitto, Angela Lindsay, and Jordan Tozer

There are many conditions that can affect the testes and scrotum, some of which are more concerning than others. The most severe, testicular torsion occurs when blood supply to one testicle is blocked, resulting in death of the testicle if not diagnosed in a timely manner. For other conditions, such as malignancy, hydrocele, epididymitis, and orchitis, while not imminently threatening, it is important that there is a timely diagnosis and treatment to prevent sequelae of disease. Ultrasound has proven to be an important imaging modality to evaluate for and diagnose these conditions as it is quick and easy to perform. This chapter will review indications for performing a testicular ultrasound, basic testicular and scrotal anatomy, image acquisition, normal ultrasound anatomy, and interpretation of pathology.

Clinical Application and Indications

- Acute testicular pain or concern for testicular torsion.
- Palpable mass or scrotal swelling.
- Evaluation for possible infection such as epididymitis or orchitis.

Supplementary Information The online version contains supplementary material available at https://doi.org/10.1007/978-3-032-27643-8_15.

M. J. Vitto (✉) · A. Lindsay · J. Tozer
Department of Emergency Medicine, Virginia Commonwealth University Health, Richmond, VA, USA
e-mail: Michael.vitto@vcuhealth.org; Angela.creditt@vcuhealth.org; jordan.tozer@vcuhealth.org

A. Lindsay et al. (eds.), *Clinical Ultrasound*,
https://doi.org/10.1007/978-3-032-27643-8_15

Normal Testicular Anatomy

- Testicles are oval-shaped structures that measure approximately 4 × 3 × 2.5 cm in size [1] and are found suspended within the scrotum.
- The tunica vaginalis surrounds the testes [2].
- Along the posterior aspect of each testicle is the epididymis, which consists of a head, body, and tail:
  - The epididymis head is typically positioned posterolateral to the upper pole of the testicle [2].
- In most males, one or both testicles will have a testicular appendix, which represents a developmental remnant. It is typically found on the upper pole of the testis near the epididymal head.
- Some males may also have an epididymal appendix, also a developmental remnant that can be found as an appendage off the epididymal head.
- The spermatic cord contains the neurovascular supply to the testicle.

Image Acquisition

(a) Transducer Selection
  - Linear transducer.

(b) Patient Position
  - The patient should be supine.
  - Support the testicles in a sling-like fashion with a towel draped over the patient's legs and the scrotum sitting on top of the towel.
  - Cover sensitive areas that are being scanned with a second towel.

(c) Standard Exam Views
  - Obtain an image of both testicles side-by-side to demonstrate any echogenicity differences between the asymptomatic and symptomatic testicle.
  - Examine the asymptomatic testicle first in transverse and longitudinal planes:
    - A normal testicle is an oval-shaped homogenous mildly echogenic structure.
    - Note the echogenicity, texture, and size:
      - Figure 15.1—Normal testicle
      - Video 15.1—Normal testicle
    - Use color Doppler and note flow patterns:
      - Figure 15.2—Color Doppler
      - Video 15.2—Color Doppler
  - Examine the symptomatic testicle in transverse and longitudinal planes:
    - Compare echogenicity, texture, and size to the unaffected side.
    - Compare color Doppler flow patterns to the unaffected side.
  - Attempt to image the appendix testis and appendix epididymis:
    - Figure 15.3—Appendix testis.
  - Image each epididymis by placing the transducer posterior to each testis:

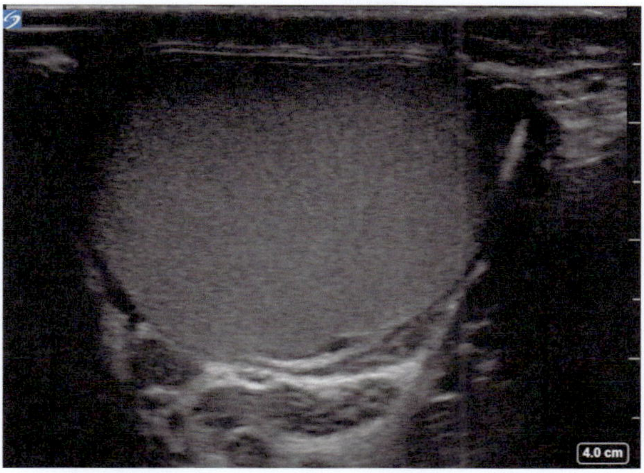

Fig. 15.1 Normal testicle. Longitudinal view of normal testicle using linear probe showing homogenous testicular architecture

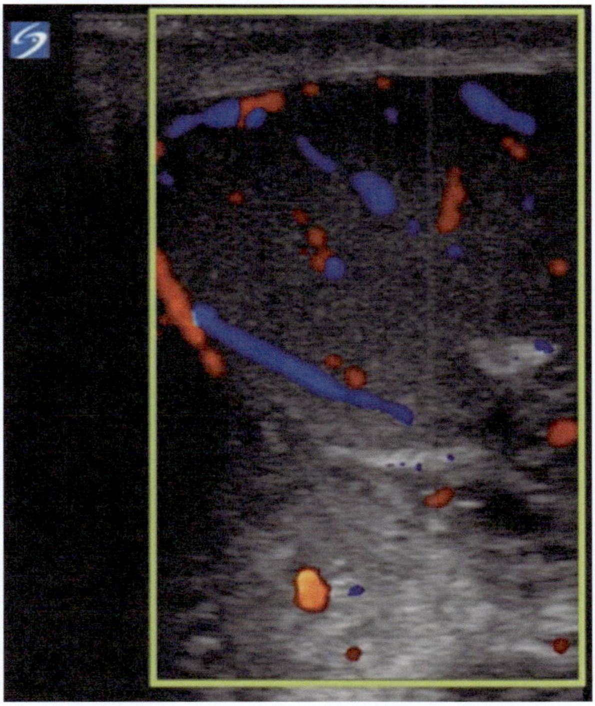

Fig. 15.2 Color Doppler. Longitudinal view of normal testicle showing normal blood flow with color Doppler

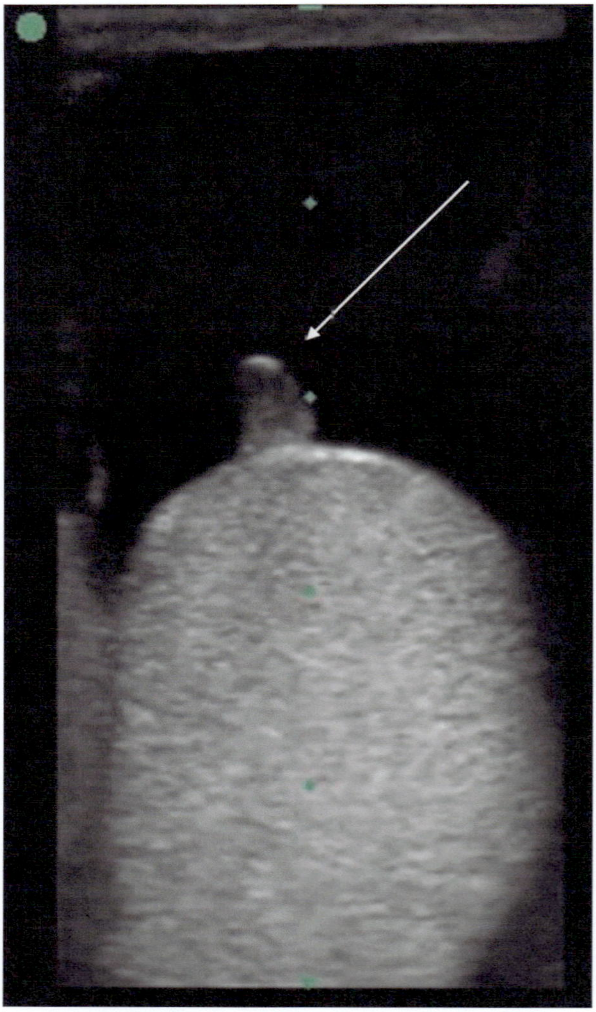

Fig. 15.3 Appendix testis. Testicular appendix (arrow), which represents a developmental remnant, is typically found on the upper pole of the testis near the epididymal head

- The epididymis has similar homogenous echogenicity to the testes, though slightly brighter.
  - Figure 15.4—Normal epididymis
  - Video 15.3—Normal epididymis
- Obtain color Doppler if there is concern for epididymitis.

- Obtain images of each inguinal canal, if indicated, to evaluate for a hernia.

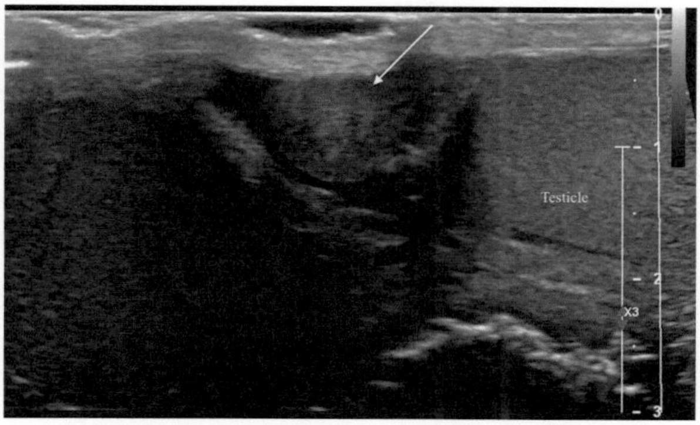

Fig. 15.4 Normal epididymis. Normal epididymis (arrow) seen adjacent to the testicle

Testicular Pathology

1. Hydrocele
   (a) Hydrocele is a collection of fluid between the visceral and parietal layers of the tunica vaginalis.
   (b) Congenital hydrocele is common and occurs due to a direct communication with the peritoneum [1].
   (c) Acquired hydroceles are typically associated with infection, tumor, trauma, torsion, or radiation therapy [1].
   (d) Hydrocele will appear as anechoic fluid surrounding the testicle without layering or septations:
   - Figure 15.5—Hydrocele.
   - Video 15.4—Hydrocele.
   - Figure 15.6—Hydrocele near testes and epididymis.

   (e) A complex hydrocele, such as hematocele or pyocele, will contain internal echoes with septations or loculations.
2. Varicocele
   (a) Varicocele is an abnormal enlargement of the pampiniform venous plexus within the spermatic cord [1].
   - Usually idiopathic and caused by valvular incompetence of the internal spermatic vein resulting in retrograde flow into the pampiniform plexus [1].
     - Ninety-nine percent of idiopathic varicoceles occur on the left [1] due to anatomical differences in between the right and left spermatic veins.
       - The right spermatic vein drains directly into the inferior vena cava [1].
       - The left spermatic vein drains into the left renal vein at almost a 90° angle [1].
   - Secondary causes are usually due to compression of the spermatic vein due to various pathologies such as a mass, hydronephrosis, or hepatomegaly [1]. Malignancy should also be considered.

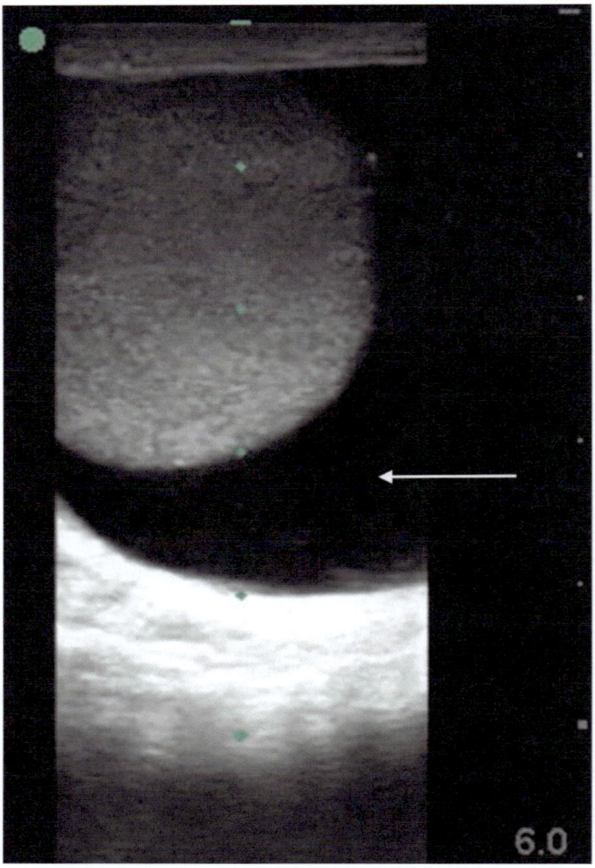

Fig. 15.5 Hydrocele. Moderate-sized hydrocele (arrow) seen adjacent to a normal testicle

   (b) Varicoceles appear as a cluster of hypoechoic vascular structures adjacent to the testicle.
      - Figure 15.7—Varicocele.
      - Video 15.5—Varicocele.
   (c) Color Doppler will demonstrate pronounced vascular flow to these hypoechoic areas.
      - Figure 15.8—Varicocele with color Doppler.
      - Video 15.6—Varicocele with color Doppler.
   (d) Valsalva maneuver can increase size and flow pattern of varicoceles.
3. Testicular Torsion
   (a) Twisting of the spermatic cord results in venous congestion and obstruction, followed by decreased arterial flow, and eventually complete arterial obstruction leading to ischemia and infarction [1, 2].
   (b) Severity of torsion ranges from 180 to 720°, and complete occlusion of blood flow is thought to occur after 450° of torsion [2].

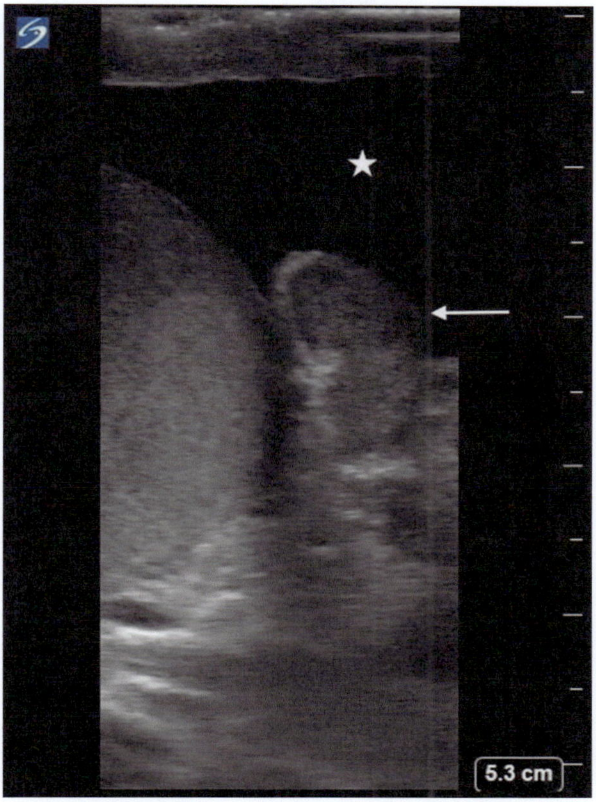

Fig. 15.6 Hydrocele near testes and epididymis. Normal epididymis (arrow) within small hydrocele (star) adjacent to a normal testicle

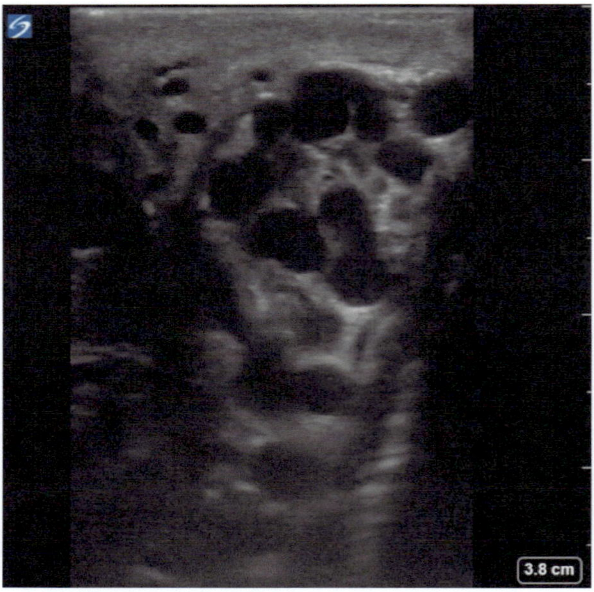

Fig. 15.7 Varicocele. Varicoceles appear as a cluster of enlarged or engorged vascular structures in the pampiniform plexus adjacent to the testicle. Having the patient perform the Valsalva maneuver will increase the size

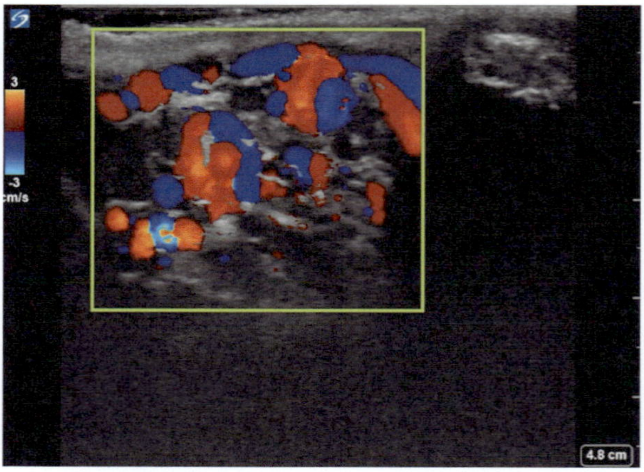

Fig. 15.8 Varicocele with color. Varicocele shown in this case with pronounced color flow. This can be augmented with by having the patient perform the Valsalva maneuver

(c) B-mode (2D) imaging:
- Affected testicle will appear enlarged and hypoechoic with less homogeneity compared with the unaffected testicle.
  - Figure 15.9—Testicular torsion.
  - Figure 15.10—Advanced testicular torsion.
  - Video 15.7—Testicular torsion.
- The epididymis may appear hypoechoic and enlarged, similar to how it appears in epididymitis.

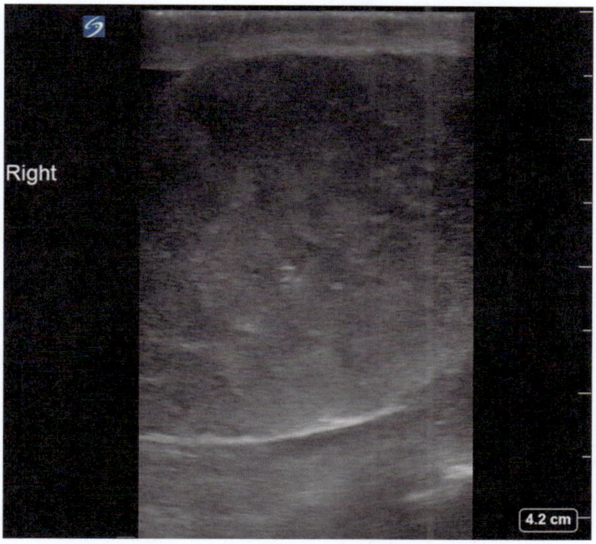

Fig. 15.9 Testicular torsion. The affected testicle will appear enlarged, as compared with the normal testicle, with loss of the typical homogenous architecture

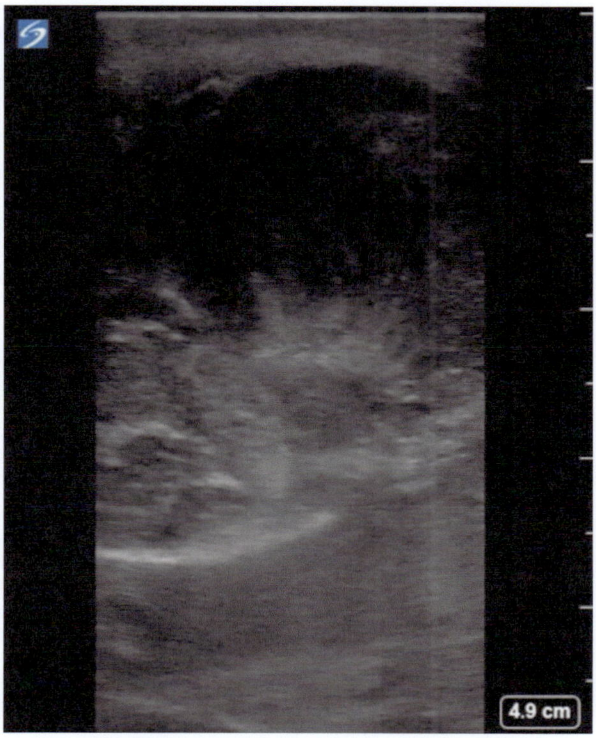

Fig. 15.10 Advanced testicular torsion. This testicular image shows delayed presentation of torsion. There is loss of normal architecture and variable echogenicity within the parenchyma

(d) Color Doppler:
- Decreased color Doppler signal will be seen or, in cases of complete torsion, the absence of color Doppler signal.
  - Figure 15.11—Color Doppler of a normal testicle.
  - Figure 15.12—Color Doppler testicular torsion.
  - Video 15.8—Color Doppler testicular torsion.
- Always compare the color Doppler signal to the unaffected side.

(e) Power Doppler, which can identify low-flow states, should also be used to evaluate for torsion. The absence of flow within the testicle using power Doppler is diagnostic of testicular torsion [1].
- Figure 15.13—Power Doppler of a normal testicle.
- Video 15.9—Power Doppler of a normal testicle.
- Figure 15.14—Power Doppler in testicular torsion.
- Figure 15.15—Power Doppler in testicular torsion long axis.
- Video 15.10—Power Doppler in testicular torsion.

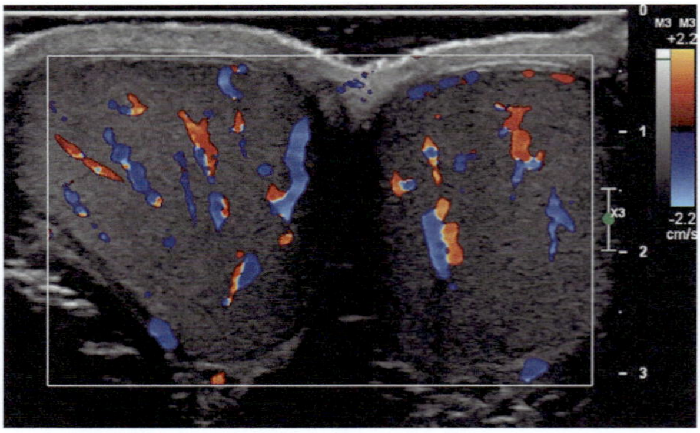

Fig. 15.11 Color Doppler of a normal testicle. This sunrise view shows normal color Doppler signal to both testicles. Not also the equal signal between each side

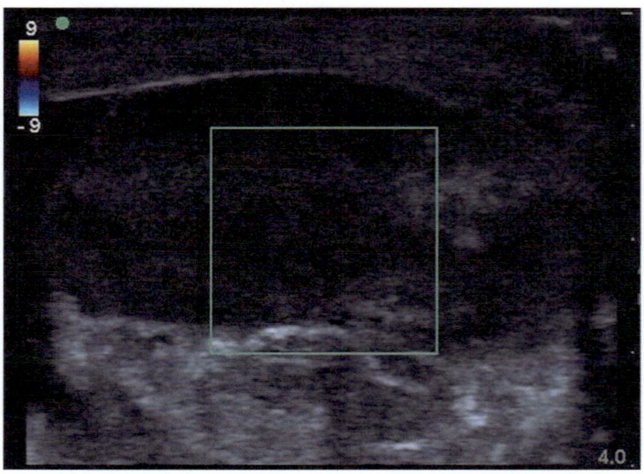

Fig. 15.12 Color Doppler testicular torsion. Loss of normal testicular architecture with absent flow on color Doppler indicating testicular torsion

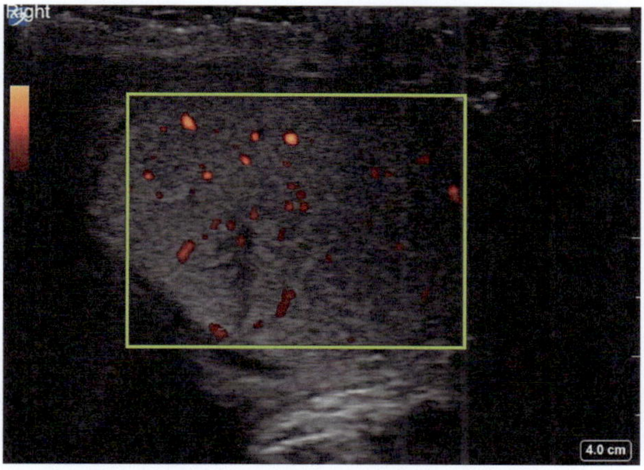

Fig. 15.13 Power Doppler of a normal testicle. Single testicle in longitudinal view showing normal flow by power Doppler

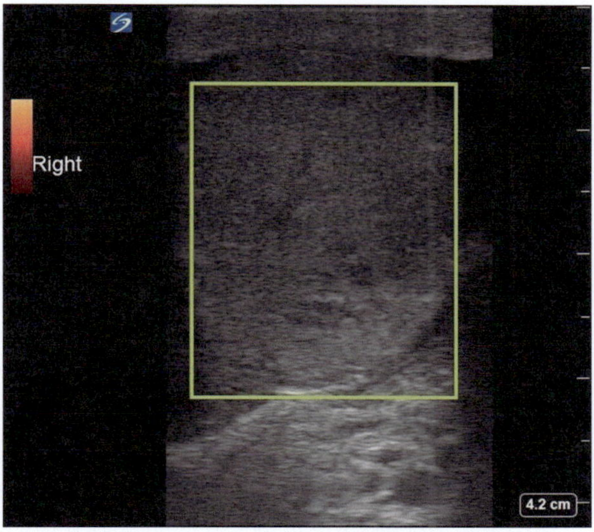

Fig. 15.14 Power Doppler in testicular torsion. Right testicle with the absence of flow using color Doppler, indicating testicular torsion

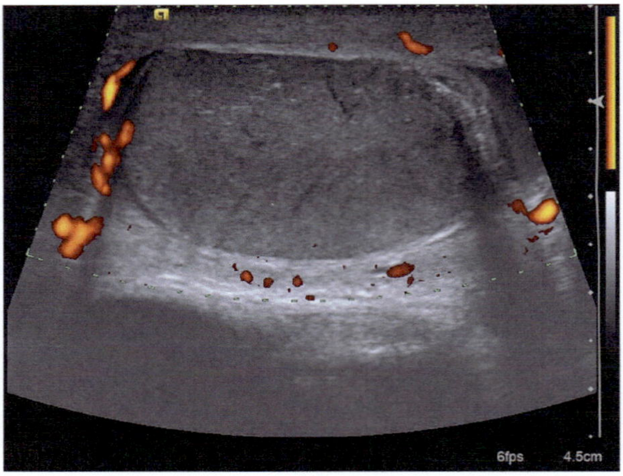

Fig. 15.15 Power Doppler in testicular torsion. Longitudinal view of testicle with power Doppler showing absence of flow

   (f) Ultrasound may also demonstrate the twisted spermatic cord just superior to the testis and epididymis with the transducer oriented in a sagittal plane [1].
      - This may have a "whirlpool" like appearance [2].
4. Torsion of Appendix Testis or Appendix Epididymis
   (a) Self-limiting and does not threaten testicular viability [2].
   (b) Palpable nodule with a bluish discoloration near the testicle [2].
   (c) Ultrasound will show a hyperechoic mass with a central hypoechoic area adjacent to the testis or epididymis [2].
   (d) Can result in inflammation of the epididymis and characteristic ultrasound findings of epididymitis [1].
5. Epididymitis
   (a) Epididymitis is characterized by a tender epididymis, dysuria, and occasionally a fever due to retrograde spread of an infection from the bladder or prostate.
   (b) Most common cause of acute scrotal pain in postpubertal males [2].
   (c) Epididymis will be enlarged compared to the unaffected side.
   (d) Color Doppler will demonstrate increased vascularity and blood flow to the infected epididymis.
      - Figure 15.16—Epididymitis color Doppler.
      - Video 15.11—Epididymitis color Doppler.
   (e) Reactive hydrocele can also be present [2].
6. Orchitis
   (a) Infection of the testicle that typically begins as epididymitis.
   (b) Ultrasound will show an enlarged testicle with decreased echogenicity [1].
   (c) On color Doppler, increased blood flow will be seen.
      - With B-mode imaging, torsion and orchitis will appear similar. Color Doppler must be used to differentiate between torsion and orchitis [1].
   (d) Scrotal wall thickening and a reactive hydrocele may also be present.

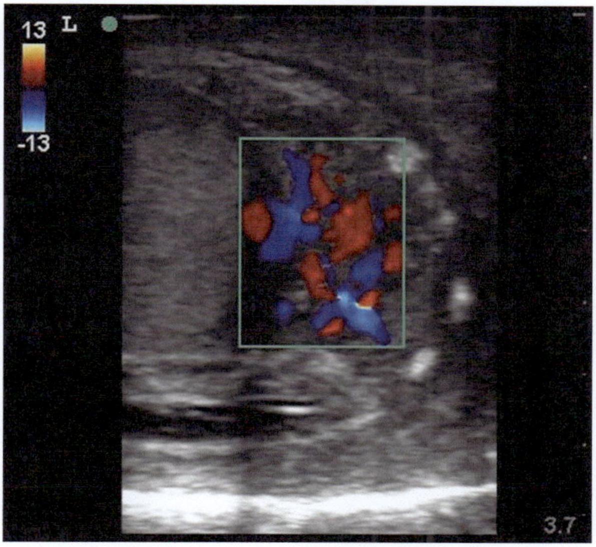

Fig. 15.16 Epididymitis color Doppler. Color Doppler will demonstrate increased vascularity and blood flow to the infected epididymis

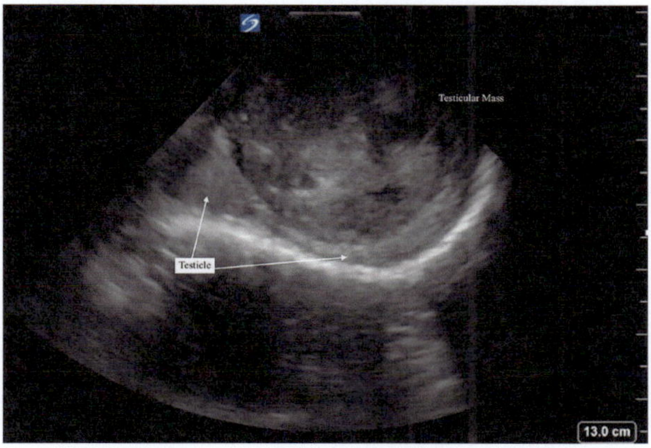

Fig. 15.17 Testicular mass or neoplasm. Large testicular mass with various echogenicity distorting normal testicular architecture

7. Testicular Neoplasm
   (a) Typically, a painless mass within the testicle or scrotum. Approximately 10% of cases may be associated with testicular pain [2].
   (b) Ultrasound will most often show a homogeneous, well-defined hypoechoic lesion within the testicular parenchyma.
   (c) Figure 15.17—Testicular mass or neoplasm.
   (d) Video 15.12—Testicular mass.
8. Fournier's Gangrene
   (a) Severe necrotizing soft tissue infection of the scrotum and perineum.
   (b) Thickening of the scrotal wall with scattered foci of dirty shadowing indicating subcutaneous air [1].
   (c) Figure 15.18—Fournier's gangrene.

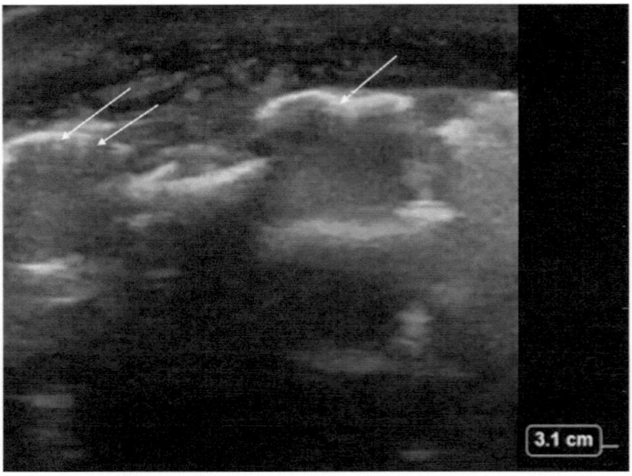

Fig. 15.18 Fournier's gangrene. Fournier's gangrene will appear similar to necrotizing fasciitis by ultrasound. In the presence of gas-forming bacteria, it will be visualized by identifying dirty shadowing (arrows) caused by air-tissue interface

Key Points

- Once full torsion has occurred and there is no blood flow, infarction and loss of the testicle occur rapidly. Salvage rates are approximately 100% at 3 hours, 90% at 6 hours, 50% at 12 hours, and 10% at 24 hours [2]
- Sonographic findings of testicular torsion are variable depending on the duration and extent of vascular compromise.
- Torsion remains a clinical diagnosis, and ultrasound cannot rule out torsion [2] especially in cases of partial torsion and intermittent torsion.
- If obtaining color Doppler flow is difficult, switch to power Doppler mode:
  - Set the gain to the highest setting that allows a distinct signal within vessels without surrounding artifact.
  - See Chap. 1 for details on power Doppler.
- A sunrise view can be used to image both testicles simultaneously by placing the transducer on to the scrotum from an inferior location:
  - If available, use a wider linear transducer or, as an alternative, use the curvilinear transducer.
  - Figure 15.19—Sunrise view.

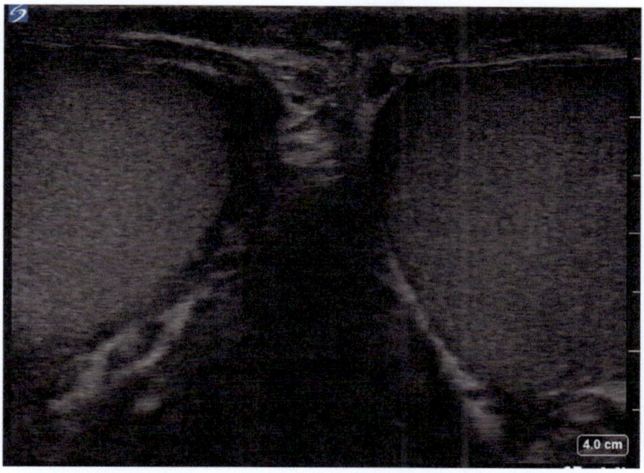

Fig. 15.19 Sunrise view. Sunrise view shows both testicles side-by-side allowing for comparison

References

1. Adhikari S. Chapter 13: testicular. In: Ma OJ, Mateer JR, Reardon RF, Joing SA, editors. Emergency ultrasound. 3rd ed. New York: McGraw-Hill Education; 2014. p. 353–80.
2. Goldenberg E, Gilbert BR. Chapter 4: scrotal ultrasound. In: Gilbert BR, editor. Ultrasound of the male genitalia. New York: Springer; 2015. p. 75–124.

Lower Extremity Venous Ultrasound 16

Jason Jennings, Michael J. Vitto, Lindsay Taylor, and Angela Lindsay

Venous thromboembolism is a common condition, with a global annual incidence of over 10 million cases [1]. While many episodes are provoked by hypercoagulability, venous stasis, and/or endothelial injury, in up to half of cases, no known risk factor is identified [2]. Point-of-care ultrasound allows for the rapid diagnosis of deep vein thrombosis in patients who may present in both the outpatient and inpatient settings. While there are a multitude of etiologies of a painful or swollen leg, it is critical to identify the diagnosis of deep vein thrombosis, as this can become life-threatening if the clot dislodges, causing a pulmonary embolism. This chapter will review basic lower extremity venous anatomy, image acquisition, normal ultrasound anatomy, and interpretation of pathology.

Clinical Application/Indications

- Lower extremity pain or swelling.
- Evaluation for deep vein thrombosis (DVT).

Supplementary Information The online version contains supplementary material available at https://doi.org/10.1007/978-3-032-27643-8_16.

J. Jennings (✉)
Department of Emergency Medicine, Virginia Commonwealth University Medical Center, Richmond, VA, USA
e-mail: jason.jennings@vcuhealth.org

M. J. Vitto · L. Taylor · A. Lindsay
Department of Emergency Medicine, Virginia Commonwealth University Health, Richmond, VA, USA
e-mail: Michael.vitto@vcuhealth.org; Lindsay.Taylor@vcuhealth.org; Angela.creditt@vcuhealth.org

A. Lindsay et al. (eds.), *Clinical Ultrasound*,
https://doi.org/10.1007/978-3-032-27643-8_16

- Evaluate for DVT in a hemodynamically stable patient in whom pulmonary embolism is suspected but is unable to undergo CT angiography for diagnosis.

Lower Extremity Venous Anatomy

(a) The common femoral vein is located just inferior to the inguinal ligament:
- The common femoral vein runs parallel with the common femoral artery and femoral nerve:
  - From medial to lateral: vein, artery, and nerve.
- Branches of the common femoral vein include:
  - Greater saphenous vein, femoral vein, and deep femoral vein.
  - From proximal to distal:
    - Greater saphenous vein branches from the medial aspect of the common femoral vein.
    - Common femoral vein then bifurcates into the femoral (previously known as superficial femoral) and deep femoral veins.

(b) The popliteal vein can be found just proximal to the popliteal fossa and trifurcates into the posterior tibial, anterior tibial, and peroneal veins before entering the proximal calf.
- The popliteal vein is most often located superficial to the popliteal artery.

(c) Under ultrasound, veins are thin walled with an anechoic (black) lumen. In the absence of pathology, they are easily compressible under pressure.

(d) Comparatively, arteries are thick walled and pulsate, and arteries will not collapse.

(e) Figure 16.1—Comparison between vein and artery.

(f) Video 16.1—Comparison between vein and artery.

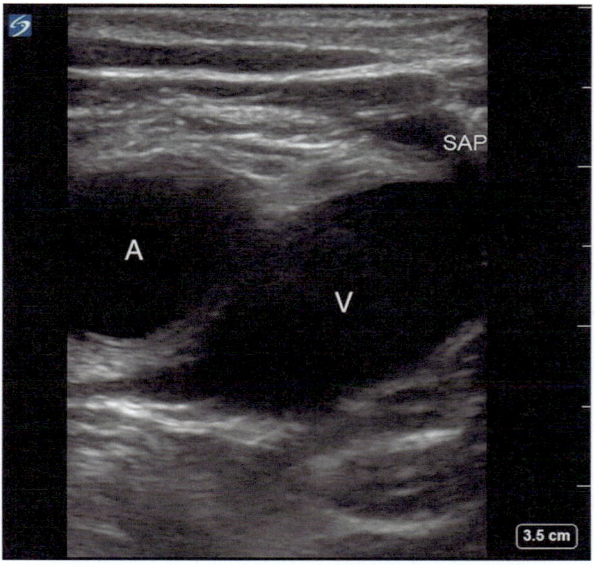

Fig. 16.1 Comparison between vein and artery. Arteries (A) have a thick muscular wall that is pulsatile and maintains its circular structure with compression. Veins (V) have a thin wall with increased compliance and therefore lack a specific shape; veins are easily compressible under pressure

Image Acquisition

- Transducer Selection.
  - Linear array.
  - Curvilinear transducers may be needed for obese patients.
- Patient Positioning
  - For imaging the proximal lower extremity veins including common femoral, saphenous, femoral, and deep femoral:
    - The patient should be placed in a supine position with their leg externally rotated, knee slightly flexed, and the head of the bed elevated or with the bed in reverse Trendelenburg.
    - Figure 16.2—Patient position for proximal veins.
  - For imaging the popliteal vein and popliteal trifurcation:
    - With the patient supine, slightly externally rotate the leg, then flex the knee.
    - Figure 16.3—Patient position for popliteal vein imaging.
    - Alternatively, the patient can lay in a lateral recumbent position with their knee slightly flexed [3].

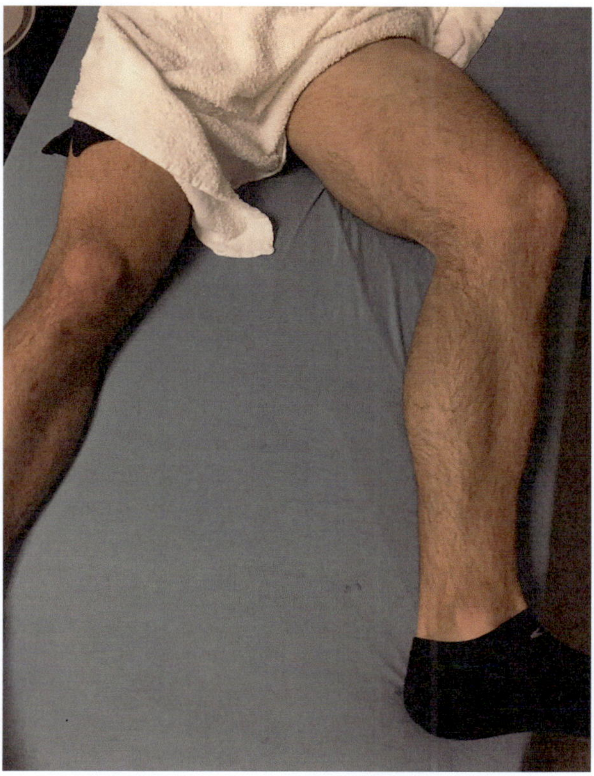

Fig. 16.2 Patient position for proximal vein imaging. To assess the proximal lower extremity veins, externally rotate the patient's leg and slightly flex the knee

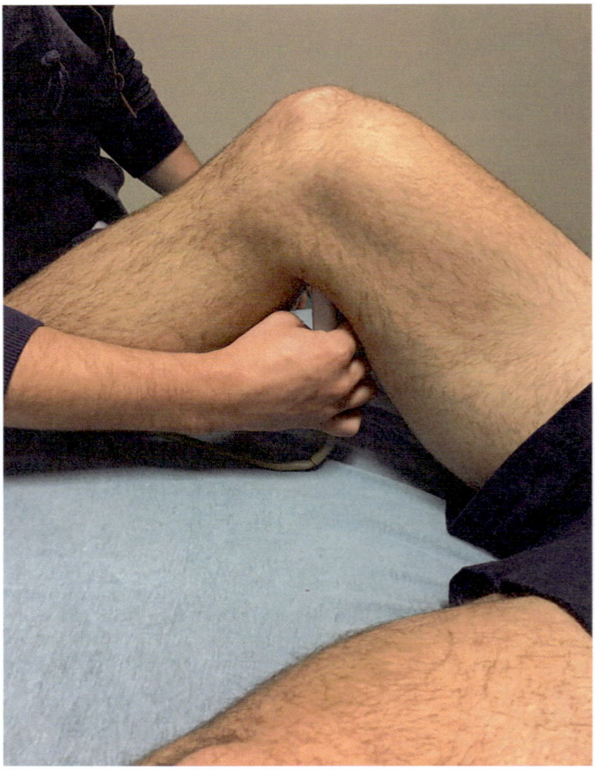

Fig. 16.3 Patient position for popliteal vein imaging. Flex the knee with slight external rotation of the patient's leg

- Standard Exam Views
  - Place the transducer just inferior to the inguinal ligament on the anteromedial thigh to visualize the common femoral vein:
    - Figure 16.4—Common femoral vein
    - Video 16.2—Common femoral vein
  - With the transducer perpendicular to the vein, apply direct and even downward pressure with the transducer and observe for compressibility of the vein with complete apposition of the vessel walls:
    - Figure 16.5—Common femoral vein compressed
  - Slowly move the transducer distally tracing the common femoral vein until the area where the greater saphenous vein drains into the common femoral vein can be seen:
    - Figure 16.6—Common femoral vein with greater saphenous vein
    - Video 16.3—Common femoral vein with greater saphenous vein
    - Apply pressure and observe for collapse of the greater saphenous vein and the common femoral vein.
    - The greater saphenous vein is technically a superficial vein. However, it can easily travel into the common femoral vein and therefore will need anticoagulation [4].

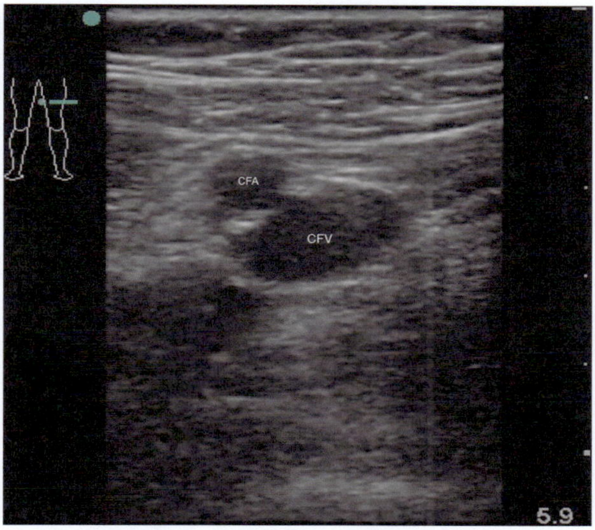

Fig 16.4 Common femoral vein. The common femoral vein (CFV) runs parallel with the common femoral artery (CFA) and femoral nerve. Commonly, the CFV will sit medial to the femoral artery and nerve, respectively

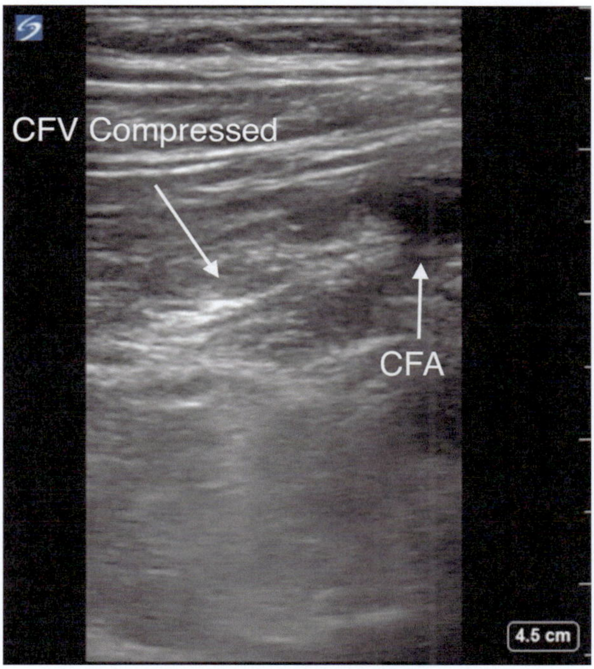

Fig. 16.5 Common femoral vein compressed. Common femoral vein is completely compressed under direct pressure

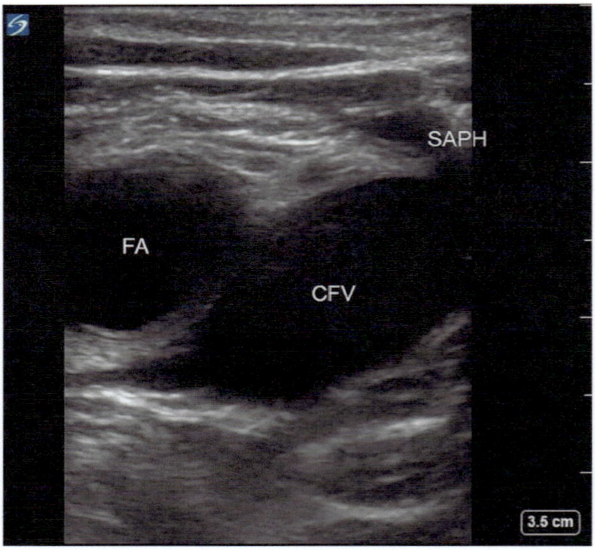

Fig. 16.6 Common femoral vein with greater saphenous vein. Greater saphenous vein (SAPH) drains into the common femoral vein from the medial side of the vessel. The femoral artery (FA) is located lateral, or to the left, of the common femoral vein in this image

- Again, move the transducer distally until the bifurcation of the common femoral vein into the femoral and deep femoral veins is visualized:
  - Apply compression with the transducer; both veins should collapse under pressure.
  - Figure 16.7—Bifurcation into femoral and deep femoral veins
  - Video 16.4—Bifurcation into femoral and deep femoral veins
  - Figure 16.8—Bifurcation viewed in long axis
- Trace the femoral vein distally compressing every 2 cm until just proximal to the knee.
- Next, place the transducer within the popliteal fossa and image the popliteal vein:
  - The popliteal vein will be located superficial or posterior to the popliteal artery.
  - Compress the popliteal vein and visualize complete occlusion of the vessel.
  - Figure 16.9—Popliteal vein
  - Video 16.5—Popliteal vein
- Complete the scan by fanning the transducer distally to image the trifurcation of the popliteal vein into the anterior tibial, posterior tibial, and peroneal veins:
  - Apply pressure with the transducer and visualize compression of each vein.
  - Figure 16.10—Trifurcation
  - Video 16.6—Trifurcation

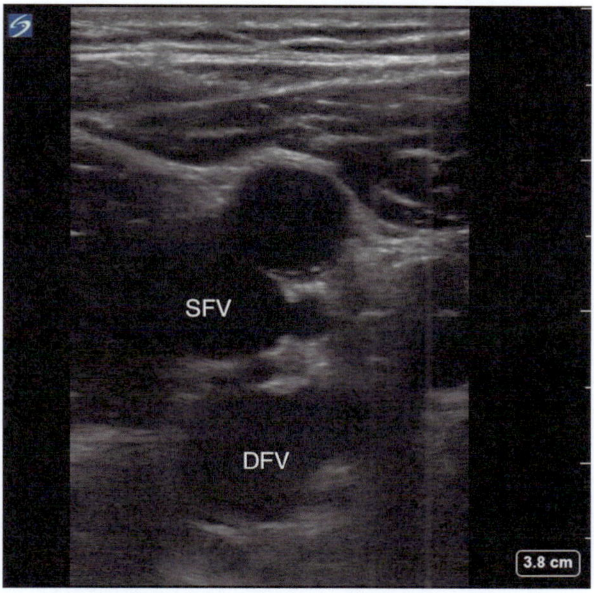

Fig. 16.7 Bifurcation with femoral and deep femoral veins. The common femoral vein bifurcates into the femoral (previously superficial femoral SFV) and deep femoral vein (DFV). The femoral vein is in the near field and the deep femoral vein is in the far field

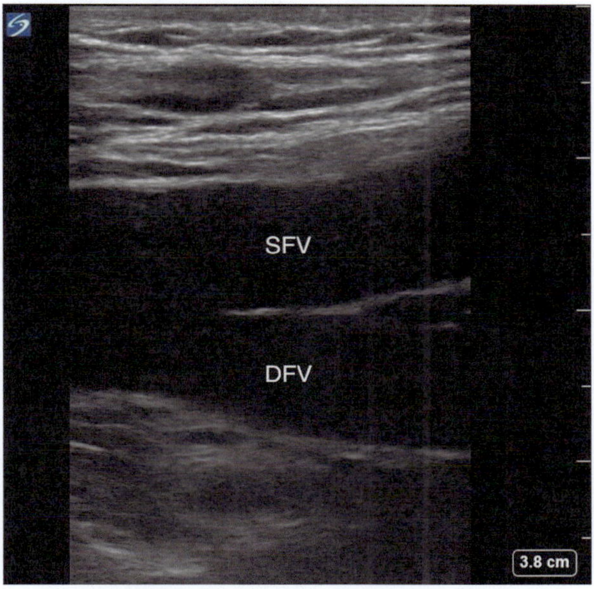

Fig. 16.8 Bifurcation in the long axis. Long axis view of the common femoral vein bifurcating into the femoral vein (previously superficial femoral vein SFV) and deep femoral vein (DFV)

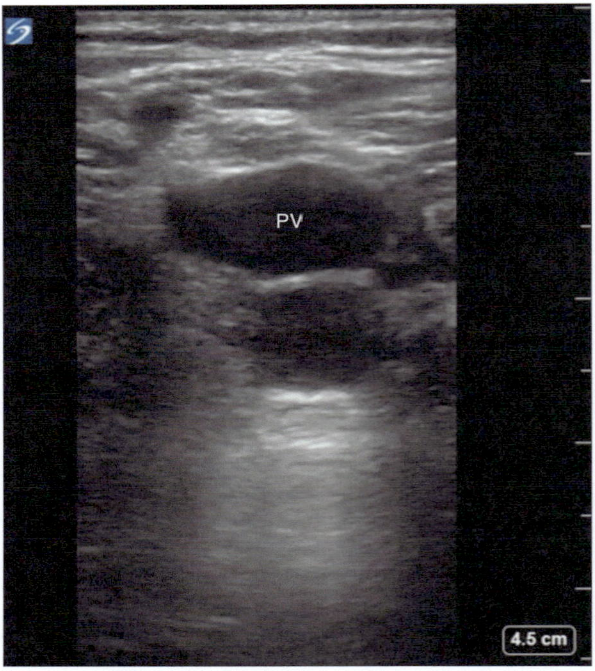

Fig. 16.9 Popliteal vein. Popliteal vein is in the near field above the popliteal artery

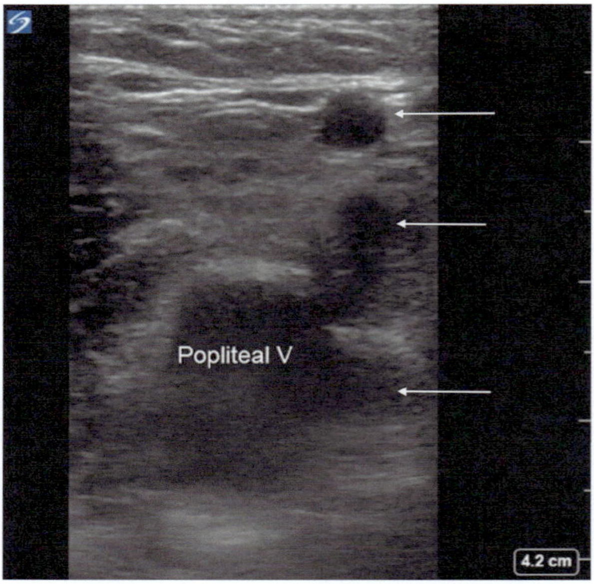

Fig. 16.10 Trifurcation. The popliteal vein trifurcates into the anterior tibial, posterior tibial, and peroneal veins within the distal popliteal fossa just before entering the proximal calf

Lower Extremity Venous Pathology

(a) Deep Vein Thrombosis
- Blood clot within one of the deep veins of the lower extremity.
- When assessing for compressibility of the deep veins, the walls of the vein must completely collapse and touch to be considered normal:
  - Figure 16.11—Completely compressed vein.
  - Video 16.7—Completely compressed vein.
- A deep vein thrombosis (DVT) will be diagnosed when the walls of the vein cannot be completely compressed:
  - Figure 16.12—Noncompressible vein.
  - Video 16.8—Noncompressible common femoral vein.
  - Video 16.9—Noncompressible deep and femoral veins.
- At times, a thrombus will be noted within the vein prior to performing a compression test:
  - An acute thrombus will most often appear hypoechoic and may be indistinguishable from a normal vein until compression testing is done.
    - Figure 16.13—Acute thrombus
    - Video 16.10—Acute thrombus

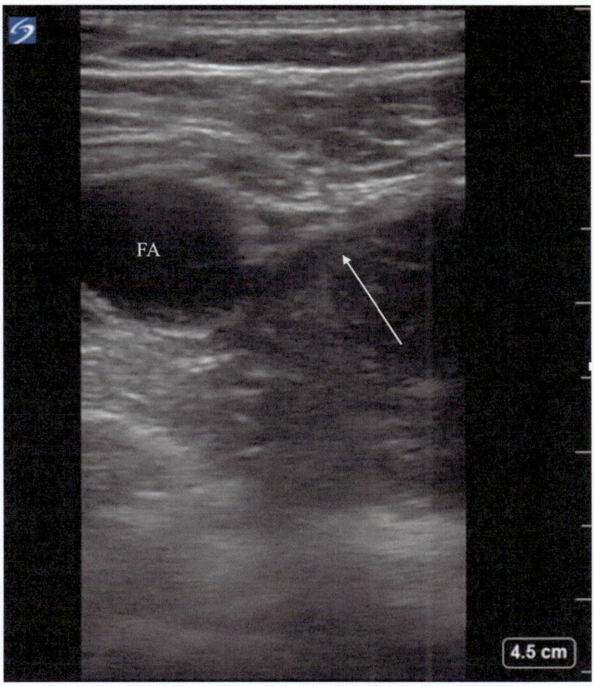

Fig. 16.11 Completely compressed vein. In the absence of a deep venous thrombosis (DVT), a vein will completely compress with direct and even pressure. The common femoral vein (CFV) here is actively collapsing under pressure. The femoral artery (FA) is seen with a slight flattening

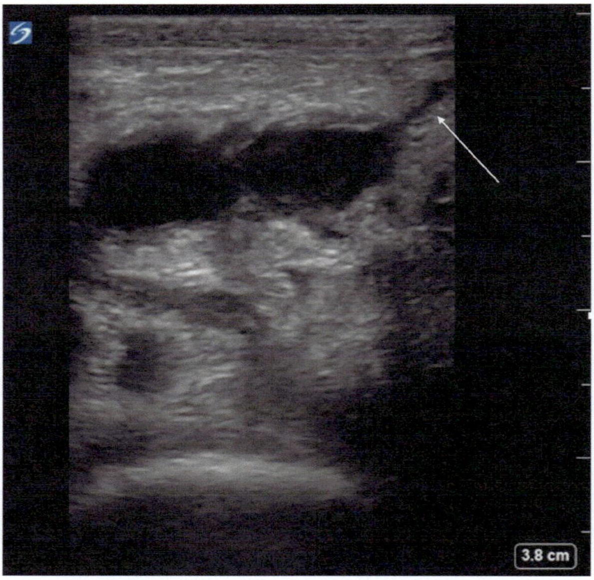

Fig. 16.12 Noncompressible vein. This vein does not collapse under pressure. Notice flattening to the top of the common femoral vein and an obvious vessel lumen, demonstrating an inability to compress the vein. This is a finding concerning for a deep vein thrombosis (DVT), especially when there is echogenic material inside the lumen of the vessel. Of note, the greater saphenous vein (arrow) is completely compressed which means enough pressure is applied to collapse the vein and there is no clot burden in this portion of the vessel

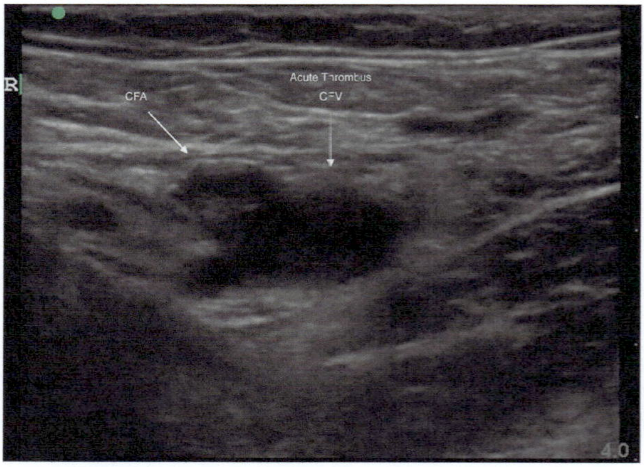

Fig. 16.13 Acute thrombus. An acute thrombus appears as a noncompressible vein with hypoechoic material within the lumen of the vein

– A chronic thrombus will appear more hyperechoic than an acute DVT:
  - It can also have a more irregular appearance than an acute thrombus [3].
  - Over time, a chronic thrombus will become recanalized centrally allowing blood to flow through the DVT [3]. This can cause the vein walls to appear thickened and irregular [5].
  - Figure 16.14—Chronic thrombus.
  - Video 16.11—Chronic thrombus.

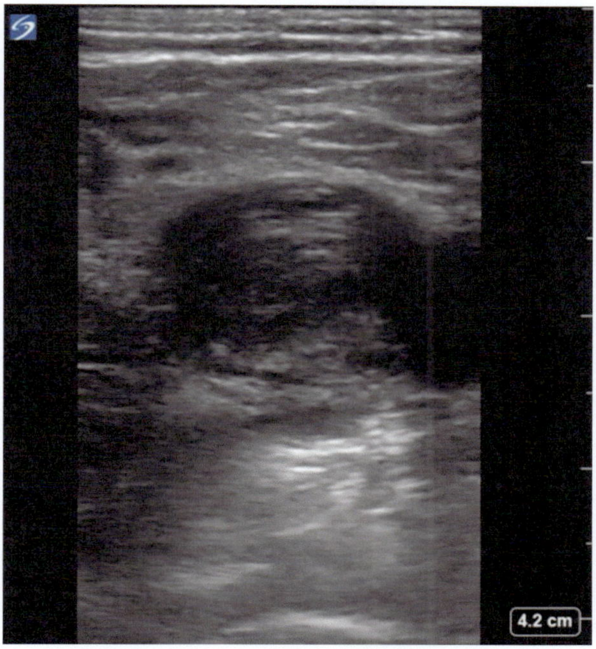

Fig. 16.14 Chronic thrombus. A chronic deep vein thrombus appears a noncompressible vein with hyperechoic material within the lumen of the vein

(b) Superficial Vein Thrombosis
  - Blood clot within a superficial vein of the lower extremity.
  - Appears similar to a DVT.
  - No indication for anticoagulation; it is recommended patients follow up for reevaluation within 1 week [3].

Key Points

- Using point-of-care ultrasound to evaluate patients in the emergency department has been shown to decrease length of stay when compared with patients who receive studies performed by the radiology department [6].
- Classically, the femoral vein lies medial to the femoral artery; however, a common anatomic variant is for the femoral artery to travel anterior to the femoral vein, though this may be dependent on patient positioning [3].
- Veins collapse easily with pressure. If you cannot visualize a vein, apply less pressure with the transducer.
- Apply direct and even pressure over the vein to assess its compressibility.
  - A false-positive DVT can be diagnosed if uneven pressure is applied, therefore, resulting in an inability to completely compress the vein.
  - This can also occur with patients who have larger body habitus, as it is harder to apply direct and even pressure.

- Noncompressible veins can also be seen with chronic DVTs; when a DVT recannulates, it can cause the walls of the vein to become stiffer and less responsive to compression.
- Do not rely on visualization of the clot for diagnosis of a DVT as the appearance changes with maturation; if a vein does not completely compress, this is diagnostic of a DVT even if no thrombus is visualized within the lumen [4].
- While a chronic DVT may appear more echogenic with thickened irregular walls, these findings may not be present, and it may not be possible to distinguish an acute from a chronic thrombus [5].
- Point-of-care ultrasound for DVT without the use of color Doppler can be less reliable in patients with recurrent DVT; approximately half of ultrasounds may remain abnormal for up to a year after initial diagnosis of a DVT [7].

References

1. Di Nisio M, van Es N, Buller HR. Deep vein thrombosis and pulmonary embolism. Lancet. 2016;388:3060–73.
2. Kearon C, Ageno W, Cannegieters SC, Cosmi B, Geersing G-J, Kyrle PA, for The Subcommittees on Control of Anticoagulation and Predictiev and Diagnostic Variables in Thrombotic Disease. Categorization of patients as having provoked or unprovoked VTE: guidance from the SSC of ISTH. J Thromb Haemost. 2016;14:1–4.
3. Costantino TG, Goett HJ, Peterson MA. Chapter 17: deep venous thrombosis. In: Ma OJ, Mateer JR, Reardon RF, Joing SA, editors. Emergency ultrasound. 3rd ed. Beijing: McGraw-Hill Education; 2014. p. 479–502.
4. Del Rios M, Lewiss RE, Saul T. Focus on: emergency ultrasound for deep vein thrombosis. ACEP News website March 2009. https://www.acep.org/clinical-practice-management/focus-on-emergency-ultrasound-for-deep-vein-thrombosis/.
5. Katz DS, Fruauff K, Kranz AO, Hon M. Imaging of deep venous thrombosis: a multimodality overview. Applied Radiology website. http://appliedradiology.com/articles/imaging-of-deep-venous-thrombosis-a-multimodality-overview. 5 March 2014.
6. Lewiss RE, Kaban NL, Saul T. Point-of-care ultrasound for a deep venous thrombosis. Glob Heart. 2013;8(3):329–33. http://www.sciencedirect.com/science/article/pii/S2211816013001646
7. Bassi B, Nickels LC, Flach FE, DePortu G, Ganti L. Acute on chronic venous thromboembolism on therapeutic anticoagulation. Case Rep Emerg Med. 2013;2013:295261. 3 pages. https://doi.org/10.1155/2013/295261.

17 Skin and Soft Tissue Ultrasound

Holly Farkosh, Angela Lindsay, Michael Joyce, and Jordan Tozer

Ultrasonography is routinely used for the evaluation of skin and soft tissue complaints. It is relatively easy to perform due to the superficial location of each structure, allowing for high-frequency imaging, thereby producing high-resolution, detailed images. Commonly, ultrasound is used to evaluate for abscess, cellulitis, and foreign bodies within the skin and soft tissue, as well as to determine the optimal location for and real-time guidance of bedside aspiration or incision and drainage procedures. Ultrasound is useful and efficient in the diagnosis of necrotizing fasciitis, a life-threatening condition that requires timely recognition. This chapter will review basic skin and soft tissue anatomy, image acquisition, normal ultrasound anatomy, and interpretation of pathology.

Clinical Application and Indications

- Evaluate for soft tissue infections or septic thrombophlebitis.
- Evaluate soft tissue mass for abscess, hematoma, lymph nodes, or cyst.
- Identify foreign bodies.

Supplementary Information The online version contains supplementary material available at https://doi.org/10.1007/978-3-032-27643-8_17.

H. Farkosh (✉)
Department of Emergency Medicine, Virginia Commonwealth University Medical Center, Richmond, VA, USA
e-mail: Holly.Farkosh@vcuhealth.org

A. Lindsay (✉) · M. Joyce · J. Tozer
Department of Emergency Medicine, Virginia Commonwealth University Health, Richmond, VA, USA
e-mail: Angela.Creditt@vcuhealth.org; John.Joyce@vcuhealth.org; jordan.tozer@vcuhealth.org

A. Lindsay et al. (eds.), *Clinical Ultrasound*,
https://doi.org/10.1007/978-3-032-27643-8_17

Normal Skin and Soft Tissue Anatomy

- From superficial to deep: epidermis, dermis, and hypodermis (also called subcutaneous fascia) containing fat and blood vessels, fascia, muscle, and bone.
  - Deeper tissues (muscle and bone) are described in the musculoskeletal chapter.

Image Acquisition

(a) Transducer Selection
  - Linear array transducer for most applications.
    - High-frequency transducers provide better-resolution images of superficial structures of interest.
  - Curvilinear for evaluation of deeper structures in larger habitus patients.

(b) Patient Position
  - Depends on the location to be evaluated.
  - Utilization of a water bath is ideal for hand, finger, foot, or toe evaluation.
    - Place the area of interest within a basin filled with just enough water to submerge the area entirely, and then place just the tip of the transducer into the water over the affected area.
    - This will allow you to visualize the structure without having to apply direct pressure to the area, as well as visualize very superficial findings [1].
    - Figure 17.1—Water bath positioning.
    - Figure 17.2—Water bath ultrasound.

(c) Standard Exam Views
  - Scan through the area in two planes 90° apart to obtain both transverse and sagittal views.
  - Begin the exam over normal tissue (either adjacent to or on the opposite side of the area of interest) to identify normal anatomy.
    - From superficial to deep.

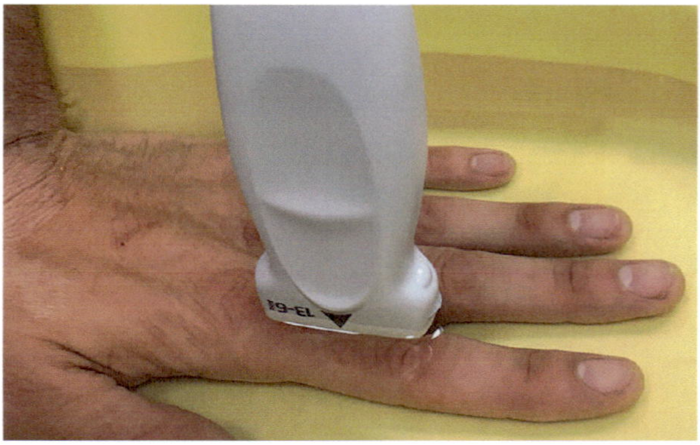

Fig. 17.1 Water bath positioning. To facilitate visualization of small parts, have the patient place the affected area in a container of water, and hover the probe over the area of interest

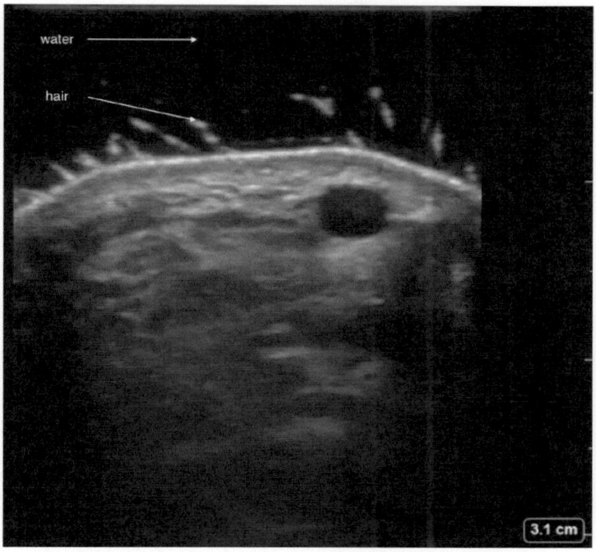

Fig. 17.2 Water bath ultrasound. Dorsal hand ultrasound using a water bath showing separation of transducer from the tissue of interest

    - Epidermis and dermis will appear as thin hyperechoic bands at the top of the screen [2].
    - Hypodermis, containing subcutaneous tissue, is more anechoic and thicker [2]; on occasion, blood vessels can be seen within this layer
    - Fascia will appear as a thin hyperechoic line [2].
    - Muscle will be visualized as a hypoechoic striated band; depending on this location, this can be thick or thin.
    - Bone will have a brightly echogenic surface with posterior acoustic shadowing.
  - Figure 17.3—Soft tissue layers.
  - Video 17.1—Normal skin and soft tissue ultrasound.
- Scan toward the affected area to evaluate for pathology.
- Obtain size measurements of any abnormal mass or fluid collection using the caliper ruler function.

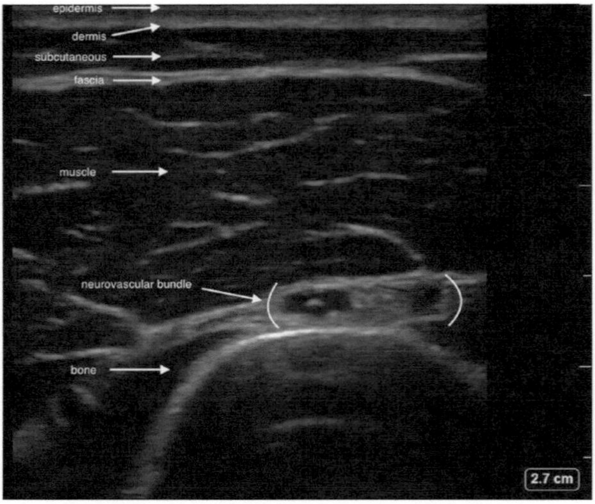

Fig. 17.3 Soft tissue layers. Soft tissue layers identified from superficial to deep including epidermis, dermis, subcutaneous tissue (hypodermis), fascia, muscle, and bone

Skin and Soft Tissue Pathology

- Cellulitis
  - Disruption of the skin with invasion of bacteria causing an infection of the dermis and subcutaneous fat.
  - Cellulitis can be identified by increased echogenicity and thickening of the subcutaneous tissue with hyperechoic areas of inflamed soft tissue outlined by hypoechoic fluid between these areas [1, 2].
    - This is referred to as cobblestoning [1], and these findings are due to the accumulation of subcutaneous edema.
    - It is important to note that cobblestoning alone is not diagnostic of cellulitis as it is nonspecific and may be seen with abscess, necrotizing fasciitis, and lymphedema.
  - Figure 17.4—Cellulitis.
  - Video 17.2—Cellulitis.
  - Figure 17.5—Cellulitis with increased soft tissue edema.
  - Video 17.3—Cellulitis with increased soft tissue edema.
- Abscess
  - Walled off bacterial infection resulting in a collection of purulent fluid.
  - Will be identified most commonly as an irregularly shaped hypoechoic fluid collection containing debris [1].
    - Figure 17.6—Abscess
    - Video 17.4—Abscess
  - Internal swirling of the fluid will typically occur with compression and can help distinguish a fluid-filled collection from solid mass.
    - Video 17.5—Abscess with internal swirling from compression

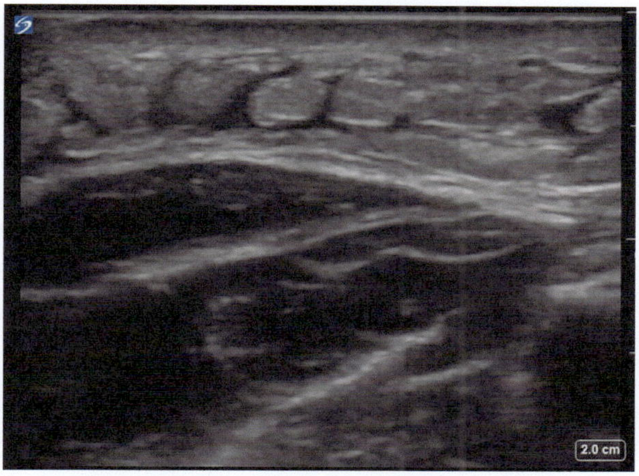

Fig. 17.4 Cellulitis. Cellulitis typically appears as cobblestoning of the subcutaneous tissue with associated thickening of the dermal layers

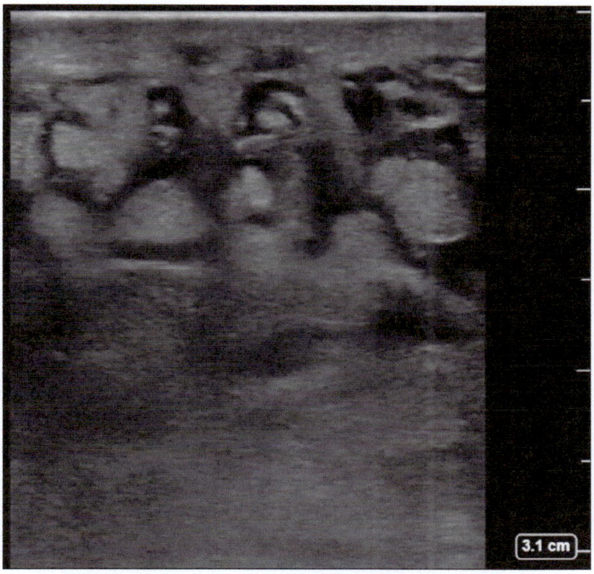

Fig. 17.5 Cellulitis with increased soft tissue edema. As cellulitis becomes more severe or with concomitant edema, there will be increased fluid within the subcutaneous tissue visualized by thicker anechoic pockets

- Abscesses will not exhibit internal Doppler flow, which can help distinguish an abscess from mimics such as lymph nodes, pseudoaneurysms, and solid tumors.
- It can be helpful to utilize US for guidance in approach to bedside incision and drainage (I&D) or needle aspiration in order to choose the optimal entrance site and avoid surrounding structures such as blood vessels.
- Air in the abscess cavity is significant for gas-forming organisms and will need emergent treatment.

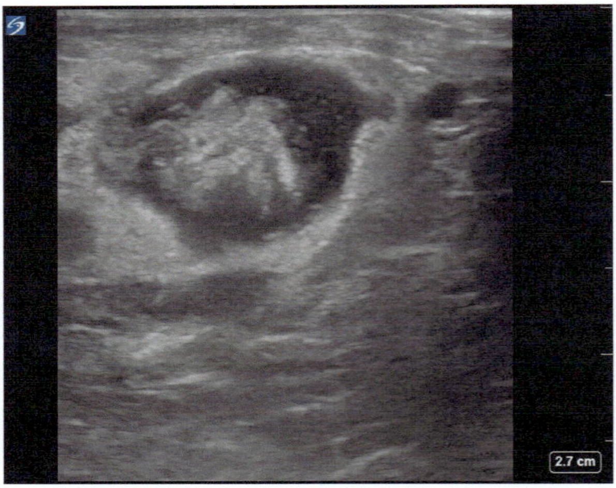

Fig. 17.6 Abscess. Hypoechoic fluid collection with thick echogenic material representing a small abscess

    - This can be identified as echogenic areas within the abscess cavity [2] with dirty posterior shadowing and posterior reverberations.
  - Ultrasound can also be used to diagnose and treat peritonsillar abscess. Please see Chap. 7: Head and Neck Ultrasound.
- Necrotizing Fasciitis
  - Severe infection that causes death of tissue and spreads rapidly along the fascial planes with associated significant morbidity and mortality.
  - Standard confirmatory imaging includes CT and MRI; however, these are time consuming and/or may be unavailable, in a situation where time to diagnosis matters [3].
  - Early necrotizing fasciitis will often resemble cellulitis with a cobblestone appearance, though overlying skin changes may not always be present, requiring high clinical suspicion to evaluate.
  - A helpful proposed mnemonic in ultrasound diagnosis of necrotizing fasciitis is to look for STAFF: Subcutaneous Thickening, Air, and Fascial Fluid [4].
  - In advanced cases, the skin will be thickened, and the fascia will appear thickened and brightly echogenic with adjacent accumulation of fluid [2, 5, 6].
    - A fluid layer measuring greater than 4 mm deep to the fascia greatly increases the likelihood for the diagnosis of necrotizing fasciitis [2, 5].
    - Figure 17.7—Necrotizing fasciitis with perifascial fluid
    - Video 17.6—Necrotizing fasciitis with perifascial fluid
  - The presence of air in the soft tissue only occurs if gas-forming organisms are present and is the key ultrasound finding for this process; air will appear as dirty shadowing with reverberation artifact [2].
    - Figure 17.8—Necrotizing fasciitis with dirty shadowing
- Hematoma
  - Collection of blood, usually due to trauma or in patients who have had a recent procedure, such as cardiac catheterization.

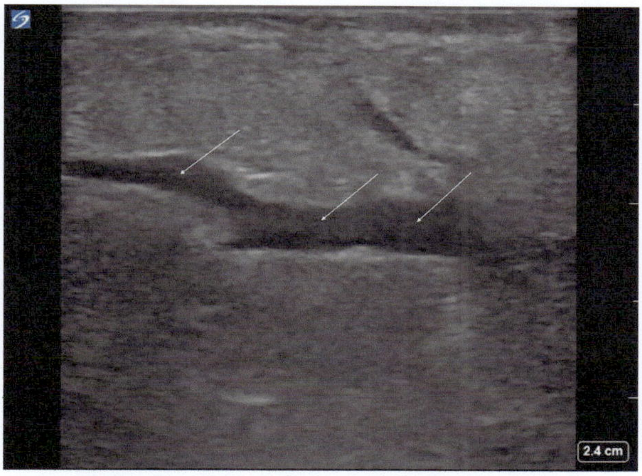

Fig. 17.7 Necrotizing fasciitis with perifascial fluid. Fluid tracking along the fascial plane with thickened subcutaneous tissue and a loss of normal architecture. Perifascial fluid greater than 4 mm likely indicates a diagnosis of necrotizing fasciitis

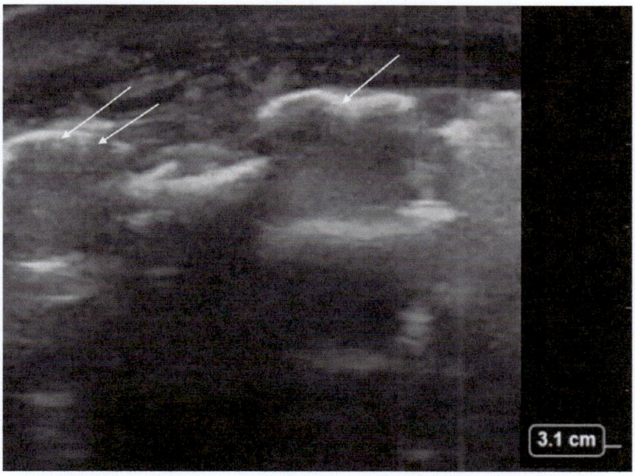

Fig. 17.8 Necrotizing fasciitis with subcutaneous air. Necrotizing fasciitis can be a subtle entity to diagnose with ultrasound. In the presence of gas-forming bacteria, it will be visualized by identifying dirty shadowing (arrows) caused by air-tissue interface

  - Hypoechoic fluid collection, often with a layered appearance [7].
  - May resemble an abscess, but clinical history can help differentiate soft tissue fluid collections.
  - Figure 17.9—Hematoma.
  - Video 17.7—Hematoma.
- Foreign Body
  - Use the linear transducer for the highest resolution. Often easiest to see when the foreign body is in the longitudinal axis, which allows visualization of the foreign body's entire length. Can be subtle and easily missed when foreign bodies are very small or mistaken for similarly appearing structures [8].
  - Will appear as hyperechoic as compared with the surrounding structures.
  - Wood or plastic foreign bodies will generally have posterior shadowing [2].
    - Figure 17.10—Wood or plastic foreign body with posterior shadowing
  - Metal objects will have comet tail artifacts or posterior reverberations [2].

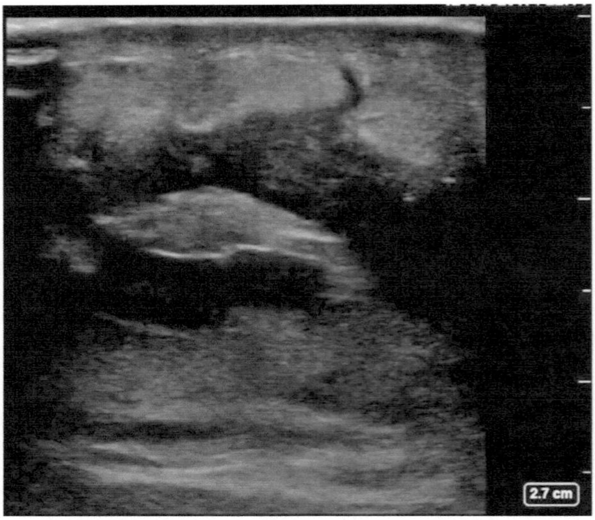

Fig. 17.9 Hematoma. Hypoechoic fluid collection representing abdominal hematoma. On ultrasound, may be indistinguishable from abscess

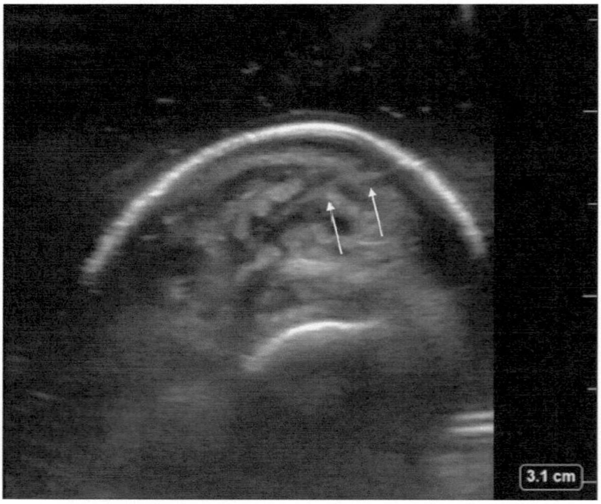

Fig. 17.10 Foreign body. Finger ultrasound in water bath with embedded foreign body (arrows)

  - Figure 17.11—Metal foreign body
  - Video 17.8—Metal foreign body long axis
  - Video 17.9—Metal foreign body short axis
- Pyomyositis
  - An uncommon deep infection where an abscess forms in the belly of muscle, between fascial layers.
  - Often difficult to diagnose clinically as patients may not have overlying skin changes or a palpable area of fluctuance [9].
  - The gold standard imaging modality for diagnosis is MRI; however, ultrasound provides a more timely diagnosis and expedition of management in a setting where MRI may not always be available [9, 10].

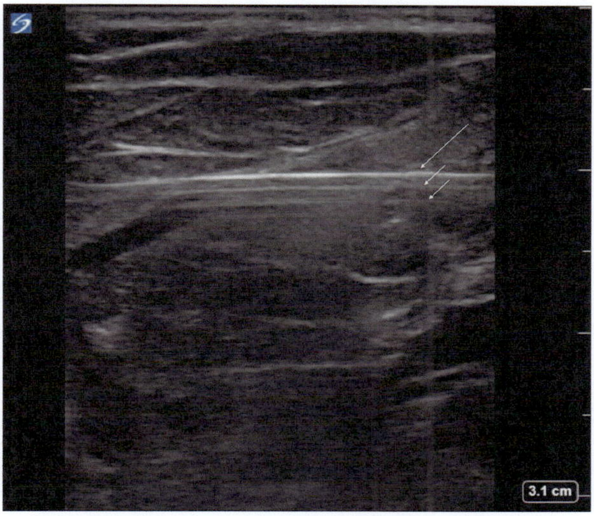

Fig. 17.11 Metal foreign body. Brightly echogenic foreign body represents a broken needle within the neck of a patient from intravenous drug abuse

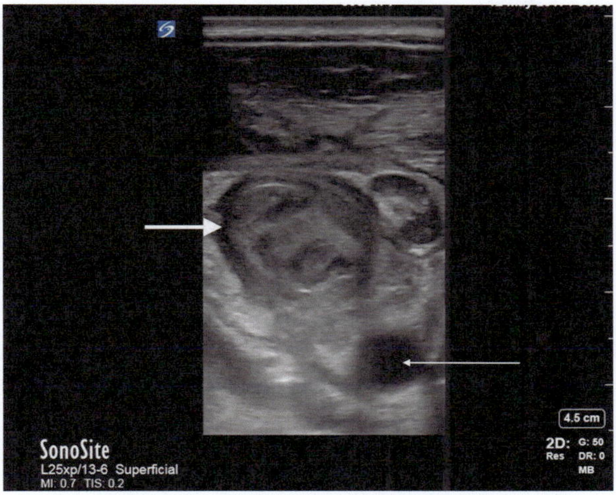

Fig. 17.12 Septic Thrombophlebitis. Internal jugular (IJ) vein containing thrombus (large arrow) with surrounding cobblestoning consistent with septic thrombophlebitis. The carotid artery (small arrow) can also be visualized deep to the IJ vein

  - These will appear similarly to subcutaneous abscesses as described above, with a complex hypoechoic structure noted between fascial layers with associated myofascial inflammation [10].
- Septic Thrombophlebitis
  - Infected peripheral vein thrombosis.
  - Ultrasound findings include identification of an intravascular thrombus (anechoic or echogenic structure that is noncompressible and lacks Doppler flow) with evidence of inflammation such as vessel wall thickening, perivascular inflammation, purulence, or cobblestoning [10].
  - Figure 17.12 Septic thrombophlebitis.

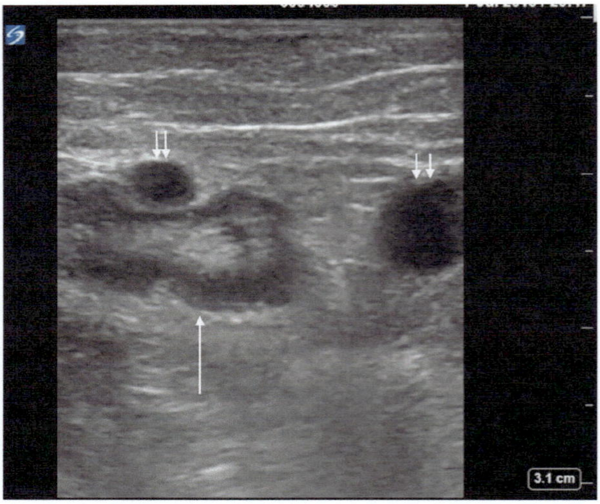

Fig. 17.13 Lymph node. Lymph node (single arrow) with hyperechoic medulla surrounded by hypoechoic cortex. Vascular structures denoted by double arrows

Key Points

- Cobblestoning can occur with other disease processes that cause edema of the soft tissue; therefore, ultrasound cannot be used to determine the presence of cellulitis in areas of existing edema.
- Soft tissue ultrasound is best used to rule in an abscess, not to rule out or diagnose cellulitis.
- Be sure to image the base of the abscess—if you are unable to visualize this, it is likely that this is not a simple superficial abscess and will require further imaging or surgical consult.
- Ultrasound cannot rule out necrotizing soft tissue infections.
- Lymph nodes can appear similar to an abscess, especially in the axilla, neck, and groin. Abscesses, unlike lymph nodes, will have swirling on compression and will not have internal color flow with application of a Doppler window:
  - Figure 17.13—Lymph node
  - Video 17.10—Lymph node

References

1. SonoSim ultrasound training solution [video]. Santa Monica: SonoSim Inc.; 2017.
2. Dewitz A. Chapter 18: musculoskeletal, soft tissue, and miscellaneous applications. In: Ma OJ, Mateer JR, Reardon RF, Joing SA, editors. Emergency ultrasound. 3rd ed. New York: McGraw-Hill Education; 2014. p. 503–68.
3. Gan RK, Sanchez Martinez A, Abu Hasan MAS, Castro Delgado R, Arcos González P. Point-of-care ultrasonography in diagnosing necrotizing fasciitis—a literature review. J Ultrasound. 2023;26(2):343–53.
4. Castleberg E, Jenson N, Dinh VA. Diagnosis of necrotizing fasciitis with bedside ultrasound: the STAFF exam. West J Emerg Med. 2014;15(1):111–3.

5. Yen Z, Wang H, Ma H, Chen S, Chen W. Ultrasonographic screening of clinically-suspected necrotizing fasciitis. Acad Emerg Med. 2002;9(12):1448–51. http://onlinelibrary.wiley.com/doi/10.1197/aemj.9.12.1448/epdf. Accessed 17 Apr 2017
6. Wronski M, Slodkowski M, Cebulski W, Karkocha D, Krasnodebski I. Necrotizing fasciitis: early sonographic diagnosis. J Clin Ultrasound. 2011;39(4):236–9. http://edus.ucsf.edu/sites/edus.ucsf.edu/files/wysiwyg/Necrotizing%20fasciitis%3A%20Early%20sonographic%20diagnosis.pdf. Accessed 17 Apr 2017
7. Jacobson JA. Chapter 6: hip and thigh ultrasound. In: Jacobson JA, editor. Fundamentals of musculoskeletal ultrasound. 2nd ed. Philadelphia: Sanders; 2013. p. 162–211.
8. Rooks VJ, Shiels WE, Murakami JW. Soft tissue foreign bodies: a training manual for sonographic diagnosis and guided removal. J Clin Ultrasound. 2020;48(6):330–6.
9. Kumar MP, Seif D, Perera P, Mailhot T. Point-of-care ultrasound in diagnosing Pyomyositis: a report of three cases. J Emerg Med. 2014;47(4):420–6.
10. Situ-LaCasse E, Adhikari S. Soft tissue infections. In: Ma OJ, Mateer JR, Reardon RF, Byars DV, Knapp BJ, Laudenbach AP, editors. Emergency ultrasound. 4th ed. New York: McGraw Hill Education; 2021. Available from: https://accessemergencymedicine.mhmedical.com/content.aspx?bookid=2966&sectionid=249987740.

Ocular Ultrasound

18

Noah Hillerbrand, Angela Lindsay, and Lindsay Taylor

Ultrasound now gives clinicians the ability to evaluate patients with acute vision changes more efficiently and accurately. It allows the sonographer to see behind the superficial structures and assess the lens, retina, vitreous body, ocular nerve, and ocular vasculature for pathology. Some disease processes, such as retinal detachment or central retinal artery occlusion, need to be treated in a timely manner to prevent sequelae of disease and ultrasound can facilitate prompt recognition. In addition to ocular pathology, using the same technique, one can evaluate for neurologic conditions such as increased intracranial pressure. This chapter will review indications for performing an ocular ultrasound, basic ocular anatomy, image acquisition, normal ultrasound anatomy, and interpretation of pathology.

Clinical Application and Indications

- Vision loss.
- Ocular pain.
- New flashes or floaters.
- Ocular trauma.

Supplementary Information The online version contains supplementary material available at https://doi.org/10.1007/978-3-032-27643-8_18.

N. Hillerbrand
VCU Health, Department of Emergency Medicine, Richmond, VA, USA
e-mail: noah.hillerbrand@vcuhealth.org

A. Lindsay (✉) · L. Taylor
Department of Emergency Medicine, Virginia Commonwealth University Health, Richmond, VA, USA
e-mail: Angela.creditt@vcuhealth.org; Lindsay.taylor@vcuhealth.org

A. Lindsay et al. (eds.), *Clinical Ultrasound*, https://doi.org/10.1007/978-3-032-27643-8_18

- Evaluate for vitreoretinal disorders such as foreign body, vitreous hemorrhage, vitreous detachment, retinal detachment, and lens dislocation or subluxation.
- Evaluate for increased intracranial pressure (ICP) or papilledema.

Normal Ocular Anatomy

- Superficial Ocular Anatomy.
  - Conjunctiva is a transparent membrane that covers the surface of the eye and inner surface of the eyelids.
  - Sclera covers almost the entire surface of the eye (except for the cornea) and is white in appearance.
  - Cornea is located on the central portion of the eye and is confluent with the sclera.
- Intraocular Anatomy.
  - Anterior chamber is a fluid-filled space bordered by the cornea anteriorly and the iris and pupil posteriorly.
  - Iris is a disc-shaped structure located posterior to the cornea that gives color to the eye with a hole in the middle giving rise to the pupil.
  - Posterior to the pupil is the lens, a biconvex structure.
  - Vitreous body encompasses a large space between the lens and retina; it is composed of vitreous humor, which is a gelatinous substance.
  - Retina is a thin membrane that courses along the posterior inner wall of the orbit and is adhered at the optic disc and the ora serrata.
  - Optic nerve originates posterior to the globe and is surrounded by the optic nerve sheath.
  - Macula is lateral to the optic nerve.
  - Central retinal artery arises from the ophthalmic artery and courses in the middle of the optic nerve.

Image Acquisition

(a) Transducer Selection.
  - Linear array transducer.

(b) Patient Position.
  - Patient should be supine with the head of the bed at approximately 30°.
  - The patient's head should be tilted upward, so the plane of the orbit is relatively horizontal to the ground.
  - Apply at least a centimeter of gel on the patient's eye to prevent compression of the globe. A recent study showed significantly decreased image quality with use of a transparent adhesive membrane over the eye, without a difference in patient-rated discomfort [6].
  - Be careful not to apply pressure on the patient's eye—you can rest your hand on the patient's face or nose for ease of scanning.
  - Figure 18.1—Patient position.

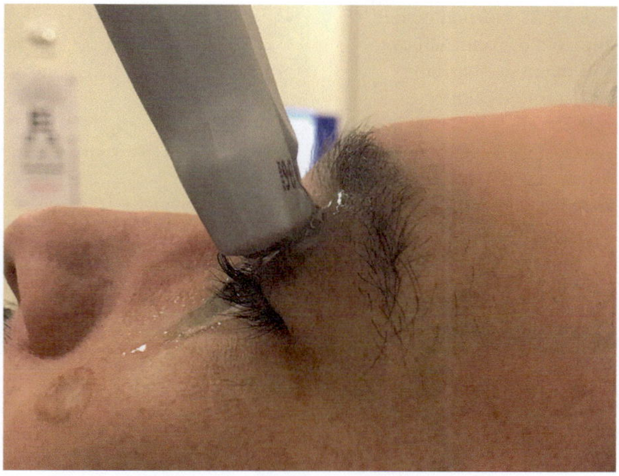

Fig. 18.1 Patient position. Lean the patient's head back and apply a copious amount of gel on top of a closed eyelid

(c) Standard Exam Views
- Image the eye in both transverse and sagittal planes.
- Place the transducer on the patient's eye with the transducer marker pointed toward the patient's right to obtain a transverse view:
  - Visualize the eye with the anterior chamber seen superficially, and the lens posterior to this followed by the posterior chamber and retina.
  - Vitreous body, which makes up most of the posterior chamber, is anechoic.
  - Optic nerve courses from the posterior globe and is surrounded by the optic nerve sheath.
  - The central retinal artery and central retinal vein can be seen in the center of the optic nerve; these structures can be identified by using color Doppler.
  - Have the patient look from side to side with their eyes closed for dynamic imaging; this will enable visualization of otherwise subtle findings such as vitreous detachment, retinal detachment, or vitreous hemorrhage.
  - Figure 18.2—Normal eye and normal eye with labels.
  - Video 18.1—Normal eye.
- Rotate the transducer 90° so the transducer marker is pointed cephalad:
  - Visualize the same anatomy as in the transverse view.
  - Have the patient look up and down with their eyes closed.
- Obtain an optic nerve sheath diameter (ONSD) measurement bilaterally:
  - This measurement is used to assess for increased intracranial pressure.
  - Identify the optic nerve and its accompanying nerve sheath:
    - The nerve is hypoechoic and will be flanked on both sides by its more hyperechoic sheath.
    - Figure 18.3—Optic nerve
  - Measure the diameter 3 mm posterior to the optic disc [1] and obtain the measurement from inner-edge to inner-edge.
  - Normal ONSD is up to 5.7 mm in diameter [2, 3].
  - Figure 18.4—ONSD measurement.

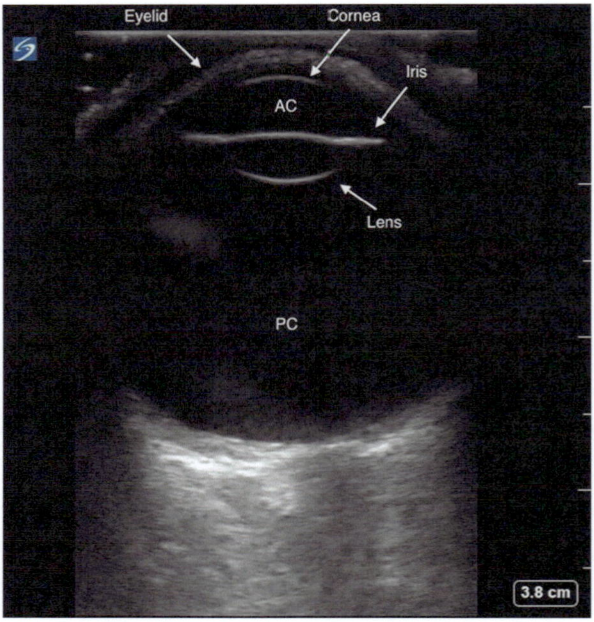

Fig. 18.2 Normal ocular ultrasound. A normal eye will maintain its shape with a round cornea, anterior chamber, iris, lens, and posterior chamber. Adjust the depth to visualize the entire globe and optic nerve

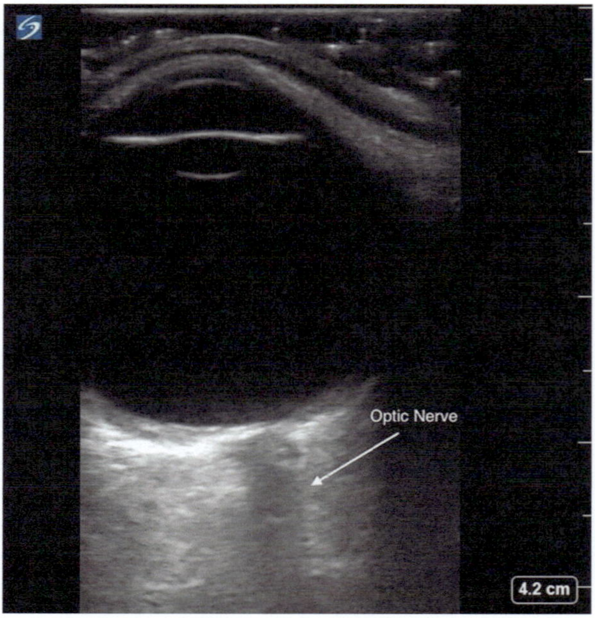

Fig. 18.3 Optic nerve. The nerve is hypoechoic and will be flanked on both sides by its more hyperechoic sheath

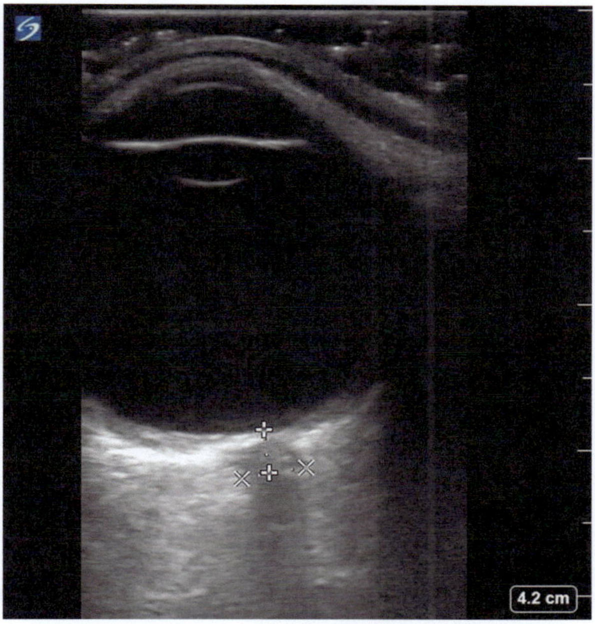

Fig. 18.4 ONSD measurement. Measure the diameter 3 mm posterior to the optic disc

Ocular Pathology

- Globe Rupture
  - While suspected globe rupture was previously considered a contraindication to ocular ultrasound, expert opinion now suggests that with ample gel, no applied pressure, and great care, it is reasonable to evaluate for changes in globe shape suggestive of open globe in cases when physical exam is limited (e.g., severe, traumatic periorbital edema). Research has shown that increases in IOP from ocular POCUS are minimal, transient, and less than diurnal variation in the healthy subjects studied [8].
  - Sonographic signs consistent with globe rupture include flattening of the anterior chamber, decreased globe size compared to contralateral side, scleral buckling, and asymmetric volume loss leading to nonspherical shape.
  - Globe rupture is often associated with vitreous hemorrhage.
- Vitreous Hemorrhage
  - Extravasation of blood into the posterior chamber.
  - Most commonly due to posterior vitreous detachment (PVD), however, it can also be due to trauma or even be idiopathic.
  - Appears as echogenic debris within the posterior chamber, which may appear as layering of echogenic material posteriorly [2].
  - May only be visualized during dynamic eye imaging as swirling of echogenic debris while the eye is moving, known as "washing machine sign".
  - Figure 18.5—Vitreous hemorrhage.
  - Video 18.2—Vitreous hemorrhage.

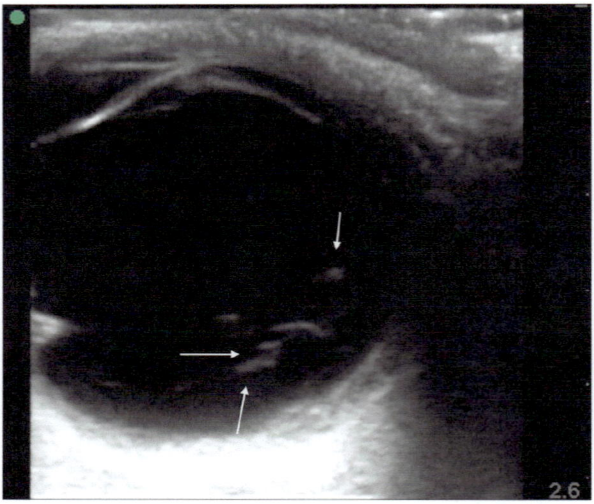

Fig. 18.5 Vitreous hemorrhage. During dynamic movement of the eye, echogenic debris (*arrows*) swirls in the posterior chamber of the eye

- Retinal Detachment (RD)
  - Separation of the retina from the underlying epithelium, resulting in ischemia and photoreceptor damage.
  - Appears as a thick echogenic/hyperechoic band floating in the posterior chamber.
  - Associated retinal hemorrhage can appear as additional hyperechoic material posterior to the detached retinal flap.
  - With dynamic eye movements, there will be little movement of the echogenic band, which will remain attached to an area near the optic nerve and the ora serrata [1]. The presence of these attachment points helps to differentiate a retinal detachment from a posterior vitreous detachment.
  - It is important to attempt to identify if the retina is still attached at the macula, as this impacts management by the consulting ophthalmology service.
    - When the retina remains attached at the macula, "mac on", emergent repair is required to save central and high-acuity vision and prevent progression of the detachment to include the macula, "mac off".
    - The macula is located temporally/laterally from the optic nerve.
  - Figure 18.6—Retinal detachment.
  - Video 18.3—Retinal detachment.
- Posterior Vitreous Detachment (PVD)
  - Degenerative process in which the vitreous gel loses its attachment to the membrane.
  - Increase the gain to identify PVD, which will appear as a smooth, thin membrane and echogenic material within the posterior chamber.
  - With dynamic movements of the eye, echogenic material will swirl within the posterior chamber [2].
  - Can be confused with retinal detachment.
    - The retina will remain attached at the optic nerve or ora serrata.

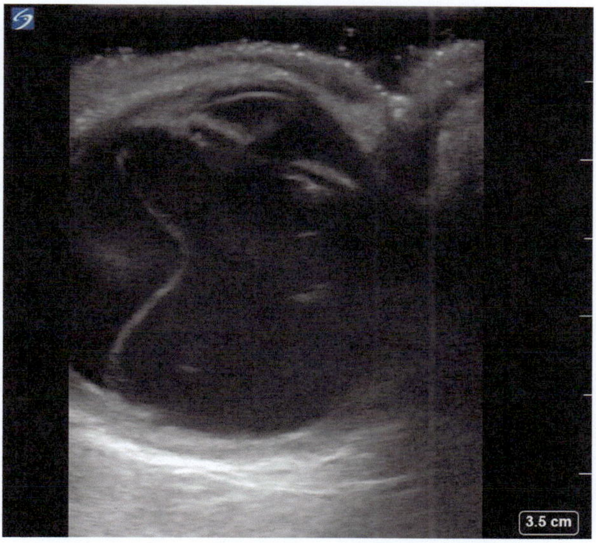

Fig. 18.6 Retinal detachment. Thick echogenic band posteriorly. With dynamic eye movements, you will see that the retina is attached to an area near the optic nerve and the ora serrata

  - Figure 18.7—Posterior vitreous detachment.
  - Video 18.4—Posterior vitreous detachment.
- Retrobulbar Hematoma
  - Collection of blood posterior to the globe that appears hypoechoic compared to the surrounding tissue.
  - Retrobulbar hematoma can distort the globe due to pressure caused by the hematoma on the eye [1]. Coined the "guitar pick sign", as it results from the conical deformation of the posterior ocular globe. Globe shape has been shown to normalize after appropriate therapy (i.e., lateral canthotomy/cantholysis) and return to appropriate spherical shape [7].
  - Figure 18.8—Retrobulbar hematoma.
- Lens Dislocation
  - With a complete dislocation, the lens will not be seen in its usual central location just posterior to the anterior chamber.
  - Figure 18.9—Lens dislocation.
  - Video 18.5—Lens dislocation.
  - Lens subluxation, or partial dislocation, can also occur.
    - Lens may appear to be in its normal location; however, with eye movement the lens will move independently of other ocular structures [1].
    - Video 18.6—Lens subluxation
- Foreign Body
  - Foreign bodies appear as hyperechoic structures located within the vitreous body or embedded in the superficial structures of the eye.
  - Likely accompanied by a vitreous hemorrhage with posterior acoustic shadowing.

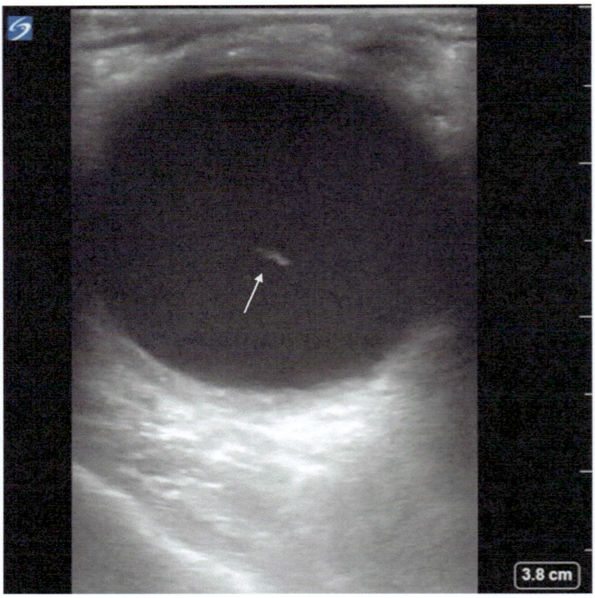

Fig. 18.7 Posterior vitreous detachment. With increased gain the PVD (*arrow*) will appear as a smooth, thin membrane. This echogenic membrane is freely mobile with dynamic movements of the eye without attachment to the optic disc, such as with retinal detachment

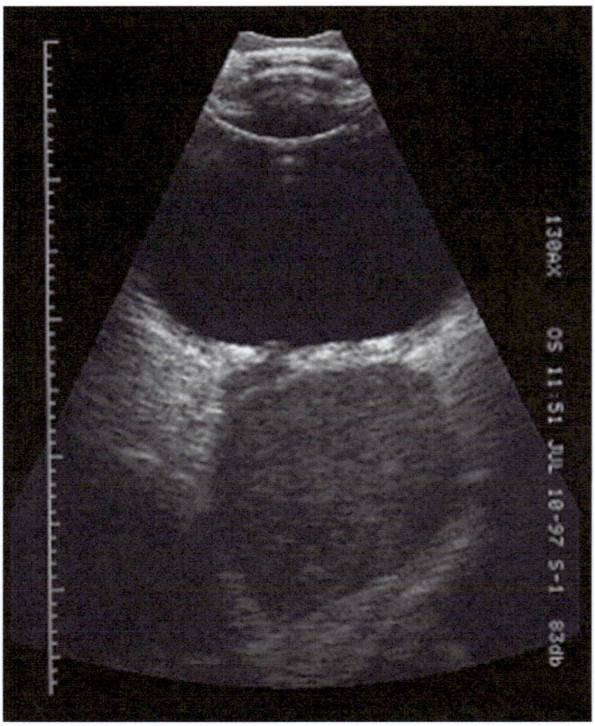

Fig. 18.8 Retrobulbar hematoma. Echolucency posterior to the globe. It often takes the shape of a guitar pick

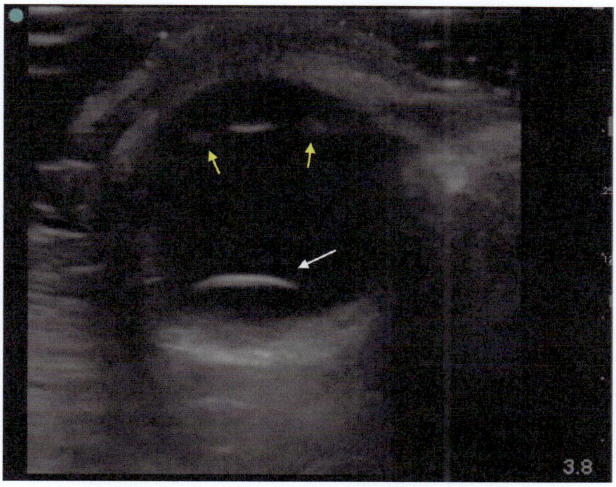

Fig. 18.9 Lens dislocation. In this complete dislocation, the lens is seen at the bottom of the posterior chamber (*white arrow*). Note absence of the lens in its typical location near the ciliary bodies (*yellow arrows*)

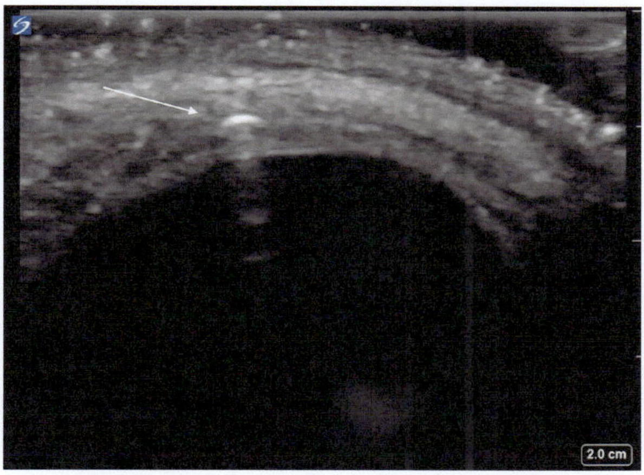

Fig. 18.10 Foreign body. Hyperechoic material within the outer surface of the eye (*arrow*). Metal objects will demonstrate reverberation artifact posterior to the foreign body

  - May be superior to x-ray examination for recognition of non-radiopaque objects (wood, plastic).
    - Figure 18.10—Foreign body
    - Video 18.7—Foreign body
- Central Retinal Artery Occlusion
  - Utilize color Doppler just posterior to the globe to evaluate blood supply.
  - Figure 18.11—Central retinal artery color and pulsed wave Doppler may also visualize an area of echogenicity centrally within the optic nerve sheath just posterior to the optic disc, termed retrobulbar spot sign [4]
    - Figure 18.12—Central retinal artery occlusion, B-mode
- Increased Optic Nerve Sheath Diameter
  - Defined as greater than 5.7 mm in diameter, however, this measurement can vary depending on source [2, 3]. More commonly, up to 5.0 mm in diameter

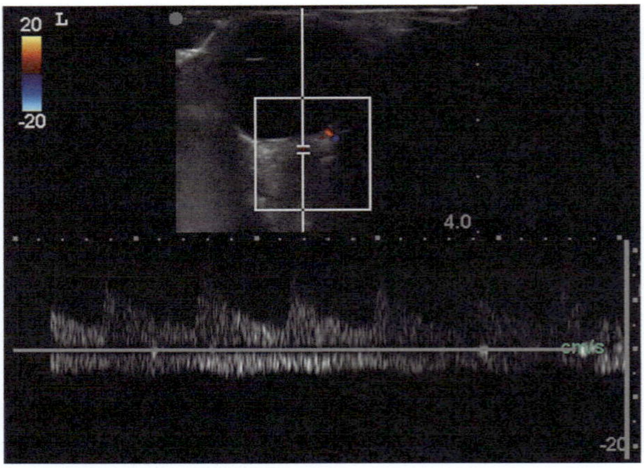

Fig. 18.11 Central retinal artery color and pulsed wave Doppler. Utilize color and/or pulsed wave Doppler just posterior to the globe to evaluate blood supply. Color is present within the Doppler gates. This is an example of central retinal artery waveform

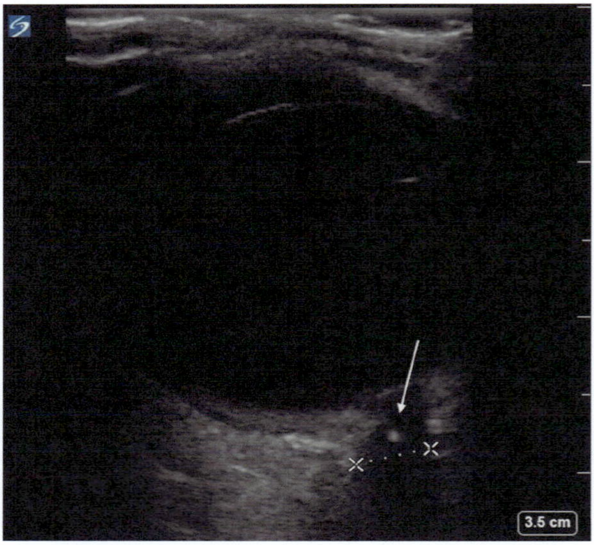

Fig. 18.12 Central retinal artery occlusion, B-mode. A hyperdense echogenicity located in the center of the retinal artery just posterior to the optic disc; commonly termed retrobulbar spot sign (*arrow*)

is considered normal and greater than 6.0 mm in diameter is considered abnormal, with between 5.0 mm and 6.0 mm being somewhat of a "grey zone."

- Above 5.0 mm in diameter, ONSD appears to increase linearly with increased ICP.
- Predicts an increased intracranial pressure of greater than 20 mmHg [2].
- With severe increases in ICP, the optic nerve sheath can separate from the optic nerve. This will appear as a hyperechoic circle within the optic nerve sheath, called the "crescent sign" and is more commonly seen in chronic ICP elevation rather than acute [1].

– Increased ONSD bilaterally can indicate increased intracranial pressure of greater than 20 mmHg [2]; if unilateral, it may indicate optic neuritis.

- In children greater than 1 year of age, increased intracranial pressure can be identified by ONSD greater than 4.5 mm [1, 2]; in children less than 1 year of age, ONSD greater than 4.0 mm suggests increased ICP [1].
- Figure 18.13—Increased ONSD.
- Elevation of the Optic Disc.
- Most commonly defined as 0.6 mm elevation, maximizing sensitivity.
- Similar to ONSD, elevation of the optic disc can represent a direct transmission of elevated ICP through subarachnoid space to the anterior optic nerve [5].
- Elevation of the optic disc may also be seen in optic neuritis [3].
- When combined with measurement of ONSD (as above), yields increased sensitivity and specificity of elevated ICP.
- Figure 18.14 Elevation of the Optic Disc [5]

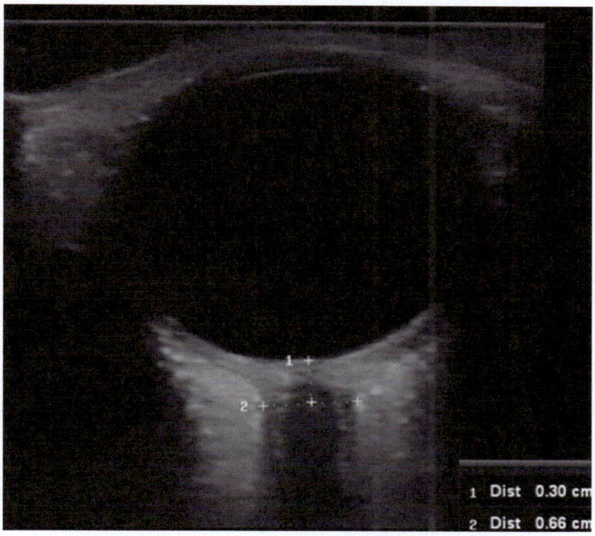

Fig. 18.13 Increased ONSD. Greater than 5.7 mm in diameter is considered pathologic

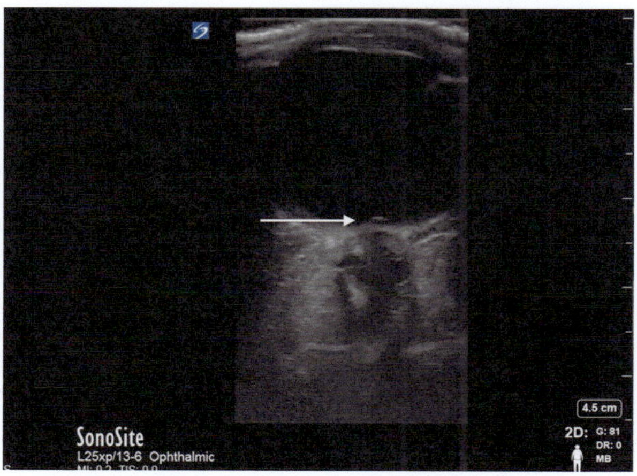

Fig. 18.14 Elevation of the optic disc (arrow). Greater than 0.6 mm suggests elevated ICP. Can be combined with measurement of the ONSD for increased specificity

Image of Papilledema GOES Here

- Pseudopapilledema: optic nerve edema caused by etiologies other than elevated ICP presents on ultrasound as increased ONSD or optic disc elevation in the absence of elevated ICP.
  - Optic Disc Drusen: Genetic disorder leading to deposition of proteins within the optic disc that become calcified with age. Patients are typically asymptomatic. On ultrasound, it commonly presents with elevated optic disc, but asymmetric in severity. Typically presents with normal ONSD and can be distinguished by the presence of hyperechoic calcifications within the optic disc and associated posterior shadowing.
- Optic Neuropathy
  - Commonly presents as unilateral increased ONSD or elevation of the optic disc; however, this may be bilateral in systemic disease. Similar to cases of elevated ICP, ONSD >5.0 mm is considered abnormal, or in the case of unilateral symptoms, a difference of >0.3 mm between the affected and unaffected eyes may include acute optic neuritis, optic neuropathy secondary to systemic disease such as lupus or sarcoidosis, or primary demyelinating conditions like multiple sclerosis.

Key Points

- Ocular ultrasound allows for prompt evaluation of both anterior and posterior chamber ocular pathology.
- Ultrasound can be performed in almost all clinical scenarios as concern for globe rupture is no longer a contraindication to ocular ultrasound when performed with extreme care.
- It is important to use a liberal amount of gel to obtain optimal images as well as to avoid compression of the globe. The eye can be examined in both static position and with voluntary eye movements.
- Always increase the gain to identify artifact, hemorrhage, PVD, or RD within the posterior chamber.
- Both increased ONSD and optic disc elevation can indicate elevated intracranial pressure however caution and clinical picture should be used with interpretation as there are also non-ICP-related causes of both, which may mimic elevated ICP.

References

1. Lyon M, von Kuenssberg JD. Chapter 19: ocular. In: Ma OJ, Mateer JR, Reardon RF, Joing SA, editors. Emergency ultrasound. 3rd ed. Beijing: McGraw-Hill Education; 2014. p. 569–86.
2. SonoSim ultrasound training solution [video]. Santa Monica: SonoSim Inc.; 2017.
3. Tran V, Irwin Z. Chapter 22: ocular ultrasound. In: Fox JC, editor. Clinical emergency radiology. 2nd ed. Cambridge: Cambridge University Press; 2017. p. 324–30.
4. Nedelmann M, Graef M, Weinand F, Wassill K, Kaps M, Lorenz B, Tanislav C. Retrobulbar spot sign predicts thombolytic treatment effects and etiology in Central Retinal Artery Occlusion.

Stroke. 2015;46(8):2322–4. June 25, 2015. https://doi.org/10.1161/STROKEAHA.115.009839. Accessed 14 Apr 2017

5. Ghanem G, Haase D, Brzezinski A, Ogawa R, Asachi P, Chiem A. Ultrasound detected increase in optic disk height to identify elevated intracranial pressure: a systematic review. Ultrasound J. 2023;15(1):26. Published 2023 May 25. https://doi.org/10.1186/s13089-023-00324-7
6. Marks A, Patel D, Chottiner M, Kayarian F, Peksa GD, Gottlieb M. Covered or uncovered: a randomized control trial of Tegaderm versus no Tegaderm for ocular ultrasound. Am J Emerg Med. 2022;61:87–9. https://doi.org/10.1016/j.ajem.2022.08.044.
7. Theoret J, Sanz GE, Matero D, et al. The "guitar pick" sign: a novel sign of retrobulbar hemorrhage. CJEM. 2011;13(3):162–4. https://doi.org/10.2310/10.2310/8000.2011.110279.
8. Berg C, Doniger SJ, Zaia B, Williams SR. Change in intraocular pressure during point-of-care ultrasound. West J Emerg Med. 2015;16(2):263–8. https://doi.org/10.5811/westjem.2015.1.24150.

Pediatric Ultrasound

19

Ashley Haggerty, Angela Lindsay, Lindsay Taylor, and Michael J. Vitto

Point-of-care ultrasound has become an integral tool in pediatric emergency departments, offering a rapid, noninvasive method of assessment for common conditions. Ultrasound enables clinicians to expedite care and diagnose pathology without the use of harmful radiation. This chapter will review indications, image acquisition, normal ultrasound anatomy, and interpretation of pathology for various pediatric conditions encountered in the acute care setting.

Appendicitis

(a) Indications
- Right lower quadrant or periumbilical abdominal pain.
- Anorexia.
- Fever.
- Vomiting.

Supplementary Information The online version contains supplementary material available at https://doi.org/10.1007/978-3-032-27643-8_19.

A. Haggerty (✉)
Department of Emergency Medicine, Division of Pediatric Emergency Medicine, Shady Grove Medical Center, Rockville, MD, USA
e-mail: HaggertyA@usacs.com

A. Lindsay · L. Taylor · M. J. Vitto
Department of Emergency Medicine, Virginia Commonwealth University Health, Richmond, VA, USA
e-mail: Angela.creditt@vcuhealth.org; Lindsay.taylor@vcuhealth.org; michael.vitto@vcuhealth.org

A. Lindsay et al. (eds.), *Clinical Ultrasound*,
https://doi.org/10.1007/978-3-032-27643-8_19

- Sterile pyuria (often accompanied by a dull ache, dysuria, urinary frequency) which can indicate a retrocecal appendicitis.

(b) Image Acquisition
- Transducer selection.
  - Linear array: preferred transducer for evaluation of the appendix on thinner patients.
  - Curvilinear: preferred transducer for evaluation of the appendix on larger patients or in patients with concern for retrocecal or ruptured appendix.
- Patient position
  - The patient should be supine with the head of the bed flat and their knees flexed to allow abdominal muscles to relax.
- Have the patient point to the site of maximal pain and begin with transducer at this site in a transverse plane with the marker pointed toward the patient's right.
  - Scan both inferior and superior to try to identify the appendix.
  - The appendix will be visualized originating from the cecum, anterior to the external iliac vessels.
    - Normally, the appendix is a compressible tubular structure with a blind end and an outer diameter of less than 6 mm. The upper limit of normal in the pediatric population is 5.7 mm and 6 mm in adults.
  - Rotate the transducer 90° with the marker pointed toward the patient's head to obtain views in a sagittal plane.
- Alternatively, place the transducer at the hepatic flexure, and trace the ascending colon down to the cecum.
- Use graded compression by exerting gentle pressure over the area of interest with the ultrasound transducer in effort to displace bowel gas to better visualize intra-abdominal structures.
- A normal appendix will typically exhibit peristalsis and have compressibility [1].
- Pediatric patients with certain inflammatory conditions may have an enlarged appendix without other sonographic signs of acute appendicitis. These conditions include cystic fibrosis (the appendix dilates due to mucoid contents), Crohn's disease, pelvic inflammatory disease, and patients with an inflamed Meckel diverticulum.

(c) Pathology
- Aperistaltic, noncompressible, fluid-filled, blind-ended tubular structure with an outer diameter of greater than 6 mm [1–3]; for pediatric patients, consider a diameter greater than 5.7 mm to diagnose acute appendicitis [2].
  - Figure 19.1—Appendicitis.
  - Figure 19.2—Diameter greater than 5.7 mm.
  - Video 19.1—Appendicitis in long axis.
- The following may also indicate acute appendicitis.
  - Target sign appearance (in an axial plane).
    - Figure 19.3—Target sign
    - Video 19.2—Target sign

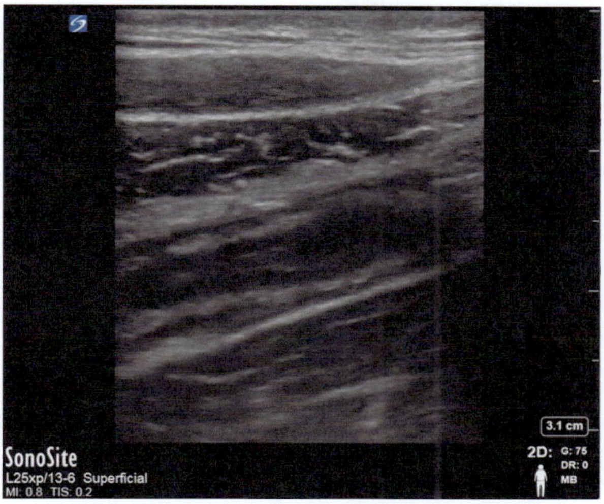

Fig. 19.1 Appendicitis. A blind-ended tubular structure with an outer diameter of greater than 5.7 mm

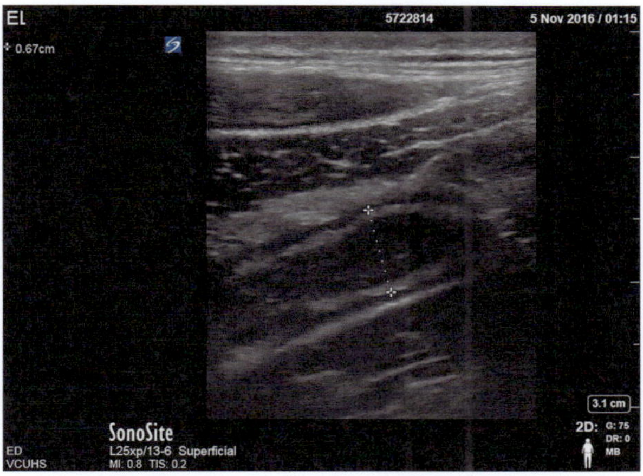

Fig. 19.2 Diameter greater than 5.7 mm. The diameter in pediatric appendicitis is greater than 5.7 mm as measured in this figure

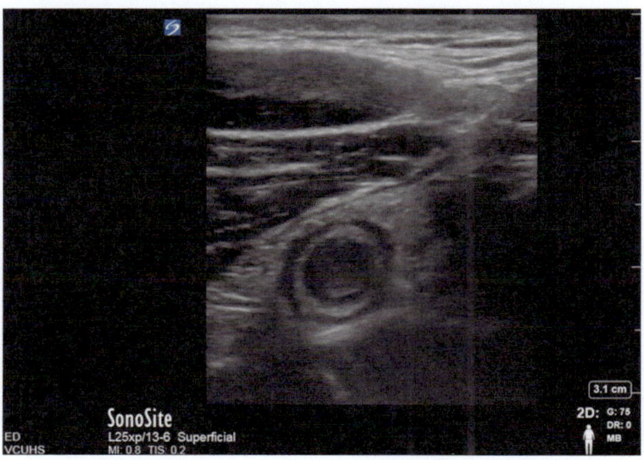

Fig. 19.3 Target sign. When the appendix is inflamed, it can resemble a target with hypoechoic and hyperechoic concentric rings

- Wall thickness greater than 3 mm [4]
- Appendicolith with posterior acoustic shadowing [3, 5]
  - Figure 19.4—Appendicolith
  - Video 19.3—Appendicolith
- Periappendiceal fluid collection [5]
  - Figure 19.5—Appendicitis with periappendiceal fluid
  - Video 19.4—Appendicitis with periappendiceal fluid
  - Video 19.5—Appendicitis with periappendiceal fluid in a different patient
- Increased periappendiceal echogenicity due to fat stranding [6].
- Color Doppler can be used to demonstrate increased vascularity in the setting of acute appendicitis, often termed "ring of fire" [1].

- Perforation may be identified by a fluid collection, hypoechoic mass, or thickening of adjacent bowel wall.
  - Complex abscess fluid collections may be present.
    - Video 19.6—Ruptured appendicitis with loculated fluid collections.

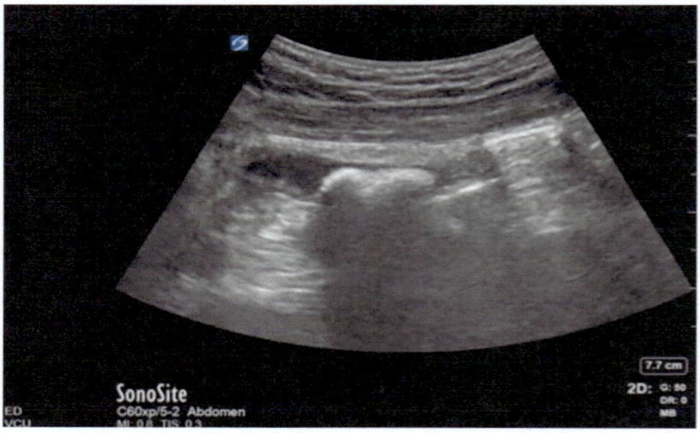

Fig. 19.4 Appendicolith. Hyperechoic foci within the lumen of the appendix that causes posterior shadowing

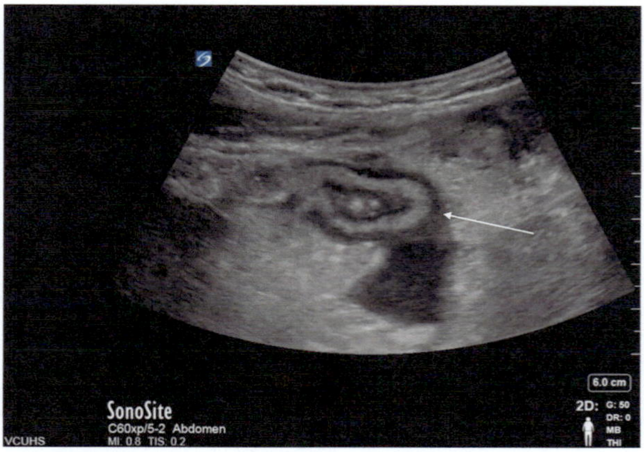

Fig. 19.5 Appendicitis with periappendiceal fluid. Inflammatory fluid surrounds the appendix depicted by the arrow

Key Points

- A normal appendix is only seen less than 15% of the time [1] due to its small size and lack of inflammatory findings.
- Inability to visualize a normal appendix does not rule out the presence of appendicitis.
- Point-of-care ultrasound is accessible and offers high diagnostic accuracy [13].

Intussusception

(a) Indications
- Colicky abdominal pain or intermittent fussiness.
- Vomiting (bilious or non-bilious).
- Currant jelly stool.
- Lethargy.
- Common age is 3 months to 3 years with the peak in cases presenting 6–9 months and the majority occurring before the second birthday.

(b) Image Acquisition
- Transducer selection.
  - Curvilinear.
  - Linear array: can be used with thinner patients.
- Patient position
  - The patient should be supine with the head of the bed flat and their knees flexed to allow abdominal muscles to relax.
- Place the transducer in the right lower quadrant, and follow the path of the large intestine.
  - It is rare to have a pathologic intussusception of the small intestine, though it is possible.
- Alternatively, another way to evaluate for intussusception is to slide the transducer using an up-and-down lawn mower technique to cover the entire abdomen.
- The majority of intussusceptions are located in the right upper quadrant.

(c) Pathology
- Telescoping of one section of the bowel into another.
  - Commonly occurs at the ileocecal junction.
  - Figure 19.6—Intussusception.
- In a transverse plane, there will be concentric alternating hypoechoic and hyperechoic rings representing layers of the bowel with adjacent free fluid and inner fecal matter [1, 14], known as “doughnut” or “target sign.”
  - Figure 19.7—Doughnut sign.
  - Video 19.7—Doughnut sign.
- In long axis, there will be a hypoechoic edematous intussususceptum (similar to a renal cortex) and an invaginated mesenteric fat (resembling a renal sinus); this finding is commonly referred to as “pseudo-kidney sign”.

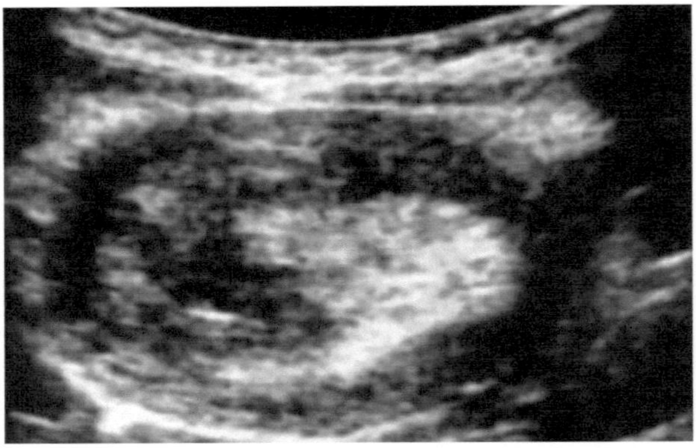

Fig. 19.6 Intussusception. In a longitudinal plane, there is an invagination of the bowel into itself causing a telescoping-like effect. This is commonly referred to as a "pseudokidney" as it looks like a kidney in appearance

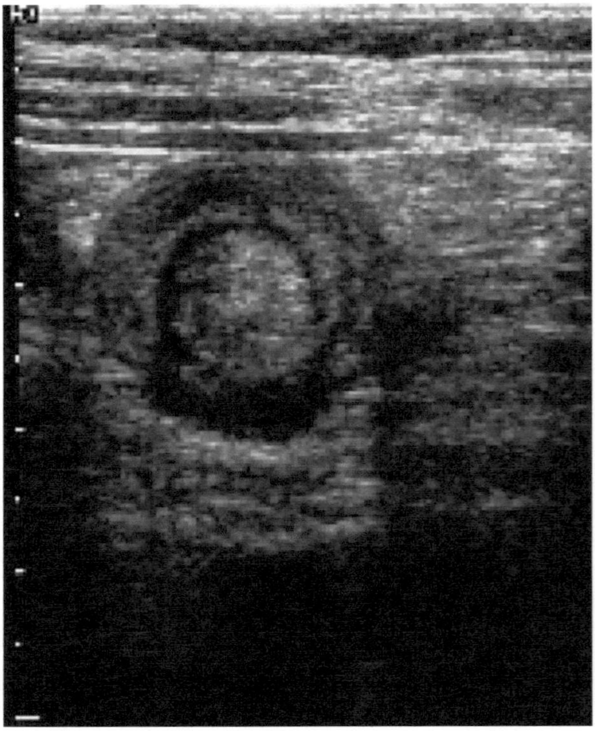

Fig. 19.7 Doughnut sign. In a transverse plane, there will be concentric alternating hypoechoic and hyperechoic rings representing layers of the bowel with adjacent free fluid and inner fecal matter

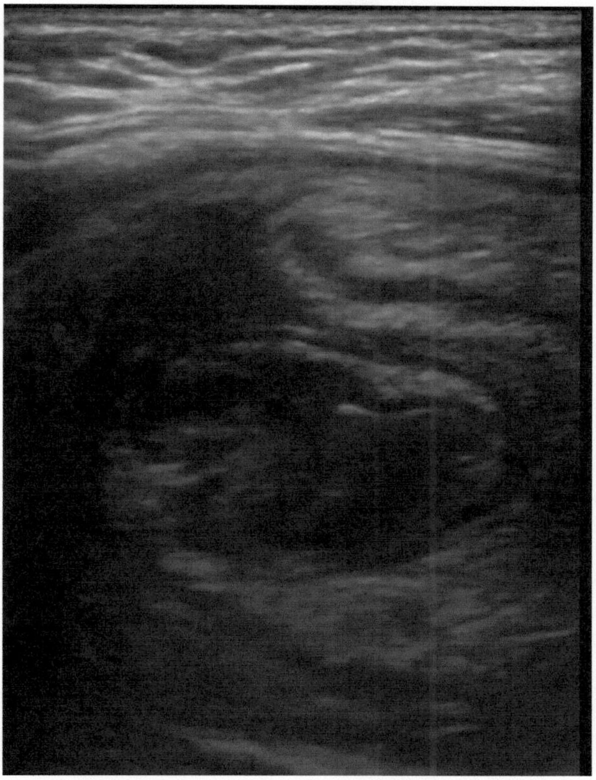

Fig. 19.8 Pseudo-kidney sign. In a long-axis plane, there will be a hypoechoic edematous intussususceptum (similar to a renal cortex) and an invaginated mesenteric fat (resembling a renal sinus) to create a pseudokidney sign

– Figure 19.8 Pseudo-kidney sign
– Video 19.8 Pseudo-kidney sign.

Pyloric Stenosis

(a) Indications
- Projectile nonbilious vomiting that commonly occurs within the first weeks of life (4–8 weeks).
- Palpable olive-shaped mass in the upper abdomen.
- Visible gastric hyperperistalsis.

(b) Image Acquisition
- Transducer.
  – Linear array.
- Patient position.
  – The patient should be supine with the head of the bed flat; alternatively, have the infant supine with the parent as the holder.

  - Overall, the goal should be to place the infant in a slightly right posterior oblique position to allow the fluid in the gastric fundus to flow into the pyloric region.
  - If the area is difficult to identify, feeding the baby a glucose solution can be helpful.
- Place the transducer in an oblique position over the epigastrium with the marker pointed toward the patient's left shoulder.
- Fan the transducer up and toward the right shoulder, and then fan the transducer down toward the right hip.
  - If the patient has a lot of bowel gas, use graded compression by exerting gentle pressure over the area of interest with the ultrasound transducer in effort to displace the bowel gas.
  - Or reposition the patient by placing them in the right lateral decubitus position to move air up into the fundus of the stomach and fluid down.

(c) Pathology

- Pyloric stenosis occurs when the pylorus becomes hypertrophied blocking food from exiting the stomach into the small intestine.
- Identify the pyloric channel.
  - The outer thick muscular wall will appear hypoechoic compared to the more hyperechoic inner mucosa.
    - Figure 19.9—Pyloric stenosis short axis
  - Measure the pyloric muscle thickness.
    - Greater than 3 mm is diagnostic [7, 8].
  - Other findings suggestive of pyloric stenosis.
    - Pyloric channel length greater than 14–20 mm [8]
    - Pyloric diameter greater than 12 mm [8]
    - Pyloric volume (fluid in the stomach) greater than 12 cc [9]
    - Antral nipple sign (prolapse of the pyloric channel mucosa into the gastric antrum)
  - Figure 19.10—Pyloric stenosis measurement.
  - Figure 19.11—Positive pyloric stenosis infant with measurements and a partially visible antral nipple sign

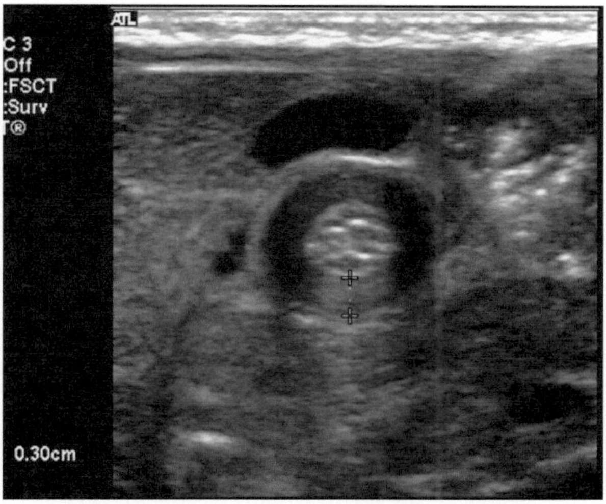

Fig. 19.9 Pyloric stenosis—short axis. The outer thick muscular wall will appear hypoechoic compared to the more hyperechoic inner mucosa

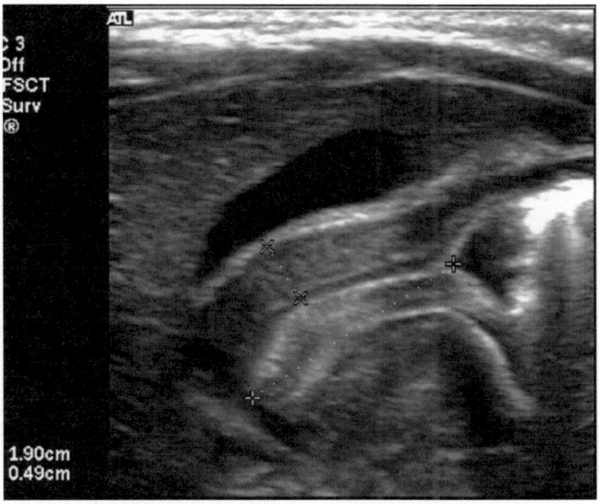

Fig. 19.10 Pyloric stenosis measurements. Measurement of the pyloric muscle thickness greater than 3 mm, channel length greater than 14–20 mm, and pyloric channel diameter greater than 12 mm. You will also see fluid in the stomach

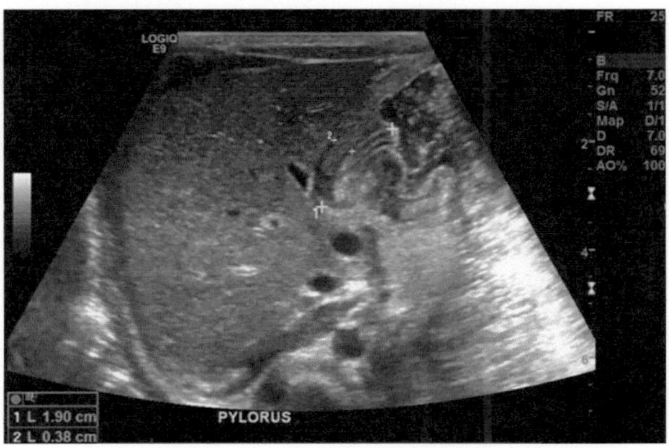

Fig. 19.11 Positive pyloric stenosis infant with measurements. Note the measurements, fluid in the stomach, and a partial view of a positive antral nipple sign partially obscured by the plus sign measuring the channel length

Testicular Torsion

(a) Indications
- Acute onset testicular pain.
- Any concern for testicular torsion.

(b) Image Acquisition
- Transducer.
  - Linear array.
- Patient position.
  - The patient should be supine.
  - Support the testicles in a sling-like fashion with a towel draped over the patient's legs and the scrotum sitting on top of the towel.
  - Cover sensitive areas that are being scanned with a towel.
- Obtain an image of both testicles side by side to demonstrate echogenicity differences between the normal and symptomatic testicles.
- Examine the asymptomatic testicle first in transverse and longitudinal planes.
  - Normal testicle is an oval-shaped homogenous mildly echogenic structure.
  - Note the echogenicity, texture, and size.
    - Figure 19.12—Normal testicle
    - Video 19.9—Normal testicle
  - Use color Doppler and note flow patterns.
    - Figrue 19.13—Color Doppler
    - Video 19.10—Normal testicle color Doppler
- Examine the symptomatic testicle in transverse and longitudinal planes.
  - Compare echogenicity, texture, and size to the unaffected side.
  - Compare color Doppler flow patterns to the unaffected side.
- See Chap. 15, Testicular Ultrasound, for complete testicular ultrasound procedure and details.

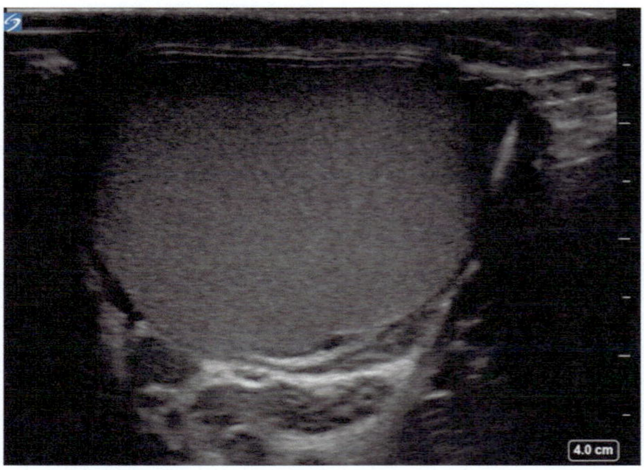

Fig. 19.12 Normal testicle. B-mode image of a normal testicle which has a homogenous echotexture

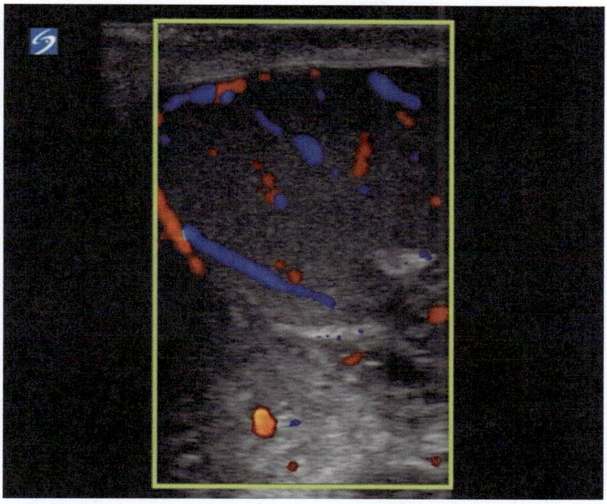

Fig. 19.13 Color Doppler. Color Doppler image of a normal testicle with normal flow

(c) Pathology
- Testicular torsion occurs when the spermatic cord twists causing venous congestion and obstruction followed by decreased arterial flow and eventually complete obstruction leading to ischemia and infarction [10, 11].
- Severity of torsion ranges from 180–720°, and complete occlusion of blood flow is thought to occur after 450° of torsion [11].
- B-mode (2D) imaging.
  - Affected testicle will appear enlarged and hypoechoic with less homogeneity compared with the unaffected testicle.
  - Figure 19.14—Testicular torsion.
  - Video 19.11—Testicular torsion.
- Color Doppler.
  - Decreased Doppler color signal will be seen or, in cases of complete torsion, the absence of Doppler color signal.
  - Always compare the Doppler color signal to the unaffected side.
  - Video 19.12—Torsion with color Doppler.
- If obtaining color Doppler flow is difficult, switch to power Doppler mode.
- Set the gain to the highest setting that allows a distinct signal within vessels without surrounding artifact.
- See Chap. 1 for more details on power Doppler.
- Power Doppler
  - Will evaluate low flow stat.
  - Absence of power Doppler is diagnostic of testicular torsion [12]
  - Figure 19.15—Testicle with power Doppler.
  - Figure 19.16—Testicular torsion with power Doppler.
- Ultrasound may also demonstrate the twisted spermatic cord just superior to the testis and epididymis with the transducer oriented in a sagittal plane; this may resemble a "whirlpool" [11].

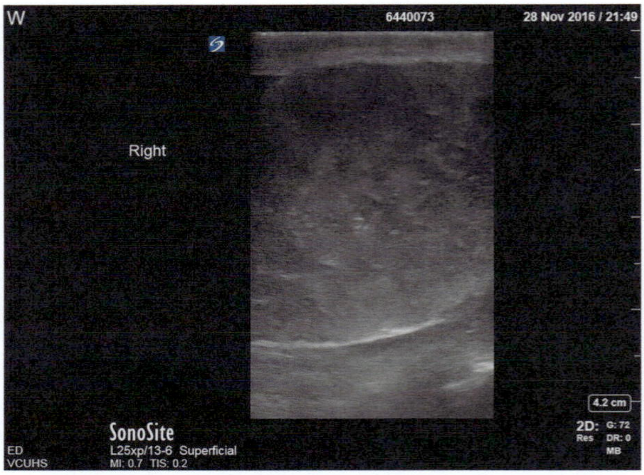

Fig. 19.14 Testicular torsion. The testicle is enlarged and hypoechoic with less homogeneity concerning for testicular torsion

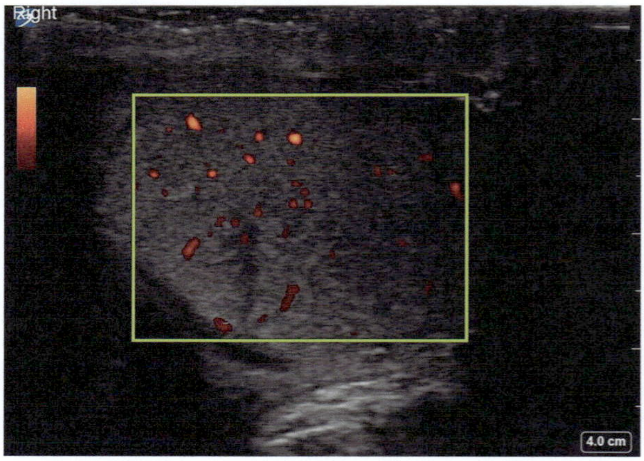

Fig. 19.15 Testicle with power Doppler. Testicle with power Doppler demonstrating a low flow state

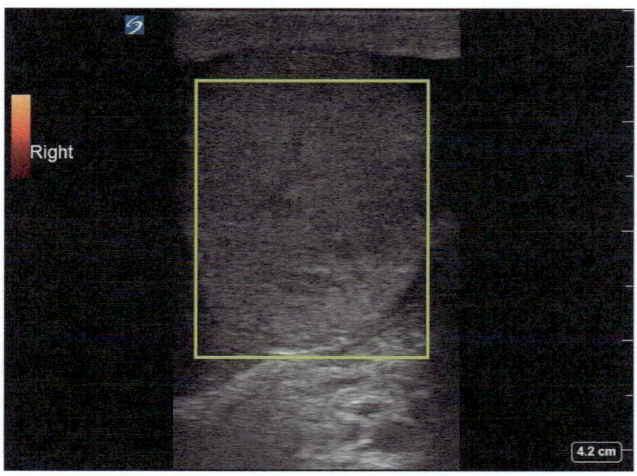

Fig. 19.16 Testicular torsion power Doppler. No flow appreciated on power Doppler as depicted by the absence of color within the testicular tissue

- Once full torsion has occurred and there is no blood flow, infarction and loss of the testicle occur rapidly; salvage rates are approximately 100% at 3 hours, 90% at 6 hours, 50% at 12 hours, and 10% at 24 hours [11].

Key Points

- Sonographic findings of testicular torsion are variable depending on the duration and extent of vascular compromise.
- Torsion remains a clinical diagnosis, and ultrasound cannot rule out torsion [11] especially in cases of partial torsion and intermittent torsion.

Skull Fracture

(a) Indications
- Presence of a scalp hematoma in <12 months old
- Concerns for non-accidental trauma
- Palpable crepitus

(b) Image Acquisition
- Transducer selection
  (i) Linear array:
    – Preferred transducer for the evaluation of superficial structures
- Patient position
  (i) The patient can be in any position of comfort, preferably with the occiput in contact with a parent or the bed.
  (ii) If the area of interest is posterior, often a parental hug with a gentle hold cradling the occipital condyles should allow for minimal movement and safe head support in infants who will either move or have poor neck control.
- Place the transducer delicately adjacent to the area of interest steadying the heel of the hand holding the probe on an uninjured part of the infant/child and begin to track over the area of interest with light pressure.
- Alternatively, if the infant or child appears uncomfortable with direct contact, the procedure can be performed with a standoff gel pad or other fluid-filled vessel such as a water-filled glove.
- Of note, suture lines can be commonly mistaken for a fracture. Suture lines are continuous with a fontanelle. They have smooth edges. There should be symmetry. In contrast, a skull fracture will have disruption of the cortex and an area of hematoma at the fracture site. Skull fractures can be jagged or smooth.
- This tool should not replace definitive imaging if the child already meets criteria for emergent imaging following PECARN criteria [15] or an infant scalp score of 5 (and sometimes 4) or more [16]. Instead, it can be used as an adjunct to help support the decision to image or not to image.

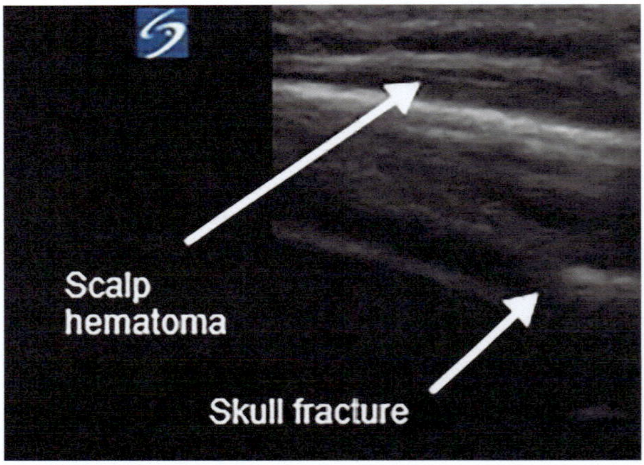

Fig. 19.17 Skull fracture: note the disruption of the echogenic bony cortex. Arrows pointing to the fracture as well as the scalp hematoma

(c) Pathology
- Normal bone will be hyperechoic with posterior shadowing and have a smooth cortex
- Skull fractures will have a disruption of the echogenic bony cortex and commonly have an adjacent, overlying hematoma [17]
  (i) Figure 19.17—Skull fracture
- Scalp hematomas that are large (>3 cm), boggy in texture, located in the temporal, parietal, or occipital areas, or that are discovered in patients <6 months old are concerning for underlying fracture and/or intracranial hemorrhage [16, 17, 20].

(d) Key Points
- Point-of-care ultrasound is highly sensitive and specific for detecting skull fractures [17, 18, 19].
- Large scalp hematomas found with or without a skull fracture in the certain areas and ages should also be concerning for intracranial hemorrhage [16, 17, 20].

Bronchiolitis

(a) Indications
- Infant <24 months old with respiratory distress or cough

(b) Image Acquisition (same as pneumonia)
- Transducer selection:
  - Linear array
    - Preferred transducer for the evaluation of thinner patients.
  - Curvilinear
    - Preferred transducer for the evaluation of larger patients or if there are concerns for parapneumonic effusions.

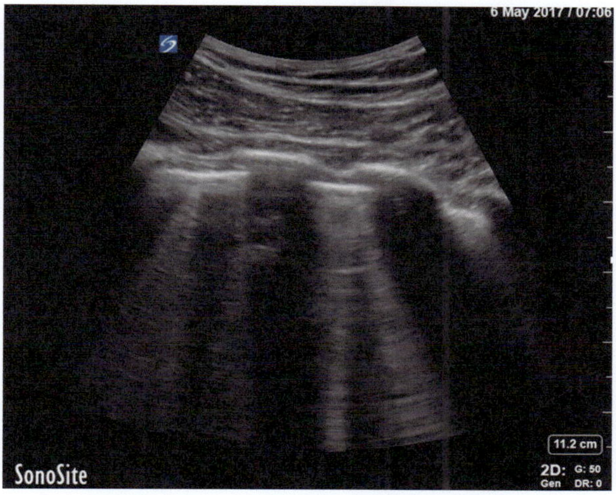

Fig. 19.18 B lines in bronchiolitis can appear as multiple comet tail artifacts that extend back from the pleural surface

- Patient position:
  - The patient can be sitting up or facing a caregiver with their back exposed.
    - Lung ultrasound will be limited to the portions of the lung scanned and so optimal positioning will include anterior (mid-clavicular), lateral (mid-axillary), and posterior (mid-scapular) views bilaterally.
- Place the transducer longitudinally (perpendicularly to the ribs) with the probe marker pointing toward the head.
  - Alternatively, the transducer can be placed with a transverse approach parallel to the intercostal space. This method does allow visualization of the pleura without interruption of the rib cage but will require imaging more areas for completion.
- Scanning can begin with the area of interest (often based on auscultation) or can start superiorly and work inferiorly. The inferior image obtained should ensure that the costophrenic angle is obtained to evaluate for possible fluid collection. This should be performed bilaterally.
- Healthy, well-aerated lungs will have a hyperechoic pleural line that is smooth. The lungs will slide with dynamic, shimmering parietal pleural over visceral pleural with each phase of respiration. The lungs will have A-lines. The A-line is a static, horizontal artifact that represents air in the alveolar spaces [21].

(c) Pathology

- The presence of numerous, possibly confluent B lines. B lines are comet tail artifacts that are hyperechoic, vertical artifacts that arise from the pleural surface and extend to the base of the screen. [21, 22].
  - Figure 19.18 B lines in bronchiolitis
- There can also be subpleural consolidations <1.5 cm [21, 22, 23].

(d) Key Points
- Bronchiolitis is a clinical diagnosis. It does not require imaging. Based on recent recommendations, chest radiographs should be avoided. Lung ultrasound is an accessible, sensitive, and specific alternative to help identify bronchiolitis if imaging is still desired.
- There are an increasing number of studies looking at the lung ultrasound findings for bronchiolitis as a prognostic tool [23, 24, 25].

Constipation

(a) Indications
- Clinical concerns for constipation

(b) Image Acquisition
- Transducer selection:
  - Curvilinear
  - Phased array is an acceptable alternative
- Patient position:
  - Lying supine
- Obtain a transverse view, place the transducer just superior to the pubic symphysis with the transducer angled inferiorly and the transducer marker pointed to the right of the patient.
- Measure the transrectal diameter.
  (i) The upper limit of normal for a transrectal diameter for 2-month-olds is: 2.3 cm.
  (ii) The upper limit of normal for a transrectal diameter for 3-12-month-old is: 2.6 cm.

(c) Pathology
  (i) The transrectal diameter of 3.8 cm or greater is indicative of constipation across all ages [26].
  - Figure 19.19 transrectal diameter of 4.2 cm in a preschool-aged child

(d) Key Points
- Imaging is never required for the diagnosis of constipation, but it can provide the patient and their families tangible evidence of constipation without resorting to a radiograph.

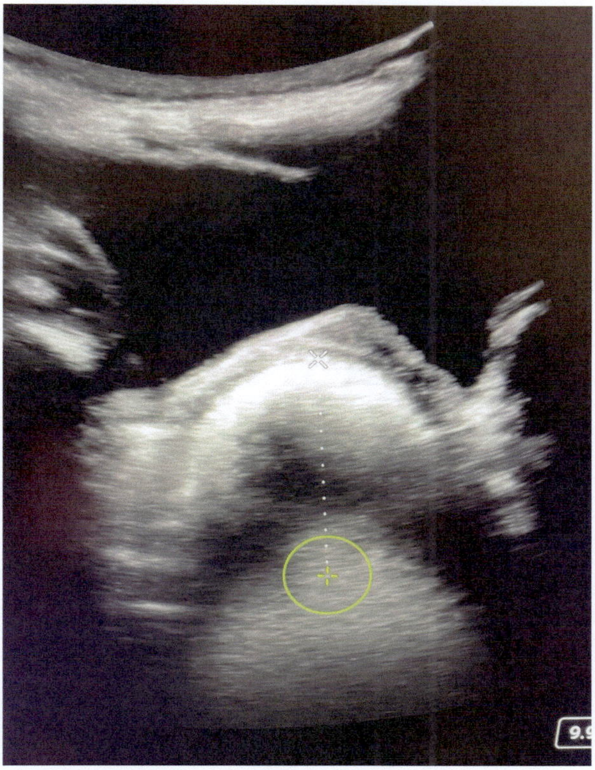

Fig. 19.19 Transrectal diameter of 4.2 cm in a preschool-aged child. There is also an altered contour of the bladder due to the stool burden. The stool, in this instance, is creating a posterior echo shadowing, which is not altogether uncommon and can make placing the calipers a bit challenging

Hip Effusion

(a) Indications
- Hip pain
- Painful limp
- Refusal to bear weight
- Warm, erythematous, or swollen hip

(b) Image Acquisition
- Transducer selection:
  - Linear array
  - Curvilinear
    - If a linear large footprint probe is not available

- Patient position:
  - Lying supine
- Measure the capsular to synovial thickness of the hip from the anterior bony cortical surface to the concavity of the femoral neck.
  - A capsular-synovial thickness <5 mm is normal [26].
  - Alternatively, comparing the thickness of both sides should measure no more than 2 mm different to also be negative [26].

(c) Pathology
- Capsule-to-bone distance greater than or equal to 5 mm, or
  - Figure 19.20: 6.7 mm hip effusion
  - Figure 19.21 Normal hip for comparison
- Capsule-to-bone distance greater than 2 mm difference between both hips.

(d) Key Points
- Hip effusion can be detected with portable ultrasound and is positive if >5 mm or if >2 mm difference than the asymptomatic side [26].
- Hip effusions can be present for both septic arthritis and for transient synovitis. To help delineate between the two pathologies, Kocher criteria should be applied to aid in the diagnosis (or exclusion) of septic arthritis. In the presence of 1 or 2 Kocher criteria, the presence of a hip effusion does not help delineate between septic arthritis and transient synovitis [27].

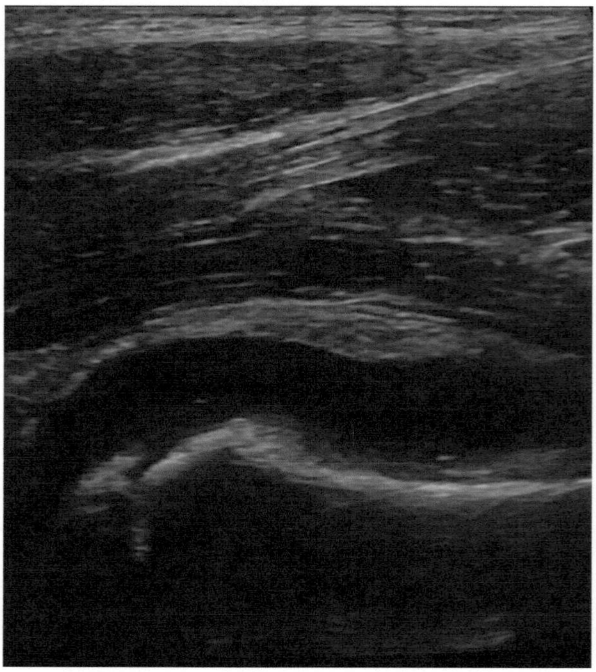

Fig. 19.20 6.7 mm hip effusion. Any effusion >5mm is positive by itself. See how the fluid also collects and begins to curve around the hip joint

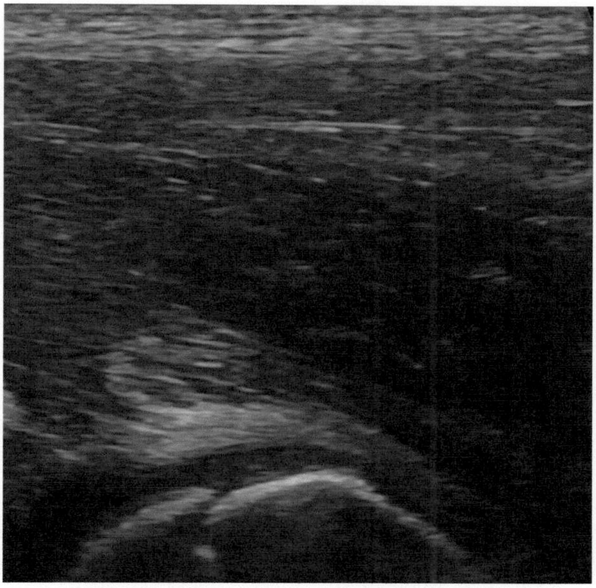

Fig. 19.21 Normal hip for comparison. This is a normal joint capsule where there is a very scant amount of fluid present. Normal hip fluid in pediatric patients can be isoechoic or anechoic

Pediatric Key Points

- Use distraction to help the patient tolerate the exam and talk to the patient (and parent/guardian) through the process.
- Whenever possible, offer the ability for the patient to view the screen.
- If available, use warm ultrasound gel to make the exam more comfortable.

References

1. SonoSim ultrasound training solution [video]. Santa Monica: SonoSim Inc.; 2017.
2. Park NH, Oh HE, Park HJ, Park JY. Ultrasonography of normal and abnormal appendix in children. World J Radiol. 2011;3(4):85–91. https://www.ncbi.nlm.nih.gov/pmc/articles/PMC3084437/. Accessed 17 Apr 2017
3. Janitz E, Naffaa L, Rubin M, Ganapathy SS. Ultrasound evaluation for appendicitis focus on the pediatric population: a review of the literature. J Am Osteopath Coll Radiol. 2016;5(1):5–14. http://www.jaocr.org/articles/ultrasound-evaluation-for-appendicitis-focus-on-the-pediatric-population-a-review-of-the-literature. Accessed 17 Apr 2017
4. Paspulati RM. Chapter 23: ultrasonography of bowel disorders. In: Dogra V, Rubens D, editors. Ultrasound secrets. London: Elsevier Health Sciences; 2004. p. 207–11.
5. Chao A, Gharahbaghian L. Tips and tricks: ultrasound in the diagnosis of acute appendicitis. American College of Emergency Physicians website April 2015. https://www.acep.org/Content.aspx?id=101803. Accessed 15 Apr 2017.
6. Old JL, Dusing RW, Yap W, Dirks J. Imaging for suspected appendicitis. Am Fam Phys. 2005;71(1):71–8. http://www.aafp.org/afp/2005/0101/p71.html. Accessed 15 Apr 2017

7. Costa Dias S, Swinson S, Torrao H, Goncalves L, Kurochka S, Vaz CP, Mendes V. Hypertrophic pyloric stenosis: tips and tricks for ultrasound diagnosis. Insights Imag. 2012;3(3):247–50. https://www.ncbi.nlm.nih.gov/pmc/articles/PMC3369120/. Accessed 17 Apr 2017
8. Hussain M. Sonographic diagnosis of infantile hypertrophic pyloric stenosis—use of simultaneous grey-scale and colour Doppler examination. Int J Health Sci. 2008;2(2):134–40. https://www.ncbi.nlm.nih.gov/pmc/articles/PMC3068743/ Accessed 17 Apr 2017
9. Rohrschneider WK, Mittnacht H, Darge K, Troger J. Pyloric muscle in asymptomatic infants: sonographic evaluation and discrimination from idiopathic hypertrophic pyloric stenosis. Pediatr Radiol. 1998;28(6):429–34. http://link.springer.com/article/10.1007%2Fs002470050377 Accessed 17 Apr 2017
10. Fischer JW, Sivitz AB, Abo AM. Chapter 20: pediatric applications. In: Ma OJ, Mateer JR, Reardon RF, Joing SA, editors. Emergency ultrasound. 3rd ed. Beijing: McGraw-Hill Education; 2014. p. 587–630.
11. Goldenberg E, Gilbert BR. Chapter 4: scrotal ultrasound. In: Gilbert BR, editor. Ultrasound of the male genitalia. New York: Springer; 2015. p. 75–124.
12. Adhikari S. Chapter 13: testicular. In: Ma OJ, Mateer JR, Reardon RF, Joing SA, editors. Emergency ultrasound. 3rd ed. Beijing: McGraw-Hill Education; 2014. p. 353–80.
13. Lawton B, Goldstein H, Davis T, et al. Diagnosis of appendicitis in the paediatric emergency department: an update. Curr Opin Pediatr. 2019;31(3):312–6.
14. Bergmann KR, Arroyo AC, Tessaro MO, Nielson J, Whitcomb V, Madhok M, Yock-Corrales A, Guerrero-Quesada G, Chaudoin L, Berant R, Shahar-Nissan K, Deanehan JK, Lam SHF, Snelling PJ, Avendano P, Cohen SG, Friedman N, Ekpenyong A, Pade KH, Park DB, Lin-Martore M, Kornblith AE, Montes-Amaya G, Thomas-Mohtat R, Jin J, Watson D, Sivitz A; P2Network. Diagnostic accuracy of point-of-care ultrasound for intussusception: a multi-center, noninferiority study of paired diagnostic tests. Ann Emerg Med. 2021;78(5):606–5. https://doi.org/10.1016/j.annemergmed.2021.04.033. Epub 2021 Jul 3. Erratum in: Ann Emerg Med. 2022 Feb;79(2):222. PMID: 34226072.
15. Gambacorta A, Moro M, Curatola A, Brancato F, Covino M, Chiaretti A, Gatto A. PECARN rule in diagnostic process of pediatric patients with minor head trauma in emergency department. Eur J Pediatr. 2022;181(5):2147–54. https://doi.org/10.1007/s00431-022-04424-9. Epub 2022 Feb 22. PMID: 35194653; PMCID: PMC9056473
16. Schutzman SA, Nigrovic LE, Mannix R. The infant scalp score: a validated tool to stratify risk of traumatic brain injury in infants with isolated scalp hematoma. Acad Emerg Med. 2021;28(1):92–7. https://doi.org/10.1111/acem.14087. Epub 2020 Aug 19. PMID: 32673432
17. Choi JY, Lim YS, Jang JH, Park WB, Hyun SY, Cho JS. Accuracy of bedside ultrasound for the diagnosis of skull fractures in children aged 0 to 4 years. Pediatr Emerg Care. 2020;36(5):e268–73. https://doi.org/10.1097/PEC.0000000000001485. PMID: 29698348
18. Parri N, Crosby BJ, Mills L, Soucy Z, Musolino AM, Da Dalt L, Cirilli A, Grisotto L, Kuppermann N. Point-of-care ultrasound for the diagnosis of skull fractures in children younger than two years of age. J Pediatr. 2018;196:230–236.e2. https://doi.org/10.1016/j.jpeds.2017.12.057. Epub 2018 Feb 28. PMID: 29499992
19. Alexandridis G, Verschuuren EW, Rosendaal AV, Kanhai DA. Evidence base for point-of-care ultrasound (POCUS) for diagnosis of skull fractures in children: a systematic review and meta-analysis. Emerg Med J. 2022;39(1):30–6. https://doi.org/10.1136/emermed-2020-209887. Epub 2020 Dec 3. PMID: 33273039; PMCID: PMC8717482
20. Burns EC, Grool AM, Klassen TP, Correll R, Jarvis A, Joubert G, Bailey B, Chauvin-Kimoff L, Pusic M, McConnell D, Nijssen-Jordan C, Silver N, Taylor B. Osmond MH; pediatric emergency research Canada (PERC) head injury study group. Scalp hematoma characteristics associated with intracranial injury in pediatric minor head injury. Acad Emerg Med. 2016;23(5):576–83. https://doi.org/10.1111/acem.12957. Epub 2016 Apr 15. PMID: 26947778
21. Rizvi MB, Rabiner JE. Pediatric point-of-care lung ultrasonography: a narrative review. West J Emerg Med. 2022;23(4):497–504. https://doi.org/10.5811/westjem.2022.3.54663. PMID: 35980421; PMCID: PMC9391004

22. Bloise S, Marcellino A, Sanseviero M, Martucci V, Testa A, Leone R, Del Giudice E, Frasacco B, Gizzone P, Proietti Ciolli C, et al. Point-of-care thoracic ultrasound in children: new advances in pediatric emergency setting. Diagnostics. 2023;13:1765. https://doi.org/10.3390/diagnostics13101765.
23. Smith J, Stone B, Shin J, et al. Association of outcomes in point-of-care lung ultrasound for bronchiolitis in the pediatric emergency department. Amer J Emerg Med. 2024;75:22–8.
24. San Sebastian Ruiz N, Rodríguez Albarrán I, Gorostiza I, Galletebeitia Laka I, Delgado Lejonagoitia C, Samson F. Point-of-care lung ultrasound in children with bronchiolitis in a pediatric emergency department. Arch Pediatr. 2021;28(1):64–8. https://doi.org/10.1016/j.arcped.2020.10.003. Epub 2020 Nov 6. PMID: 33162325
25. Supino MC, Buonsenso D, Scateni S, Scialanga B, Mesturino MA, Bock C, Chiaretti A, Giglioni E, Reale A, Musolino AM. Point-of-care lung ultrasound in infants with bronchiolitis in the pediatric emergency department: a prospective study. Eur J Pediatr. 2019;178(5):623–32. https://doi.org/10.1007/s00431-019-03335-6. Epub 2019 Feb 12. PMID: 30747262
26. Doniger SJ, Dessie A, Latronica C. Measuring the Transrectal diameter on point-of-care ultrasound to diagnose constipation in children. Pediatr Emerg Care. 2018;34(3):154–9. https://doi.org/10.1097/PEC.0000000000000775. PMID: 27299294
27. Tsung JW, Blaivas M. Emergency department diagnosis of pediatric hip effusion and guided arthrocentesis using point-of-care ultrasound. J Emerg Med. 2008;35(4):393–9. https://doi.org/10.1016/j.jemermed.2007.10.054. Epub 2008 Apr 10. PMID: 18403170

Introduction to Ultrasound-Guided Regional Anesthesia

20

Robert Stenberg, Brian Makowski, and Jordan Tozer

Ultrasound-guided regional anesthesia has revolutionized the practice of perioperative and emergency pain management by enhancing both the safety and efficacy of nerve blocks. This technique allows direct visualization of neural structures, adjacent anatomy, and needle trajectory, enabling precise local anesthetic delivery while minimizing complications. As ultrasound technology becomes increasingly accessible and portable, proficiency in its use is essential for clinicians seeking to optimize patient comfort, reduce opioid use, and improve procedural outcomes. This chapter provides a foundational overview of ultrasound-guided regional anesthesia, including core principles, techniques, and clinical applications.

Clinical Applications and Indications

- Indications/background.
  - Ultrasound-guided nerve blocks are rather safe [1, 2].
    - The injury rate of peripheral nerve blocks is around 1 in 2500; with the majority being transient and minor. [3]

Supplementary Information The online version contains supplementary material available at https://doi.org/10.1007/978-3-032-27643-8_20.

R. Stenberg (✉) · B. Makowski
Department of Emergency Medicine, Cleveland Clinic, Akron, OH, USA
e-mail: stenber@ccf.org; makowsb2@ccf.org

J. Tozer
Department of Emergency Medicine, Virginia Commonwealth University Health, Richmond, VA, USA
e-mail: jordan.tozer@vcuhealth.org

A. Lindsay et al. (eds.), *Clinical Ultrasound*,
https://doi.org/10.1007/978-3-032-27643-8_20

    - The incidence of infection is very low.
      - One retrospective review of 7476 patients with single-injection nerve blocks did not identify any block-related infections [4].
- Contraindications.
  - Anticoagulation/Coagulopathy.
    - The safety is largely driven by block type and the coagulable state of the patient [5].
    - Generally, extremity/peripheral blocks, serratus anterior, and erector spinae plane blocks are considered lower risk blocks [6, 7]; therefore, in this population, it is more of a relative contraindication [8].
    - The deeper the block, and more vital structures surrounding the path, the higher risk it is. Brachial plexus blocks are sometimes grouped into deeper, higher-risk blocks, which should generate increased pause in the setting of anticoagulation/coagulopathy [9].
    - Here are some common parameters that could indicate when to avoid a higher-risk block:
      - Warfarin (Coumadin/Jantoven) + INR >1.4.
      - Ticagrelor(Brilinta), Clopidogrel (Plavix).
      - Apixaban (Eliquis), Rivaroxaban (Xarelto), Dabigatran (Pradaxa).
      - Coagulopathy.
  - Possible compartment syndrome.
    - One factor to consider is performing a nerve block for an injury pattern at high risk for compartment syndrome. One example would be posterior tibial blocks: although they can work very well for analgesia in calcaneal fractures, if the fracture pattern is at high risk for compartment syndrome, then this block may be a concern to "mask" the pain of a developing compartment syndrome [10].
    - It is generally a good idea to review with any consulting surgery team (e.g., Orthopedics) to discuss the risks and benefits of a block relative to the concern of compartment syndrome prior to blocking if not an established pathway.
  - Recent large dose of local anesthetic.
    - One must practice caution to not cause Local Anesthetic Systemic Toxicity (LAST).
    - Consider discussing with pharmacy regarding recent doses to check pharmacokinetics and impact on the current block [11].
    - Using online apps can permit factoring in multiple local anesthetics in calculation of the safe dose, and provides a leftover safe dose for upcoming or additional procedures (e.g., trauma already administered anesthetic for separate procedure or will require anesthetic use in the OR) [12].
  - Obvious skin infection overlying desired insertion site.
  - Allergy to local anesthetic.
  - Distorted anatomy preventing appropriate visualization for a safe block.
    - Example: Significant subcutaneous emphysema obscuring the transverse process for an erector spinae block in the setting of thoracic trauma.

- Consent
  - Patients should generally be consented with written consent, ensuring patients understand risks, benefits, and alternatives for best practice and medicolegal implications [13].
  - Some programs have established pathways with ethics committees for blocks in the elderly and demented (such as fascia iliaca for hip fractures); where if a patient does not have capacity, and one attempt is made to reach power of attorney, the team may proceed with the block given the significant benefit-to-risk ratio.
- Medications
  - One must consider the local anesthetic's pharmacokinetics (primarily the onset and duration of action), patient's clinical course, and potential complications of the nerve block as a part of the anesthetic choice (Fig. 20.1).
    - Common practice is 1–2% lidocaine for shorter action and 0.25–0.5% bupivacaine for longer action.
    - Some also consider chloroprocaine [14] for even short duration of action if only using for procedural analgesia/anesthesia.
    - Order sets can improve efficiency and ease, with goals to increase number of blocks performed (Fig. 20.2).
  - There is some weak evidence that bupivacaine may have more central nervous system symptoms and cardiotoxicity than ropivacaine [15–17].
  - Dexamethasone.
    - There is strong literature in support of dexamethasone with the anesthetic to extend the duration of analgesia [18, 19].

LOCAL ANESTHETIC DOSING FOR REGIONAL ANESTHESIA

ANESTHETIC	DOSE	ONSET	DURATION	NOTES/PEARLS
Chloroprocaine	11 mg/kg (MAX 800 mg)	6-12 min	30-60 min	- For ultra-short blocks, or procedural anesthesia/analgesia - Safe in pregnancy
Lidocaine	4-5 mg/kg (MAX 300 mg)	1-3 min	30-120 min	- Ideally for short blocks, or procedural anesthesia/analgesia - Do not repeat within 2 hours
Bupivacaine	2.5 mg/kg (MAX 175 mg)	5-10 min	240-720 min	- May have more CNS systems & cardiotoxicity compared to Ropivacaine
Ropivacaine	3 mg/kg (MAX 300 mg)	10-15 min	240-720 min	- Less cardiotoxic than Bupivacaine

*Should adjust doses in patient's with renal impairment, hepatic dysfunction, advanced heart failure, and age >70
↳ If present, ***decrease dose by 10-20%*** (consider up to 50% ↓ in patients with both renal & hepatic dysfunction)

Fig. 20.1 Table showing relevant anesthetic agents. (Created by Dr. Brian Makowski (with permission to share))

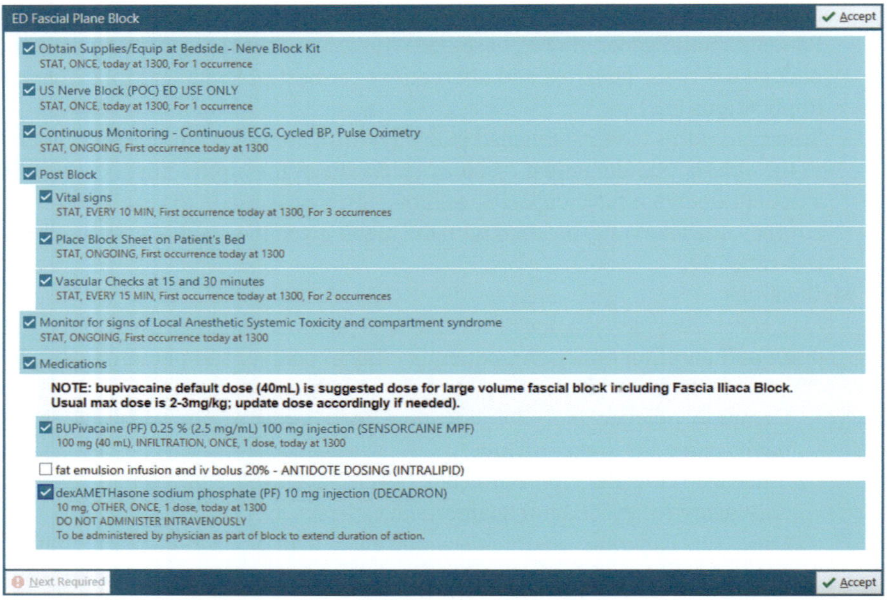

Fig. 20.2 Photo demonstrating an order set, showing multiple pieces auto-selected to reduce clicks for the end-user; also includes orders for rescue lipid emulsion therapy. (Permission to share obtained)

    - Doses in literature range from 4 mg to 10 mg, and is likely easiest to decide based on the amount provided in the vial (many locations stock 10 mg in 1 mL vials).
    - Use preservative-free dexamethasone to avoid preservative agents that can be neurotoxic [20].
    - Coadministration perineurally with anesthetic has a greater effect on duration, but if inadvertently given IV, it can still extend the duration of block [21].
  - Liposomal bupivacaine theoretically has an extended duration but comes at a significantly higher cost, and the evidence for such is weaker (especially compared to bupivacaine combined with dexamethasone) [22–24].
    - For some centers, liposomal bupivacaine comes at a cost approximately 100x the cost of standard bupivacaine.
- Complications.
  - As highlighted above, nerve blocks are rather safe procedures with low complication rates [25].
  - Intraneural injection [3].
    - Efforts should be made to avoid injecting anesthetic into the nerve (intraneural injection) due to concerns of causing nerve injury from intraneural high pressure, which can lead to decreased perfusion and nerve ischemia.

    - Ideal nerve placement is generally considered when the anesthetic is placed immediately adjacent to the epineural area [26]:
      - "Soak the bear, don't poke the bear."
    - Blunt-tipped needles reduce risk of injury, with cutting needles generally considered the least ideal [27].
      - Blunt-tipped nerve block needles > Quincke > Cutting needle.
  - Vascular puncture/hematoma.
    - Proceduralists should avoid intravascular injection given the concerns for LAST or other complications. Furthermore, if injecting anesthetic into the neck, there are also multiple case reports of small volumes of anesthetic causing seizures due to a direct load of anesthetic disrupting brain function [28–30].
    - Ultrasound guidance has significantly reduced the risk of inadvertent vascular puncture [31].
  - Local Anesthetic Systemic Toxicity (LAST).
    - It is essential when performing nerve blocks, especially large volume fascial plane blocks, that the providers have access to lipid emulsion therapy for treatment of the severe, and potential life-threatening complications of LAST.
    - Each time a block is performed, a maximum safe dose of local anesthesia should be calculated.
    - Signs symptoms of LAST include perioral numbness, metallic taste, tinnitus, dysrhythmia, seizure, coma, death [32].
    - Symptomatic treatment includes benzodiazepines for seizures, cardioversion, and sodium bicarbonate for dysrhythmias, airway protection, etcetera.
    - Mainstay treatment for adults is lipid emulsion therapy: a reasonable, easy-to-remember bolus dose is 100 mL (1.5 mL/kg) [33].
      - May repeat bolus if in cardiac arrest and no return of spontaneous circulation (ROSC).
      - Bolus is followed by a continuous infusion (0.25 mL/kg/minute), which is often ~1000 mL over 1 hour.
      - It is also worth noting the lipid emulsion is recommended to be administered with a 1.2micron filter to reduce the chance of a fat embolism.
- Equipment:
  - Consider use of nerve block kits (+/− block cart) to improve efficiency and adherence (Figs. 20.3, 20.4 and 20.5). Kits can be housemade, but there are growing premade kit options offered by companies.
  - Ultrasound with high-frequency linear probe or curvilinear probe for deeper structures; consider MSK or Nerve preset.
  - Nerve block needles (common lengths include 5 and 10 centimeters).
    - If no nerve block needles are available, spinal needles are typically less cutting (more blunt) and therefore safer.
    - If able to use shorter needles to reach the target, shorter needles tend to be easier to manipulate, easier to puncture skin with blunt tips, and also reduce risk of puncturing deep structures with inadvertent/aberrant needle advancement.

Fig. 20.3 List for nerve block supplies that can be included if making a kit. (Permission to share obtained)

Nerve Block Pack Supplies

1. 3mL Syringe (×1)
2. 20mL Syringe (×2)
3. 18G Blunt Fill Needle (×1)
4. 25G or 27G Needle (×1, for skin wheal)
5. Pajunk SonoPlex® II 21G x 100mm Nerve Block Needle (×1)
6. Chlorhexidine Swab (×1)
7. Large Tegaderm, 4" × 4¾" (×1)
8. Sterile Gel Packet (×1)
9. Skin Marker Pen (×1)
10. 10mL Normal Saline Flush (×1)
11. Band-Aid (×1)
12. Packet of Papers (including BlockAlert & Universal Protocol Sheets)

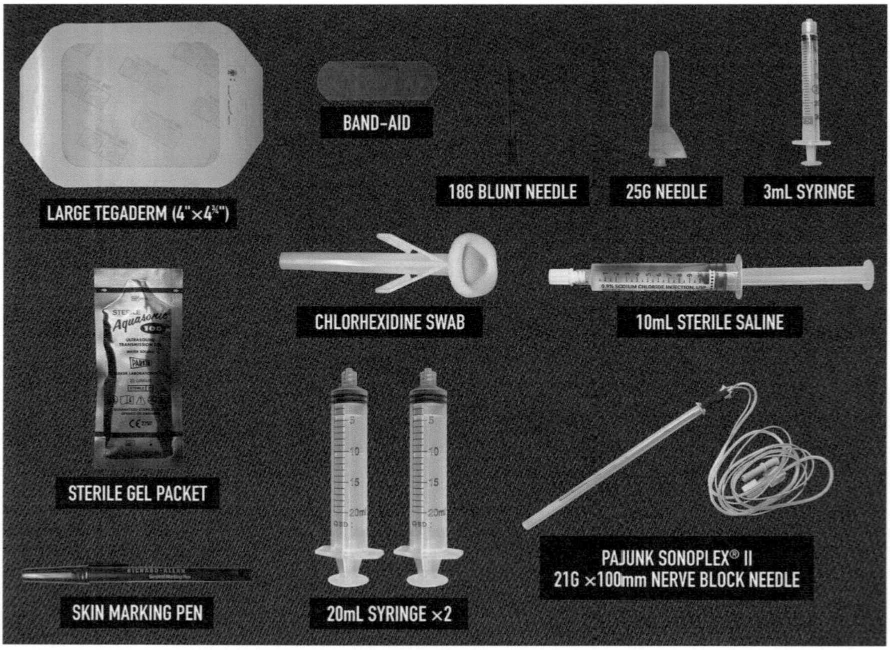

Fig. 20.4 Infographic showing equipment for a single-injection ultrasound-guided nerve block. (Created by Dr. Brian Makowski (with permission to share))

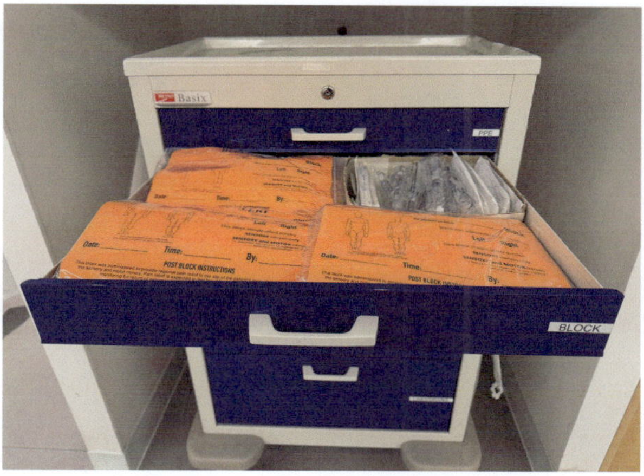

Fig. 20.5 Photograph showing a nerve block drawer in a procedure cart, conveniently located near provider desk and resuscitation rooms

- Skin cleansing (chlorhexidine, iodine, etc.)
- Sterile gel.
- Sterile gloves.
- Transducer cover (transparent dressing or sterile probe cover).
  - American Society of Regional Anesthesia (ASRA) published guidelines in 2025 recommending sterile probe cover and not using a transparent dressing [34].
  - The guidelines also highlight a large, single-center retrospective review of 7500 patients that received single-injection nerve blocks using a transparent dressing, and there were no documented infections [4]. The transparent dressing was paired with chlorhexidine with 70% isopropyl alcohol, sterile gel to the skin, and sterile gloves.
- Drawing needle.
- Saline flush(es).
- Syringes.
  - Syringe size can vary substantially based on desired block (peripheral vs high-volume fascial plane blocks).
  - Practice caution with syringes larger than 20 mL as they tend to have significantly more resistance for aspirating and injecting.
- Consider equipment for skin wheal (3 mL syringe + subcutaneous injection needle).
  - Skin wheals may improve comfort; especially for more sensitive areas of insertion, and also promote reinsertion of needle if initial poke was not ideally positioned.
- Universal protocol checklist.
- Post-block sheet (as needed by protocol; e.g., fascia iliaca).
  - If getting admitted, consider attaching a nerve block sheet to the patient's bed to communicate the block's location, duration, and any motor impairment with the inpatient team (nursing, occupational/physical therapy, etc.) (Fig. 20.6).

BLOCK ALERT

________________________________ **Block**

(For Regional Pain Relief)

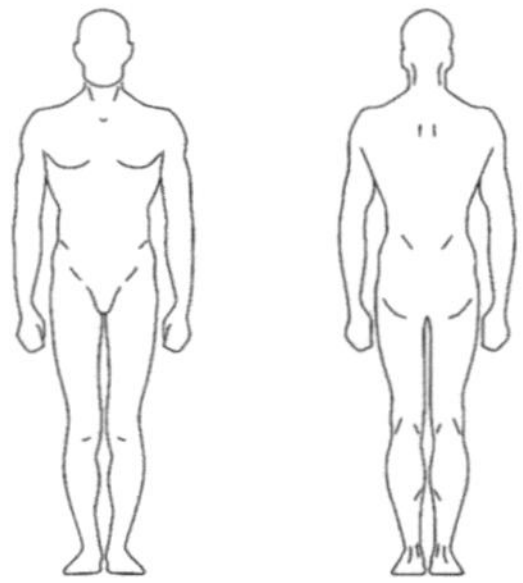

Block was administered to the (circle):

Left **Right**

This block should affect (circle):

SENSORY nerves only

SENSORY and MOTOR nerves
↳ monitor for return of motor control before mobilization

Date: __________ **Time:** __________ **By:** ____________

POST BLOCK INSTRUCTIONS

This block was administered to provide regional pain relief to the site of the patient's injury. This block can effect both the sensory and motor nerves. Pain relief is expected to last for ~12-24 hours. Ongoing assessment is important; monitoring for return of sensation and motor functions indicate that the block is wearing off.

Fig. 20.6 Figure of the block sheet that is printed, filled out at bedside, and taped to the patient's bed as a means of communication with the inpatient teams, including nursing, Anesthesia, physical therapy, and occupational therapy. (Created by Dr. Brian Makowski (with permission to share))

- Ergonomics:
  - Generally, it is worth taking the time to maximize ergonomics, and often will make the actual procedure time shorter.
  - Optimize patient positioning, bed height, machine location, bedrails, and room lighting.
  - Ideally, the room is set up in a fashion where all aspects of the procedure are in one line of view (Fig. 20.7): patient, site of interest, ultrasound screen.
- A Stepwise Two-Provider Approach.
  - Review indications and contraindications, obtain written consent, and calculate the local anesthetic safe dose. Ensure a thorough neurovascular exam has been performed prior to the block.
  - Obtain supplies and draw medications.
  - Perform time out: it is essential to confirm the correct side, especially as patient repositioning can confuse orientation. Consider reviewing any relevant imaging to further confirm such.
    - Perform universal protocol per institution policies.
  - Optimize ergonomics including operator and patient positioning, ultrasound location, and bed height.

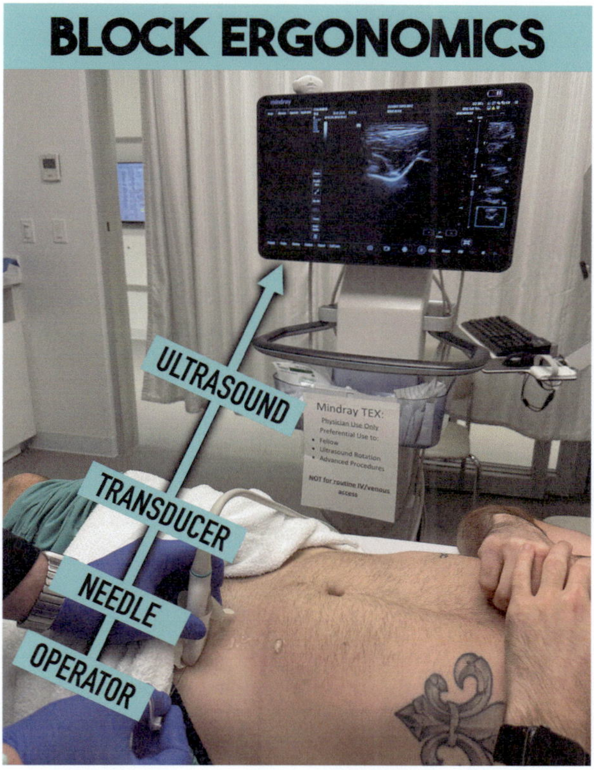

Fig. 20.7 Infographic showing all essential pieces of the procedure lined of in the field of view of the proceduralist for optimal ergonomics. (Created by Dr. Brian Makowski (with permission to share))

- Perform survey scan, consider marking site with syringe hickey technique (Fig. 20.8), or skin marker [35].
- Sterilize skin.
- Proceduralist dons gloves (typically sterile gloves), then assistant hands needle to proceduralist in a sterile fashion to detangle tubing and remove sheath.
- Assistant applies gel and transducer cover to the probe and hands to the proceduralist (may be more ideal to initially set-up transducer if using sterile probe cover).
- Consider skin wheal (performed by non-sterile assistant/supervisor while not violating sterilized skin/equipment).
  - Skin wheals may improve comfort especially more sensitive areas of insertion (e.g., neck), and also permit reinsertion of needle if initial poke was not ideally positioned.
- Perform the procedure.
  - Consider using assistant/supervisor to pull skin taught (away from insertion site) to assist with needle penetration through skin; especially with use of blunt-tipped block needles in areas of thickened skin or elderly skin.
- Post-procedure, apply bandage over the needle site, and attach post-block sheet to the patient's bed.

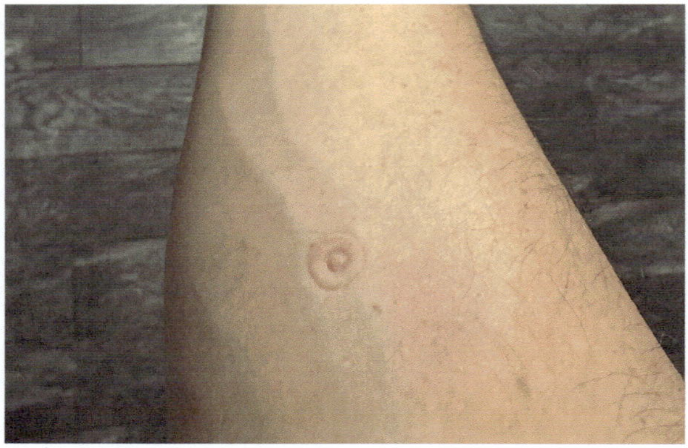

Fig. 20.8 Photo showing use of syringe hickey by contacting skin with syringe, aspirating for short period of time against intact skin, then releasing. Some studies comment using 10 mL syringe and aspirating to 5 mL mark for approximately 1 minute

- Monitor patient for at least 30 minutes after procedure, including cardiac monitoring, especially for higher volume fascial plane blocks [36]..
- Provide appropriate post-block instructions/expectations, especially if being discharged before the block wears off.

- One Provider Approach
  - There are multiple variations of a single provider approach, including using a syringe directly connected to a needle (+/− thumb slot), "Let Go Technique" where needle is released once in proper placement is achieved, and needle hand is then used to grab syringe, or other techniques, such as the Jedi hold (Fig. 20.9) [37, 38].
- Needle visualization
  - Needle visualization is an essential aspect for block success and safety.
  - In-plane approach is optimal for the majority of blocks.
    - Refer to the Ultrasound-Guided Procedures chapter for more detail on in-plane and out-of-plane approaches.
  - It is essential to line up the needle completely midline and parallel relative to the footprint of the probe (Fig. 20.10).
  - The more parallel the needle is relative to the footprint of the transducer, the more perpendicular the needle is to soundwaves, which allows more sound waves to reflect back to the transducer and improve visualization [39].
    - It's overall optimal to maintain the angle of needle relative to the transducer at greater than 55 degrees, ideally as close to 90 degrees as possible (Fig. 20.11).
    - If only able to use a steeper needle approach to reach the target, it can also be helpful to rock (also called heel) the transducer toward the needle (Fig. 20.12)·[40, 41].

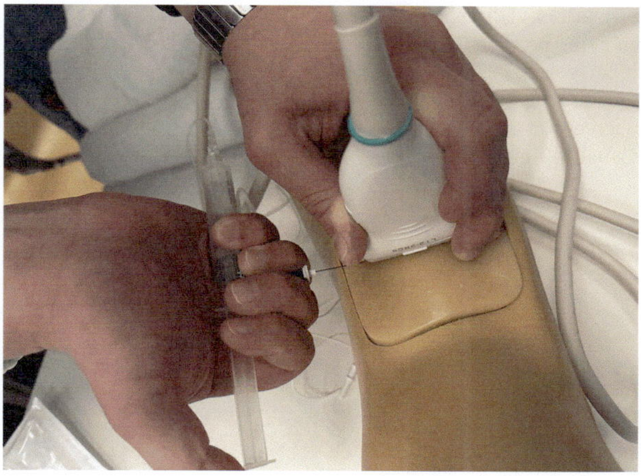

Fig. 20.9 Photo showing "Jedi" hold for single-provider nerve block technique

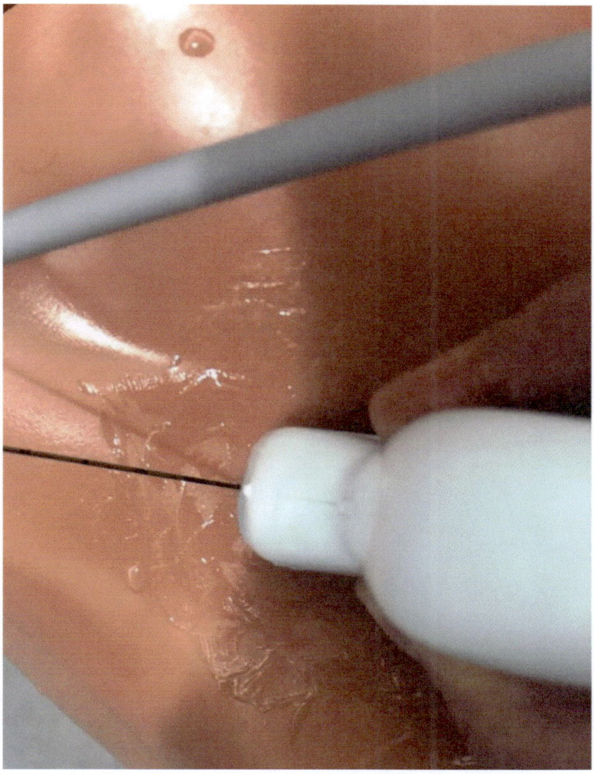

Fig. 20.10 Photograph showing the process of lining up needle midline and parallel relative to transducer to optimize needle visualization during in-plane approaches

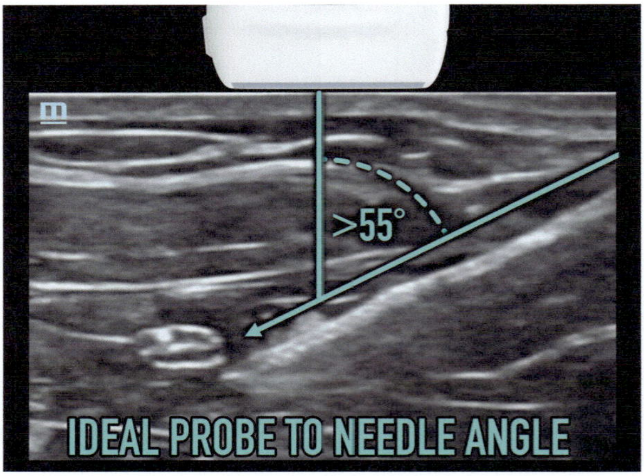

Fig. 20.11 Ultrasound showing needle angle relative to transducer, with goal to be greater than 55 degrees to improve needle visualization

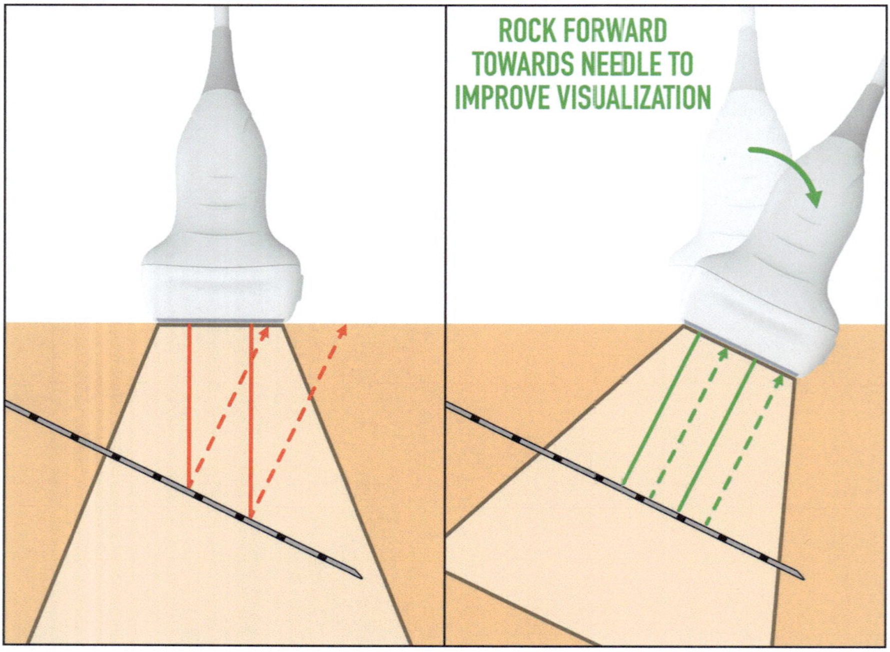

Fig. 20.12 Figure showing how rocking toward the needle can substantially improve needle visualization. (Created by Dr. Brian Makowski (with permission to share))

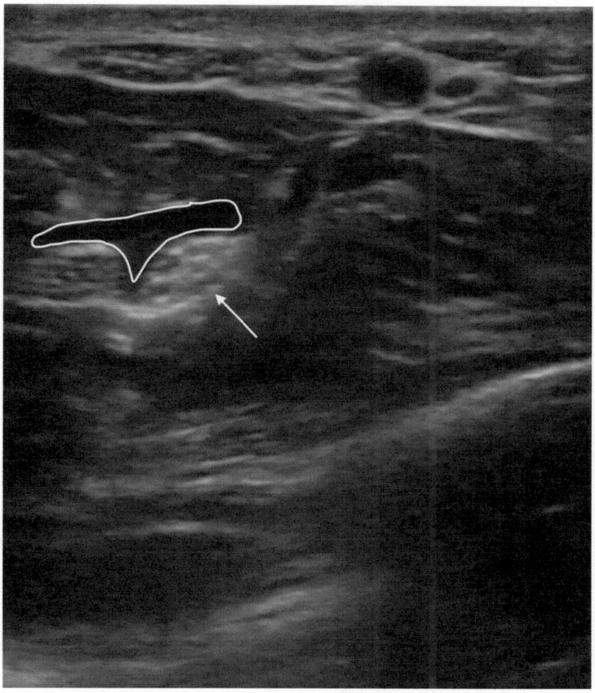

Fig. 20.13 Image demonstrating a successful nerve block. The black fluid (abstract shape) denotes the anesthetic surrounding the targeted nerve (white arrow) along the same fascial plane as the nerve

    - May also consider inserting the needle with further distance between probe and entry site, which typically permits a shallower angle.
  - Hydro-localization is a key piece to keep track of needle tip; small, somewhat brisk injections of <1 mL of sterile saline can help identify the needle tip (Fig. 20.13; Video 20.1).
  - Consider the use of nerve block needles as they are often machined in a fashion that improves needle visualization.
  - If needle visualization is lost, consider:
    - Very small fans to re-identify the needle tip.
    - Removing probe from patient and replacing the probe along the axis of the needle.
    - Completely removing the needle from the patient and restarting.
- Credits:
  - Special recognition to Dr. Arun Nagdev and his years of efforts to improve multi-modal pain control through ultrasound-guided nerve blocks in the Emergency Department.
  - Special recognition to the Blockheads Emergency-Based Regional Anesthesia Group, which is a group of Emergency Medicine providers committed to safely expanding the role of nerve blocks and improving patient care through research and education.

Key Points

- Nerve blocks have a myriad of indications, with overall low complications rates (especially with ultrasound) and nearly nonexistent infection rates with single injection blocks.
- Utilizing ergonomics (room set-up, etcetera) can drastically improve block ease and success.
- Having good in-plane needle approach skills and optimizing needle angle to >55 degrees relative to transducer footprint are key factors for block success.
- Anticoagulation/coagulopathy is typically a relative contraindication, but risks benefits should be weighed, and severity of block risk also factored (median nerve block versus interscalene brachial plexus block).
- Important safety steps include obtaining written consent, confirming correct side, calculating maximum safe dose of anesthetic, having safe needle trajectory and avoiding intraneural injection.
- Monitor for Local Anesthetic Systemic Toxicity (LAST) when using higher volumes, and have lipid emulsion therapy readily available; a reasonable first bolus in adults is 100 mL (~1.5 mL/kg).
- Preservative-free dexamethasone serves as a great perineural adjunct to extend the duration of block.

References

1. De Cassai A, et al. Complications rate estimation after thoracic erector spinae plane block. J Cardiothor Vasc Anesth. 2021;35(10):3142–3.
2. Goldsmith A, Driver L, Duggan NM, Riscinti M, Martin D, Heffler M, Shokoohi H, Dreyfuss A, Sell J, Brown C, Fung C, Perice L, Bennett D, Truong N, Jafry SZ, Macias M, Brown J, Nagdev A. Complication rates after ultrasonography-guided nerve blocks performed in the emergency department. s. 2024;7(11):e2444742. https://doi.org/10.1001/jamanetworkopen.2024.44742. Erratum in: JAMA Netw Open 2024 Dec 2;7(12):e2455847. doi:10.1001/jamanetworkopen.2024.55847. PMID: 39535792; PMCID: PMC11561692
3. Jeng CL, et al. Complications of peripheral nerve blocks. B J Anaesth. 2010;105:i97–i107.
4. Alakkad H, Naeeni A, Chan VWS, et al. Infection related to ultrasound-guided single-injection peripheral nerve blockade: a decade of experience at Toronto Western hospital. Reg Anesth Pain Med. 2015;40:82–4.
5. Tsui BCH, Kirkham K, Kwofie MK, Tran Q, Wong P, Chin KJ, Sondekoppam RV. Practice advisory on the bleeding risks for peripheral nerve and interfascial plane blockade: evidence review and expert consensus. Can J Anaesth. 2019;66(11):1356–84. https://doi.org/10.1007/s12630-019-01466-w. English. Epub 2019 Aug 26. PMID: 31452012
6. Toscano A, Capuano P, Galatà M, Tazzi I, Rinaldi M, Brazzi L. Safety of ultrasound-guided serratus anterior and erector Spinae fascial plane blocks: a retrospective analysis in patients undergoing cardiac surgery while receiving anticoagulant and antiplatelet drugs. J Cardiothorac Vasc Anesth. 2022;36(2):483–8. https://doi.org/10.1053/j.jvca.2021.05.037. Epub 2021 May 24. PMID: 34148801
7. Dultz LA, Ma R, Dumas RP, Grant JL, Park C, Alexander JC, Gasanova I, Cripps MW. Safety of erector spinae plane blocks in patients with chest wall trauma on venous thromboembolism prophylaxis. J Surg Res. 2021;263:124–9. https://doi.org/10.1016/j.jss.2021.01.020. Epub 2021 Feb 27. PMID: 33652174
8. Benzon HT, Jabri RS, Van Zundert TC. Neuraxial anesthesia and peripheral nerve blocks in patients on anticoagulants. NYSORA.

9. Ashken T, West S. Regional anaesthesia in patients at risk of bleeding. BJA Educ. 2021;21(3):84–94. https://doi.org/10.1016/j.bjae.2020.11.004. Epub 2021 Jan 26. Erratum in: BJA Educ. 2021 Jul;21(7):278. doi:10.1016/j.bjae.2021.04.001. PMID: 33664977; PMCID: PMC7892354
10. Lam D, Pierson D, Salaria O, Wardhan R, Li J. Pain control with regional anesthesia in patients at risk of acute compartment syndrome: review of the literature and editorial view. J Pain Res. 2023;16:635–48. https://doi.org/10.2147/JPR.S397428. PMID: 36891457; PMCID: PMC9987529
11. Fubini PE, Savoldelli GL, Beckmann TS, Samer CF, Suppan M. Impact of a Mobile app (LoAD Calc) on the calculation of maximum safe doses of local anesthetics: protocol for a randomized controlled trial. JMIR Res Protoc. 2024;13:e53679. https://doi.org/10.2196/53679. PMID: 38170571; PMCID: PMC10794956
12. https://apps.apple.com/ca/app/safelocal/id1440999841
13. McCombe K, Bogod D. Regional anaesthesia: risk, consent and complications. Anaesthesia. 2021;76(Suppl 1):18–26. https://doi.org/10.1111/anae.15246. PMID: 33426664
14. Tonder S, Togioka BM, Maani CV. Chloroprocaine. 2023 Jul 17. In: StatPearls [Internet]. Treasure Island (FL): StatPearls Publishing; 2025 Jan–. PMID: 30422496.
15. Scott DB, Lee A, Fagan D, Bowler GM, Bloomfield P, Lundh R. Acute toxicity of ropivacaine compared with that of bupivacaine. Anesth Analg. 1989;69(5):563–9. PMID: 2679230
16. Graf BM, Abraham I, Eberbach N, Kunst G, Stowe DF, Martin E. Differences in cardiotoxicity of bupivacaine and ropivacaine are the result of physicochemical and stereoselective properties. Anesthesiology. 2002;96(6):1427–34. https://doi.org/10.1097/00000542-200206000-00023. PMID: 12170056
17. Graf BM. The cardiotoxicity of local anesthetics: the place of ropivacaine. Curr Top Med Chem. 2001;1(3):207–14. https://doi.org/10.2174/1568026013395164. PMID: 11895138
18. Pehora C, Pearson AM, Kaushal A, Crawford MW, Johnston B. Dexamethasone as an adjuvant to peripheral nerve block. Cochrane Database Syst Rev. 2017;11(11):CD011770. https://doi.org/10.1002/14651858.CD011770.pub2. PMID: 29121400; PMCID: PMC6486015
19. Vieira PA, Pulai I, Tsao GC, Manikantan P, Keller B, Connelly NR. Dexamethasone with bupivacaine increases duration of analgesia in ultrasound-guided interscalene brachial plexus blockade. Eur J Anaesthesiol. 2010;27(3):285–8. https://doi.org/10.1097/EJA.0b013e3283350c38. PMID: 20009936
20. Knight JB, Schott NJ, Kentor ML, Williams BA. Neurotoxicity of common peripheral nerve block adjuvants. Curr Opin Anaesthesiol. 2015;28(5):598–604. https://doi.org/10.1097/ACO.0000000000000222. PMID: 26207854; PMCID: PMC4606467
21. Tan ESJ, Tan YR, Liu CWY. Efficacy of perineural versus intravenous dexamethasone in prolonging the duration of analgesia when administered with peripheral nerve blocks: a systematic review and meta-analysis. Korean J Anesthesiol. 2022;75(3):255–65. https://doi.org/10.4097/kja.21390. Epub 2021 Dec 29. PMID: 34963269; PMCID: PMC9171542
22. Kim DH, Liu J, Beathe JC, Lin Y, Wetmore DS, Kim SJ, Haskins SC, Garvin S, Oxendine JA, Ho MC, Allen AA, Popovic M, Gbaje E, Wu CL, Memtsoudis SG. Interscalene brachial plexus block with liposomal bupivacaine versus standard bupivacaine with Perineural dexamethasone: a noninferiority trial. Anesthesiology. 2022;136(3):434–47. https://doi.org/10.1097/ALN.0000000000004111. Erratum in: Anesthesiology 2023 Feb 1;138(2):233. doi:10.1097/ALN.0000000000004255. PMID: 35041742
23. Sobhani K, Hocevar M, Hanchuk S, Press B, He Z, Lin HM, Li J. Fascial plane blocks with glucocorticoids or liposomal bupivacaine versus local infiltration for laparoscopic non-donor nephrectomy: a propensity score-weighted study. Cureus. 2024;16(8):e66005. https://doi.org/10.7759/cureus.66005. PMID: 39221354; PMCID: PMC11366221
24. Truong A, Fleshner PR, Mirocha JM, Tran HP, Shane R, Zaghiyan KN. A prospective randomized trial of surgeon-administered intraoperative Transversus abdominis plane block with bupivacaine against liposomal bupivacaine: the TINGLE trial. Dis Colon Rectum. 2021;64(7):888–98. https://doi.org/10.1097/DCR.0000000000002008. PMID: 34086002

25. Suresh S, De Oliveira GS Jr. Local anaesthetic dosage of peripheral nerve blocks in children: analysis of 40 121 blocks from the Pediatric Regional Anesthesia Network database. Br J Anaesth. 2018;120(2):317–22. https://doi.org/10.1016/j.bja.2017.10.019. Epub 2017 Nov 24. Erratum in: Br J Anaesth. 2018 Sep;121(3):686. doi:10.1016/j.bja.2018.06.005. PMID: 29406181
26. McLeod G, Reina MA. Nerve block, nerve damage, and fluid injection pressure: overturning the myth. Br J Anaesth. 2024;132(5):1022–6. https://doi.org/10.1016/j.bja.2023.12.006. Epub 2024 Jan 5. PMID: 38182528
27. Maruyama M. Long-tapered double needle used to reduce needle stick nerve injury. Reg Anesth 1997;22(2):157–160. doi: https://doi.org/10.1016/s1098-7339(06)80035-0. PMID: 9089858
28. Lu F, Tian J, Dong J, Zhang K. Tonic-clonic seizure during the ultrasound-guided stellate ganglion block because of an injection into an unrecognized variant vertebral artery: a case report. Medicine (Baltimore). 2019;98(48):e18168. https://doi.org/10.1097/MD.0000000000018168. PMID: 31770265; PMCID: PMC6890314
29. Alsukhni RA, Ghoubari MS, Farfouti MT, Aboras YA. Status epilepticus following local anesthesia in a previously healthy adult. BMC Res Notes. 2016;9 300. https://doi.org/10.1186/s13104-016-2100-9. PMID: 27287503; PMCID: PMC4901442
30. Veiga D, Gomes C, Araújo R. Seizures during carotid endarterectomy under cervical plexus block: 17AP2-2. Eur J Anaesthesiol. 2012;29:218.
31. Mariano ER, Loland VJ, Bellars RH, Sandhu NS, Bishop ML, Abrams RA, Meunier MJ, Maldonado RC, Ferguson EJ, Ilfeld BM. Ultrasound guidance versus electrical stimulation for infraclavicular brachial plexus perineural catheter insertion. J Ultrasound Med. 2009;28(9):1211–8. https://doi.org/10.7863/jum.2009.28.9.1211. PMID: 19710219
32. Long B, Chavez S, Gottlieb M, Montrief T, Brady WJ. Local anesthetic systemic toxicity: a narrative review for emergency clinicians. Am J Emerg Med. 2022;59:42–8. https://doi.org/10.1016/j.ajem.2022.06.017. Epub 2022 Jun 13. PMID: 35777259
33. https://www.nysora.com/anesthesia/local-anesthetic-systemic-toxicity-last/
34. Provenzano DA, Hanes M, Hunt C, Benzon HT, Grider JS, Cawcutt K, Doshi TL, Hayek S, Hoelzer B, Johnson RL, Kalagara H, Kopp S, Loftus RW, Macfarlane AJR, Nagpal AS, Neuman SA, Pawa A, Pearson ACS, Pilitsis J, Sivanesan E, Sondekoppam RV, Van Zundert J, Narouze S. ASRA Pain Medicine consensus practice infection control guidelines for regional anesthesia and pain medicine. Reg Anesth Pain Med. 2025:rapm-2024–105651. doi: https://doi.org/10.1136/rapm-2024-105651. Epub ahead of print. PMID: 39837579.
35. Issa EC, Ware PJ, Bitange P, Cooper GJ, Galea T, Bengiamin DI, Young TP. The "syringe hickey": an alternative skin marking method for lumbar puncture. J Emerg Med. 2023;64(3):400–4. https://doi.org/10.1016/j.jemermed.2023.01.013. PMID: 37019501
36. Tsui BH, Hadzic A. Chapter 17. Equipment for peripheral nerve block. In: Hadzic A, editor. NYSORA textbook of regional anesthesia and acute pain management. The McGraw-Hill Companies; 2007. Accessed March 05, 2025. https://accessanesthesiology.mhmedical.com/content.aspx?bookid=413&sectionid=39828165.
37. Keklik N, Aytaç İ, Başkan S, Güven Aytaç B. Is Jedi grip efficient and effective in ultrasound-guided peripheral nerve blocking? A prospective, randomized, observer-blinded study. Braz J Anesthesiol. 2022;72(3):372–8. https://doi.org/10.1016/j.bjane.2021.07.016. Epub 2021 Aug 8. PMID: 34371058; PMCID: PMC9373694.
38. Singh SK, Mistry T. 'Let Go' technique in ultrasound guided regional anaesthesia. J Anaesth Crit Care Case Rep. 2019;5(3):7–9.
39. Chin KJ, Perlas A, Chan VW, Brull R. Needle visualization in ultrasound-guided regional anesthesia: challenges and solutions. Reg Anesth Pain Med. 2008;33(6):532–44. https://doi.org/10.1016/j.rapm.2008.06.002. PMID: 19258968
40. Bahner DP, Blickendorf JM, Bockbrader M, Adkins E, Vira A, Boulger C, Panchal AR. Language of transducer manipulation: codifying terms for effective teaching. J Ultrasound Med. 2016;35(1):183–8. https://doi.org/10.7863/ultra.15.02036. Epub 2015 Dec 17. PMID: 26679204
41. Prabhakar C, Uppal V, Sondekoppam RV. Effect of beam steering on echogenic and non-echogenic needle visibility at 40°, 50°, and 60° needle insertion angles. Anesth Analg. 2018;126(6):1926–9. https://doi.org/10.1213/ANE.0000000000002618. PMID: 29116966

Ultrasound-Guided Regional Anesthesia: Head and Neck

21

Robert Stenberg, Brian Makowski, and Jordan Tozer

Ultrasound-guided nerve blocks of the head and neck offer a precise, real-time approach to regional anesthesia and pain management in an anatomically complex region. By leveraging high-resolution imaging, clinicians can identify critical vascular and neural structures, enhance block efficacy, and reduce complications. This chapter provides an overview of key sonoanatomy, indications, techniques, and safety considerations for commonly performed head and neck blocks, including the superficial cervical plexus and brachial plexus blocks, among others. General considerations for approach and technique learned in the previous chapter can be applied here.

Head and Neck Blocks

- Stellate Ganglion Block (SGB)
  - Indications:
    - Electrical Storm/ Refractory ventricular tachycardia/Refractory ventricular fibrillation. [1]
      - There is growing data on its efficacy and safety [2, 3].

Supplementary Information The online version contains supplementary material available at https://doi.org/10.1007/978-3-032-27643-8_21.

R. Stenberg (✉) · B. Makowski
Department of Emergency Medicine, Cleveland Clinic, Akron, OH, USA
e-mail: stenber@ccf.org; makowsb2@ccf.org

J. Tozer
Department of Emergency Medicine, Virginia Commonwealth University Health, Richmond, VA, USA
e-mail: jordan.tozer@vcuhealth.org

A. Lindsay et al. (eds.), *Clinical Ultrasound*,
https://doi.org/10.1007/978-3-032-27643-8_21

- Significant other indications exist, but typically are not relevant to the emergency setting [4].
  - There are some scenarios in neurocritical care where it is used for severe vasospasm [5].
- Anesthetic Volume:
  - ~10 mL of anesthetic
    - Studies vary from 5 to 20 mL.
    - Doing higher doses will increase risk for complications as anesthetic diffuses into adjacent structures [6].
- Procedure [7]:
  - Position patient supine with contralateral head rotation if possible.
  - Place probe transversely along the anteromedial aspect of the left neck in the paratracheal region near the thyroid (~C6 level). May also palpate Chassaignac's tubercle (anterior tubercle of the C6 transverse process).
    - This is traditionally done first to the left neck due to some evidence showing right-sided blocks having higher incidence of hypotension and bradycardia [8].
  - Identify longus colli muscle by identifying carotid artery and finding the muscle belly deep to carotid artery (Fig. 21.1); may or may not well visualize sympathetic chain along the anterior surface of the longus colli. Locate a safe needle trajectory.
    - Consider use of Color/Power Doppler to identify any vascular structures that may be located in path of needle (particularly the vertebral and inferior thyroid arteries).
  - Insert needle posterolateral to anteromedial. Advance needle. Until tip is just superficial to the longus colli muscle, being mindful of needle

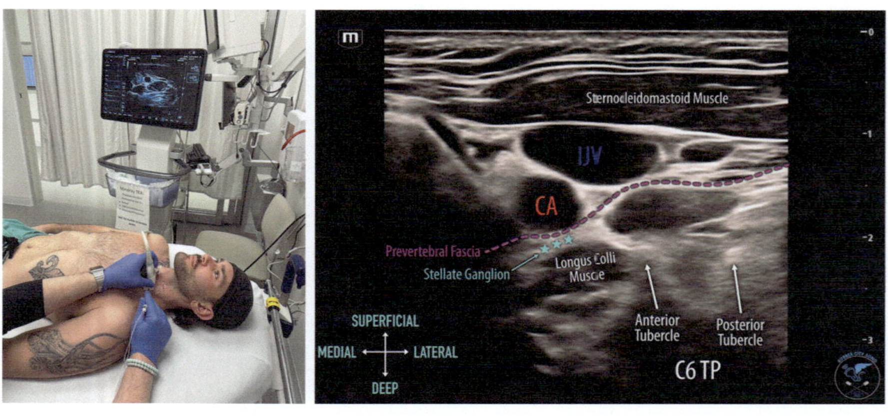

Fig. 21.1 Figure showing stellate ganglion block. Left, showing room set-up and hand positioning. Right, ultrasound image with arrow showing approximate needle approach for stellate ganglion block, with the target deep to the carotid artery along the fascial plane of longus colli muscle (circle). (Created by Dr. Brian Makowski (with permission to share))

approach to not strike vital surrounding structures. Deposit anesthetic, aspirating every 5 mL (Video 21.1). Anchoring the transducer and needle arms/hands against both patient and gurney can be crucial for stability; can also try to advance needle during pulse check if patient in cardiac arrest.
    - Reassess for need of additional stellate ganglion block to the opposite side.
    - Positive Horner's syndrome may be expected, but does not always occur, even in the setting of a successful block (defined by reduction in dysrhythmia/ectopy) [1].
    - There should be extra caution in the neck given the vital structures (thyroid artery, vertebral artery, carotid artery, esophagus, brachial plexus); and after the needle is ~1 cm in the skin, needle should NOT be advanced/adjusted unless the needle and tip are well visualized.
  - Unique Complications (percentage driven from STAR Study) [1]:
    - Horner syndrome (~39%).
    - Bradycardia (0.5%).
    - Respiratory depression (0.5%).
    - Hypotension (~0.5%).
    - Brachial plexus paralysis (1.6%).
    - Hoarseness (1.1%).
    - Neck pain/vomiting (0.5%).
- Cervical Plexus Block (intermediate, previously called superficial cervical plexus block or SCPB).
  - Indications [9]:
    - Neck abscess (anterior neck).
    - Muscular neck pain and or torticollis.
    - Midshaft clavicle fracture.
    - Adjunct to ear lobe anesthesia.
    - Anesthesia for IJ central line placement.
  - Anesthetic Volume:
    - 5-10 mL
  - Procedure [10]:
    - Position patient supine or semi-recumbent, ideally with head against bed for stability; consider contralateral head rotation to improve ergonomics.
    - Place probe transversely along anterior paratracheal neck, at approximately level of thyroid cartilage (~C4).
    - Identify the sternocleidomastoid muscle (SCM) and its surrounding fascial plane. Identify the prevertebral fascia, located on the anterior surface of the scalene muscles. (Fig. 21.2).
    - Insert needle posterolaterally to anteromedially, with the goal of placing needle tip just underneath the hyperechoic fascia on the posterior surface of the SCM.
    - After fluid is identified spreading deep to SCM, and superficial to prevertebral fascia, inject remaining anesthetic (Fig. 21.3). (Video 21.2).

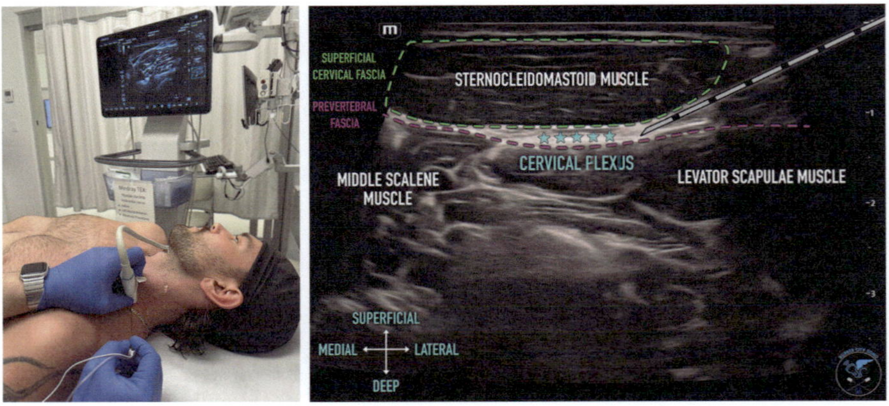

Fig. 21.2 Figure showing cervical plexus block. Left, photo showing room set-up: Head turned away, transducer approximately at C4 level. Right, ultrasound image showing target deep to sternocleidomastoid fascial plane and superficial to the prevertebral fascia overlying the scalene muscle. (Created by Dr. Brian Makowski (with permission to share))

Fig. 21.3 Image showing cervical plexus block with anesthetic infusing into the investing layer of deep cervical fascia while remaining clear/superficial to the prevertebral fascia

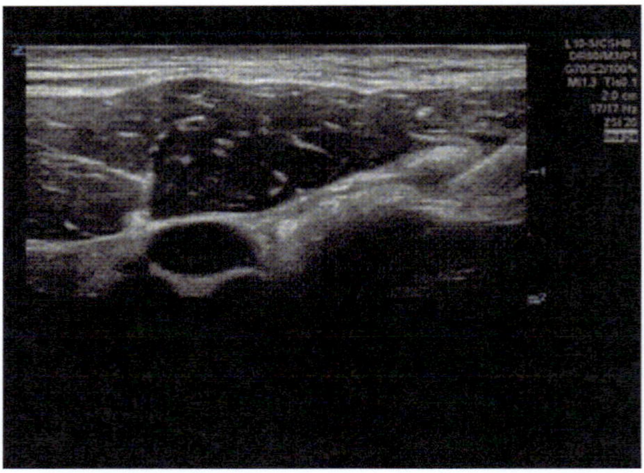

- By maintaining and infiltrating superficial to the prevertebral fascia, there is thought that this reduces the risk of phrenic nerve blockade [10].
- Be mindful of using low pressure when injecting to avoid nervous injury.
- There should be extra caution in the neck given the vital structures; and after the needle is 1-2 cm in the skin, needle should NOT be advanced/adjusted unless the needle and tip are well visualized.

- Unique Complications [11]:
  - Self-limiting hoarseness.
  - Asymptomatic hemi-diaphragmatic paresis (largely rare and mainly a complication of deep cervical plexus block).
  - Horner syndrome.

- Interscalene Brachial Plexus Block (ISPB)
  - Indications:
    - Anesthetic affecting primarily the nerve roots of C5/C6/C7.
    - Shoulder dislocation [11]
    - Humerus fractures.
    - Lacerations/abscesses at the upper arm or deltoid.
  - Contraindications [12]:
    - This block should be assumed to affect the phrenic nerve and an alternative block should be strongly considered if there is concern the patient will not tolerate phrenic nerve palsy (severe COPD, poor respiratory reserve).
    - This is a higher-risk block for patients with anticoagulation and/or coagulopathy.
  - Anesthetic Volume:
    - ~15 mL
      - 10-20 mL with old data up to 40 mL [13].
      - Anesthesia has done down to 5 mL [14].
      - Large volumes have been shown to have higher rates of temporary phrenic nerve blockade/hemidiaphragmatic paresis.
  - Procedure:
    - Position patient supine or semi-recumbent, ideally with head against bed for stability; may be helpful to rotate head away from proceduralist.
    - Identify the cervical nerve roots positioned between the anterior and middle scalene muscles. It is often easiest to place the probe in a transverse orientation in the supraclavicular fossa, and after identifying the brachial plexus, sweeping proximally until the "stoplight" appearance of the C5, C6, and C7 nerve roots is seen between the anterior and middle scalene muscles. Color and/or power Doppler can also be used to confirm nerve fascicle versus blood vessel. (Fig. 21.4).
    - Anesthesia-oriented approach [15]:
      - Insert needle in-plane, posterolaterally to anteromedially, toward the brachial plexus.
      - Needle is advanced through the middle scalene muscle belly with goal trajectory of placing needle tip between the C5 and C6 nerve fascicles, avoiding intrafascicular violation. (Fig. 21.5).

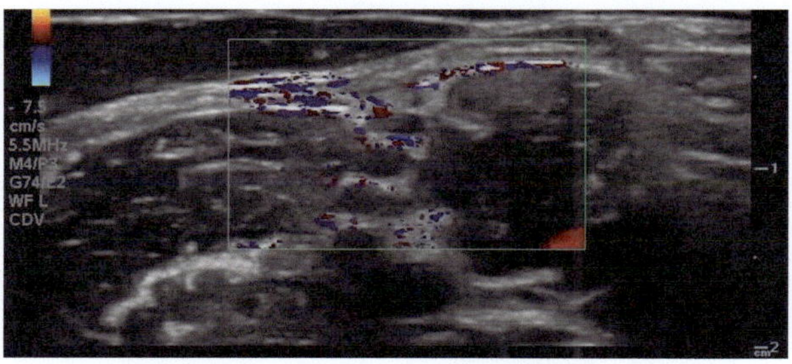

Fig. 21.4 Nerve roots seen in interscalene groove with color Doppler helping correctly recognize as nerve root/fascicle and not blood vessel

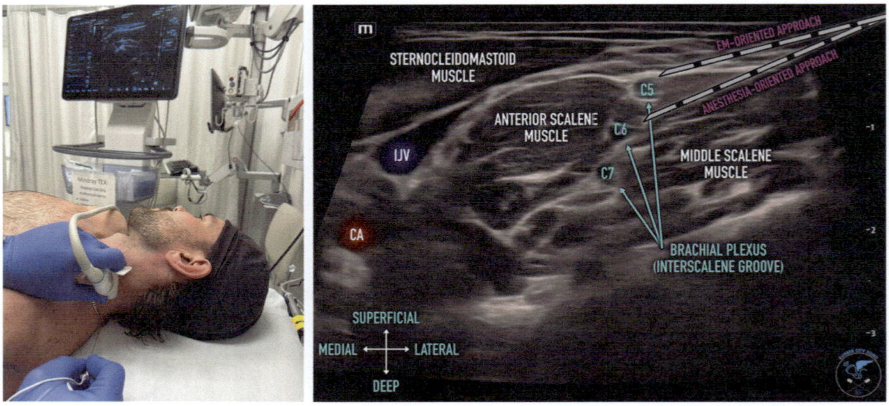

Fig. 21.5 Figure showing interscalene brachial plexus block. Left, photo showing set-up and ergonomics for block. Right, ultrasound figure showing “stoplight” C5/C6/C7 interscalene brachial plexus (oval) in between anterior and middle scalene. Both Needle approaches shown, either penetrating through middle scalene aiming between C5/C6 fascicles or along the superficial edge of C5. (Created by Dr. Brian Makowski (with permission to share))

    - Needle is carefully advanced with using hydrolocalization until the fluid is demonstrated spreading along interscalene groove, in between middle scalene and perineural tissue (Video 21.3).
  - Alternative Approach (used by some EM Providers) [16]:
    - Same set-up as standard interscalene approach.
    - Needle trajectory is now aimed toward the area between the prevertebral fascia overlying the scalene muscles and the C5 nerve fascicle (refer back to Fig. 21.5).
    - Needle is carefully advanced with using hydrolocalization until the fluid is demonstrated spreading between middle scalene and perineural tissue, and diving deep along the interscalene groove.
    - Anesthetic is deposited with low pressure (Video 21.4).
  - There should be extra caution in the neck given the vital structures; and after the needle is 1-2cm in the skin, needle should NOT be advanced/adjusted unless the needle and tip are well visualized.
- Unique Complications [17]:
  - Temporary phrenic nerve paralysis/hemidiaphragmatic paresis (high incidence) [18].
  - Major complication rate 0.35% and minor complication rate of 11.3% [19].

- Supraclavicular Brachial Plexus Block (SBP)
  - Indications [20]:
    - Large arm lacerations, abscesses, or soft tissue injuries covering multiple dermatomes in the upper extremity or deltoid.
    - Fractures and dislocations of the arm, including distal radius.
  - Anesthetic Volume:
    - 20-40 mL
      - There is evidence for higher success with higher volumes [20].

- Procedure [21, 22]:
  - Position patient in supine or semi-recumbent positioning and consider contralateral head rotation to improve ergonomics.
  - Place probe in transverse orientation in the supraclavicular fossa, parallel to the clavicle's superior border and perpendicular to skin; identify brachial plexus and center on screen.
  - To identify, sweep craniocaudally until the brachial plexus is positioned just superficial to the first rib (Fig. 21.6). May need to fan caudally to visualize optimal location for depositing anesthetic. (Video 21.5).
  - Insert needle posterolateral to anteromedially, with needle trajectory directed toward the first rib as "backstop" to prevent injury to vital structures.
  - Needle is carefully advanced until tip is adjacent to the rib and brachial plexus using hydro-localization, sometimes called the "Corner pocket". (Video 21.6).
  - Some providers, particularly in the anesthesia setting or desire to ensure superior trunk is also captured in the block, will also withdraw, redirect, and place needle superficial to the plexus closer to superior trunk fascicles [23].
    - There should be extra caution in the neck given the vital structures; and after the needle is 1-2 cm in the skin, needle should NOT be advanced/adjusted unless the needle and tip are well visualized.
    - There is also debate whether or not the brachial plexus sheath should be violated, with some noting increased concern for nerve damage by injecting into the sheath.

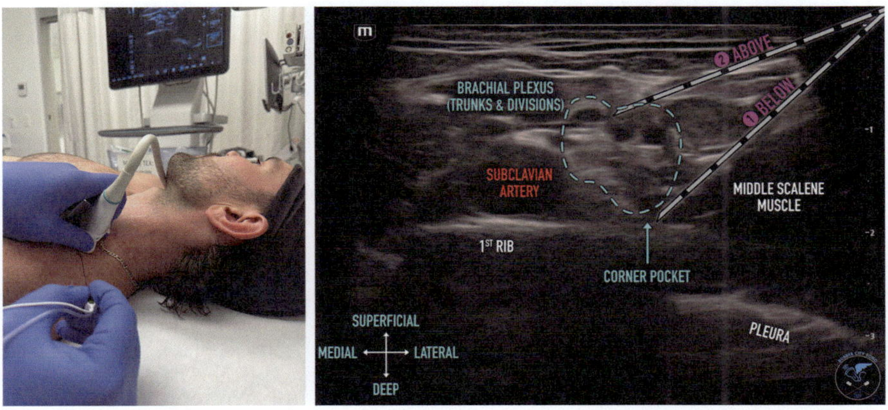

Fig. 21.6 Figure showing supraclavicular brachial plexus block. Left, photo showing set-up and ergonomics for supraclavicular brachial plexus block. Right, image showing ideal visualization with brachial plexus (oval) sitting on top of first rib lateral to the subclavian artery, and a safe approach (arrow) to reach the "corner pocket" (space between rib and nerve group). (Created by Dr. Brian Makowski (with permission to share))

- Unique Complications:
  - Incidence of complications around 1% from review of over 500 patients [24, 25].
    - Horner syndrome (~1%).
    - Hemidiaphragmatic paresis (~1%).
    - Vascular puncture (0.4%).
    - Transient sensory deficits (0.4%).
    - 0 cases of clinical significant pneumothorax.

References

1. Savastano S, Baldi E, Compagnoni S, Rordorf R, Sanzo A, Gentile FR, Dusi V, Frea S, Gravinese C, Cauti FM, Iannopollo G, De Sensi F, Gandolfi E, Frigerio L, Crea P, Zagari D, Casula M, Sangiorgi G, Persampieri S, Dell'Era G, Patti G, Colombo C, Mugnai G, Notaristefano F, Barengo A, Falcetti R, Perego GB, D'Angelo G, Tanese N, Currao A, Sgromo V, De Ferrari GM, STAR Study Group. Electrical storm treatment by percutaneous stellate ganglion block: the STAR study. Eur Heart J. 2024;45(10):823–33. https://doi.org/10.1093/eurheartj/ehae021. Erratum in: Eur Heart J. 2024 Oct 14;45(39):4235. doi:10.1093/eurheartj/ehae631. PMID: 38289867; PMCID: PMC10919918
2. Motazedian P, Quinn N, Wells GA, et al. Efficacy of stellate ganglion block in treatment of electrical storm: a systematic review and meta-analysis. Sci Rep. 2024;14:24719. https://doi.org/10.1038/s41598-024-76663-9.
3. Lobato EB, Kern KB, Paige GB, Brown M, Sulek CA. Differential effects of right versus left stellate ganglion block on left ventricular function in humans: an echocardiographic analysis. J Clin Anesth. 2000;12(4):315–8. https://doi.org/10.1016/s0952-8180(00)00158-6. PMID: 10960205
4. Feigin G, Velasco Figueroa S, Englesakis MF, D'Souza R, Hoydonckx Y, Bhatia A. Stellate ganglion block for non-pain indications: a scoping review. Pain Med. 2023;24(7):775–81. https://doi.org/10.1093/pm/pnad011. PMID: 36727500
5. Jing L, Wu Y, Liang F, Jian M, Bai Y, Wang Y, Liu H, Wang A, Chen X, Han R. Effect of early stellate ganglion block in cerebral vasospasm after aneurysmal subarachnoid hemorrhage (BLOCK-CVS): study protocol for a randomized controlled trial. Trials. 2022;23(1):922. https://doi.org/10.1186/s13063-022-06867-9. PMID: 36333751; PMCID: PMC9636713
6. Feigl GC, Rosmarin W, Stelzl A, Weninger B, Likar R. Comparison of different injectate volumes for stellate ganglion block: an anatomic and radiologic study. Reg Anesth Pain Med. 2007;32(3):203–8. https://doi.org/10.1016/j.rapm.2006.11.013. PMID: 17543814
7. Nair A, Bhoi S, Choudhary Y. Cease the storm – successful stellate ganglion block in terminating refractory electrical storm. Am J Emerg Med. 2024;81:160.e3–7. https://doi.org/10.1016/j.ajem.2024.03.003. Epub 2024 Apr 1. PMID: 38575462
8. Yokota S, Taneyama C, Goto H. Different effects of right and left stellate ganglion block on systolic blood pressure and heart rate. Open J Anesthesiol. 2013;3(3):143–7. https://doi.org/10.4236/ojanes.2013.33033.
9. Ho B, De Paoli M. Use of ultrasound-guided superficial cervical plexus block for pain Management in the Emergency Department. J Emerg Med. 2018;55(1):87–95. https://doi.org/10.1016/j.jemermed.2018.04.030. Epub 2018 May 29. PMID: 29858144
10. Kim JS, Ko JS, Bang S, Kim H, Lee SY. Cervical plexus block. Korean J Anesthesiol. 2018;71(4):274–88. https://doi.org/10.4097/kja.d.18.00143. Epub 2018 Jul 4. PMID: 29969890; PMCID: PMC6078883
11. Tran DQ, Dugani S, Finlayson RJ. A randomized comparison between ultrasound-guided and landmark-based superficial cervical plexus block. Reg Anesth Pain Med. 2010;35(6):539–43. https://doi.org/10.1097/AAP.0b013e3181faa11c. PMID: 20975470

12. Mirsch D, Jelic T, Prats MI, Dreyfuss A, Yates E, Kummer T, Stenberg B, Vlasica K, Nagdev A. Just the facts: brachial plexus blocks for upper extremity injuries in the emergency department. CJEM. 2024;26(4):228–31. https://doi.org/10.1007/s43678-023-00628-6. Epub 2023 Dec 7. PMID: 38060159
13. Hamal PK, Lamichhane B, Pokhrel N, Singh J, Yadav RK. Ultrasound-guided Interscalene brachial plexus block for pathological Humerus fracture due to multiple myeloma with systemic manifestation: useful option for Management in low-Income Countries. Case Rep Anesthesiol. 2020;2020:9892580. https://doi.org/10.1155/2020/9892580. PMID: 33123386; PMCID: PMC7586149
14. Gautier P, Vandepitte C, Ramquet C, DeCoopman M, Xu D, Hadzic A. The minimum effective anesthetic volume of 0.75% ropivacaine in ultrasound-guided interscalene brachial plexus block. Anesth Analg. 2011;113(4):951–5. https://doi.org/10.1213/ANE.0b013e31822b876f. Epub 2011 Aug 4. PMID: 21821517
15. Diwan S, Sethi D, Kamath N, Nair A. Low-volume C5–6 interscalene and supraclavicular nerve blocks for arthroscopic shoulder surgery: A case series. J Anaesthesiol Clin Pharmacol. 2021;37(4):661–4. https://doi.org/10.4103/joacp.JOACP_438_20. Epub 2022 Jan 6. PMID: 35340964; PMCID: PMC8944358
16. Nagdev A. Interscalene Nerve block. 2012. Highland Ultrasound. https://highlandultrasound.com/interscalene-block
17. Hutchins JL, Habeck J, Novaczyk Z, Campbell R, Creedon C, Spartz E, Richter M, Wolter J, Suryawanshi G, Kaizer A, Berg AA. Patient complications after Interscalene block: a retrospective comparison of liposomal bupivacaine to nonliposomal bupivacaine. Anesthesiol Res Pract. 2020;2020:6704303. https://doi.org/10.1155/2020/6704303. PMID: 32280340; PMCID: PMC7139877
18. Bergmann L, Martini S, Kesselmeier M, Armbruster W, Notheisen T, Adamzik M, Eichholz R. Phrenic nerve block caused by interscalene brachial plexus block: breathing effects of different sites of injection. BMC Anesthesiol. 2016;16(1):45. https://doi.org/10.1186/s12871-016-0218-x. PMID: 27473162; PMCID: PMC4966700
19. Moore DD, Maerz T, Anderson K. Shoulder surgeons' perceptions of interscalene nerve blocks and a review of complications rates in the literature. Phys Sportsmed. 2013;41(3):77–84. https://doi.org/10.3810/psm.2013.09.2026. PMID: 24113705
20. Shalaby M, Sahni R. Supraclavicular brachial plexus block: the unsung hero of emergency department regional anesthesia. Clin Exp Emerg Med. 2023;10(3):342–4. https://doi.org/10.15441/ceem.23.035. Epub 2023 Aug 25. PMID: 37818547; PMCID: PMC10579728
21. Ayala A, Ashworth H, Nagdev A. How to: the ultrasound-guided Supraclavicular brachial plexus block. ACEP Now, April 6, 2023.
22. Stone MB, Price DD, Wang R. Ultrasound-guided supraclavicular block for the treatment of upper extremity fractures, dislocations, and abscesses in the ED. Am J Emerg Med. 2007;25(4):472–5. https://doi.org/10.1016/j.ajem.2006.08.019. PMID: 17499669
23. D'Souza RS, Johnson RL. Supraclavicular Block. 2023 Jul 25. In: StatPearls [Internet]. Treasure Island (FL): StatPearls Publishing; 2025 Jan–. PMID: 30085598.
24. Perlas A, Lobo G, Lo N, Brull R, Chan VW, Karkhanis R. Ultrasound-guided supraclavicular block: outcome of 510 consecutive cases. Reg Anesth Pain Med. 2009;34(2):171–6. https://doi.org/10.1097/AAP.0b013e31819a3f81. PMID: 19282715
25. Kaye AD, Allampalli V, Fisher P, Kaye AJ, Tran A, Cornett EM, Imani F, Edinoff AN, Djalali Motlagh S, Urman RD. Supraclavicular vs. Infraclavicular brachial plexus nerve blocks: clinical, pharmacological, and anatomical considerations. Anesth Pain Med. 2021;11(5):e120658. https://doi.org/10.5812/aapm.120658. PMID: 35075423; PMCID: PMC8782193

Ultrasound-Guided Regional Anesthesia: Upper Extremity

22

Robert Stenberg, Brian Makowski, and Jordan Tozer

Ultrasound-guided nerve blocks of the upper extremity provide reliable and site-specific anesthesia and analgesia for a wide range of surgical, traumatic, and procedural indications. By allowing direct visualization of peripheral nerves and surrounding structures, ultrasound enhances block accuracy, onset time, and safety, while minimizing complications such as vascular puncture or nerve injury. From proximal approaches at the shoulder to more distal blocks at the terminal branches in the forearm and hand, this chapter outlines the relevant anatomy, scanning techniques, and clinical considerations essential for effective upper extremity regional anesthesia.

Supplementary Information The online version contains supplementary material available at https://doi.org/10.1007/978-3-032-27643-8_22.

R. Stenberg (✉) · B. Makowski
Department of Emergency Medicine, Cleveland Clinic, Akron, OH, USA
e-mail: stenber@ccf.org; makowsb2@ccf.org

J. Tozer
Department of Emergency Medicine, Virginia Commonwealth University Health, Richmond, VA, USA
e-mail: jordan.tozer@vcuhealth.org

A. Lindsay et al. (eds.), *Clinical Ultrasound*,
https://doi.org/10.1007/978-3-032-27643-8_22

Upper Extremity Blocks

- Shoulder Pericapsular Nerve Group (PENG) Block, also called interfascial plane block.
  - Indications [1, 2]:
    - Analgesia for proximal humeral fractures near joint capsule (humeral head, surgical neck, and very proximal humeral shaft fractures).
    - Analgesia for shoulder dislocation.
      - Note this is not a motor block so there will be no muscular relaxation from the block.
  - Anesthetic Volume:
    - ~20 mL
  - Procedure [3]:
    - Position arm abducted with some external rotation (ideally ~45°), as tolerated.
    - Place probe in a sagittal orientation (parallel to the long axis of the upper extremity), on the anterior aspect of the shoulder overlying humeral head region (superomedial aspect of anterior shoulder). Identify the subscapularis tendon located between the deltoid muscle and humeral head. May need to sweep/slide medially to identify (Fig. 22.1).
    - Insert needle, in-plane, cranial to caudal, advancing needle until tip is located in the target fascial plane between the deltoid muscle and subscapularis tendon (Video 22.1).
      - Conventionally, the technique is a needle trajectory in a cranial-to-caudal fashion. Anecdotally, it has been successful from a caudal to cranial fashion; which, depending on patient's positioning and pathol-

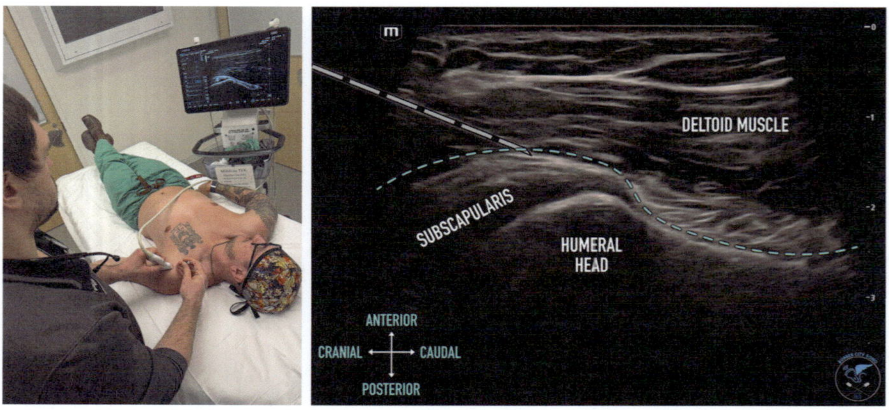

Fig. 22.1 Figure showing shoulder PENG/shoulder interfascial plane block. Left, photo showing positioning and set-up for shoulder PENG. Right, image showing needle trajectory (arrow) inserting cranially to caudally with goal to get underneath deltoid fascia adjacent to subscapularis tendon. (Created by Dr. Brian Makowski (with permission to share))

ogy, may provide a significant ergonomic advantage (Video 22.2). In theory, similar to other fascial plane blocks such as the ESP block, as long as the appropriate fascial plane is reached, the approach should not matter.
    - Inject anesthetic within this sub-deltoid fascial layer after needle is positioned in the appropriate fascial plane.
    - There is some thought and growing evidence that placing the needle and infiltrating the anesthetic deep to the subscapularis may provide better articular coverage based on cadaveric studies [4–6]. Furthermore, some clinical studies show good utility with combining an injection into the interfascial plane between the deltoid and subscapularis and injection beneath the subscapularis (also called a shoulder anterior capsular block, or SHAC block) [7, 8]. The additional injection deep to subscapularis can be facilitated with the same poke through the skin; and after the interfascial plane injection, the needle can be advanced deep to subscapularis for second injection.
- Axillary Brachial Plexus Block
  - Indications:
    - Upper extremity fractures* [9].
    - Distal radius fractures.
    - Lacerations, abscesses, or soft tissues injuries to arm distal to the elbow or lateral aspect of upper arm (proximal to the elbow) [10].
      - *Medial aspect of upper arm and axilla not anesthetized (axillary, suprascapular, and medial cutaneous of arm and forearm nerves are spared).
    - Has the benefit of avoiding any phrenic nerve paralysis or lung injury, therefore sometime is referred to as the safest brachial plexus block [11].
  - Anesthetic Volume.
    - 20 mL (split into 8 mL, 8 mL, and 4 mL separate injections at each target site)
  - Procedure [12].
    - Position patient supine, with arm abducted at 90° and external rotated (to expose axilla/medial aspect of upper arm).
    - Place probe transversely across medial aspect of the upper arm, distal to the insertion of the pectoralis major muscle [13, 14]. Scan proximally to visualize the axillary artery and surrounding target nerves (median, ulnar, radial). Musculocutaneous nerve is typically seen been the coracobrachialis and biceps muscles, however anatomic variations do exist* (Fig. 22.2).
      - Due to the axillary region's rich venous vasculature that can be variable in location and easily compressible, critical to use light probe pressure and frequent negative aspiration prior to inject when performing this block to avoid inadvertent intravascular injection.
      - Consider using Color Doppler to identify/delineate vasculature and nerves, and to map these structures for optimal trajectory planning.

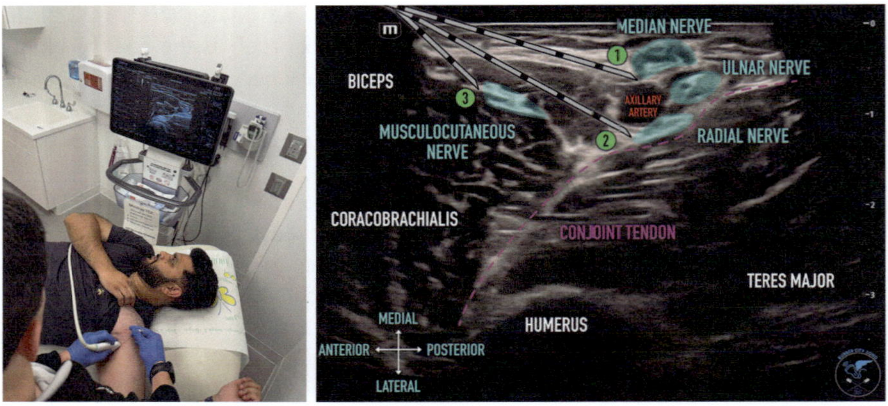

Fig. 22.2 Figure showing axillary brachial plexus block. Left, photo showing set-up and ergonomics for block. Right, ultrasound figure showing nerves surrounding axillary artery, and sites for injection for upper extremity analgesia/anesthesia. (Created by Dr. Brian Makowski (with permission to share))

        - 3 target sites exist for this block, so plan an approach that allows starting from a single-entry site. Insert needle in-plane, along the medial aspect of the arm, aiming anterior to posteriorly. After each target site is reached, retract the needle, redirect, and advanced needle to the next site (Video 22.3). Perform the block in the following order:
            - Target 1: Deep to axillary artery, deposit 8 mL of anesthetic (targets median and ulnar nerves).
            - Target 2: Superficial to axillary artery, deposit 8 mL of anesthesic (targets radial nerve).
            - Target 3: Fascial layer between the coracobrachialis and biceps muscles, deposit final 4 mL of anesthetic (targets musculocutaneous nerve).
    - Unique Complications
        - Up to 4% of cases have been noted to have dysesthesias after performing block, however, permanent nerve injury is exceedingly rare [15–18].
        - Vascular puncture has been described as the most common complication, and has been found to occur more often in obese patients vs. nonobese patients (27% vs. 9%, $P < 0.001$).* [19].
- Radial Nerve Block/Supracondylar Radial Nerve Block
    - Indications [20]:
        - Distal radius fracture
        - Dorsal hand soft tissue injuries and lacerations [21].
        - Wrist arthrocentesis (radiocarpal joint)
    - Anesthetic Volume:
        - 5–10 mL
    - Procedure [22]:

- Position affected arm internally rotated for ease ("palm on stomach"), ideally with elbow resting on bed/patient/table for stability.
- Supracondylar approach ensures all branches of the radial nerve are blocked.
  - The alternative approach is below the elbow; however, this approach will miss branches innervating the sensation to the posterolateral aspect of forearm, interosseous membrane, periosteum of radius and ulna, and extensor surfaces of the carpal joints, as well as miss the motor branches.
    - This alternative approach is typically performed by identifying radial artery; after centering on the artery, sweep transducer proximally up the forearm where the fascial plane is well seen, and there is a clear path to nerve.
- Place probe transversely near the distal third of the humerus, along the lateral aspect splitting the biceps and triceps. Identify radial nerve as it peels away from the spiral groove (also called radial groove) of the humerus, running with vessels (Fig. 22.3).
  - Since this is a more proximal area, the nerve can appear more fascicular and less honeycombed (Fig. 22.4).
  - Sweep slightly distally until nerve splits off humerus/vessels, providing an optimal window of approach.
- Insert needle in-plane toward the fascial plane adjacent to the nerve, with trajectory free of any nerves/vessels/tendons.
- Surround nerve with anesthetic. If trying for a very dense block, consider placing needle on both sides of fascial plane while injecting to have the nerve completely surrounded in anesthetic, which is often called the "donut sign" or circumferential spread (although this is debated by some) (Video 22.4) [23].

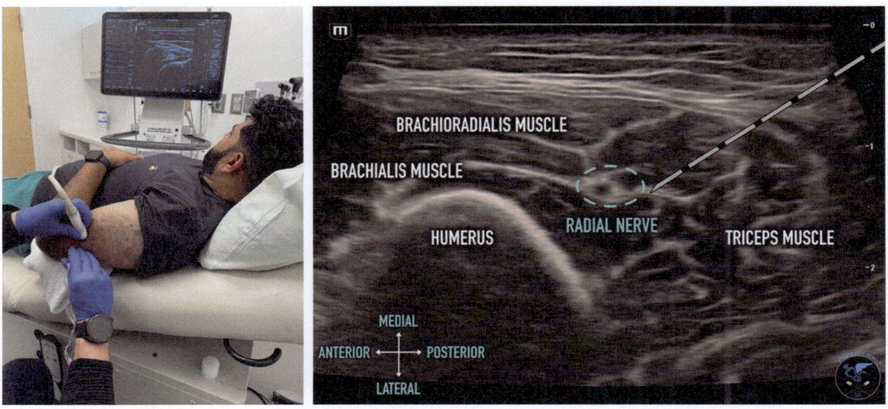

Fig. 22.3 Figure showing radial nerve block. Left, photo showing setup and room ergonomics. Right, ultrasound showing radial nerve superficial to distal humerus with needle trajectory (arrow) into fascial plane adjacent to nerve. (Created by Dr. Brian Makowski (with permission to share))

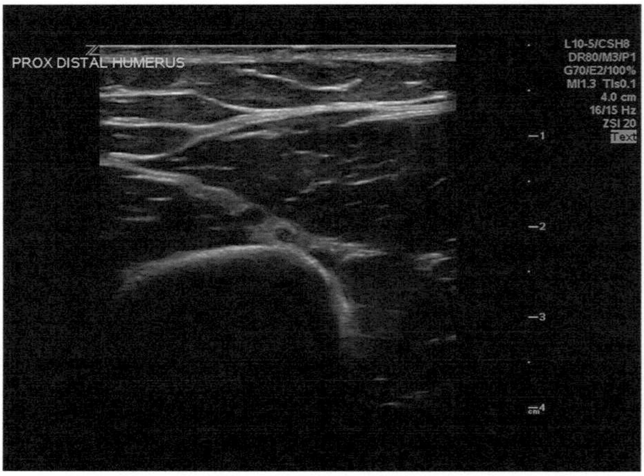

Fig. 22.4 Ultrasound image showing the radial nerve sitting superficial to the distal humerus. Given the more proximal location, the radial nerve can appear more fascicular as demonstrated. Color Doppler can be helpful to discern between nerve and vessel

- Ulnar Nerve Block
  - Indications:
    - Fifth metacarpal fracture including boxer fracture (can consider fourth metacarpal) [24].
    - Fifth digit flexor Tenosynovitis [25].
    - Hypothenar eminence and fifth digit lacerations, abscesses, and soft tissue injuries [26].
  - Anesthetic Volume:
    - 5–10 mL
  - Procedure:
    - Position affected arm supine or flexed ideally planted on bed or table for stability.
    - Place probe transversely oriented on distal wrist; Identify ulnar nerve (located medially) next to ulnar artery at wrist and sweep proximally (Fig. 22.5).
      - If tracked proximally enough, the ulnar nerve will split away from the artery to provide a safer/easier approach (Video 22.5).
      - Alternative approach:
        - Place probe transversely on distal elbow near cubital tunnel. Identify ulnar nerve exiting cubital tunnel at elbow and sweep distally until a clear needle trajectory with identifiable fascial plane is seen.
      - Attempt to perform at least mid-forearm, as injecting too distally may miss the superficial branches.
      - Insert needle in-plane toward adjacent fascial plane, with trajectory free of any nerves/vessels/tendons (Video 22.6).
      - Surround nerve with anesthetic. If trying for a very dense block, consider placing needle on both sides of fascial plane while injecting to have the nerve completely surrounded in anesthetic, which is often

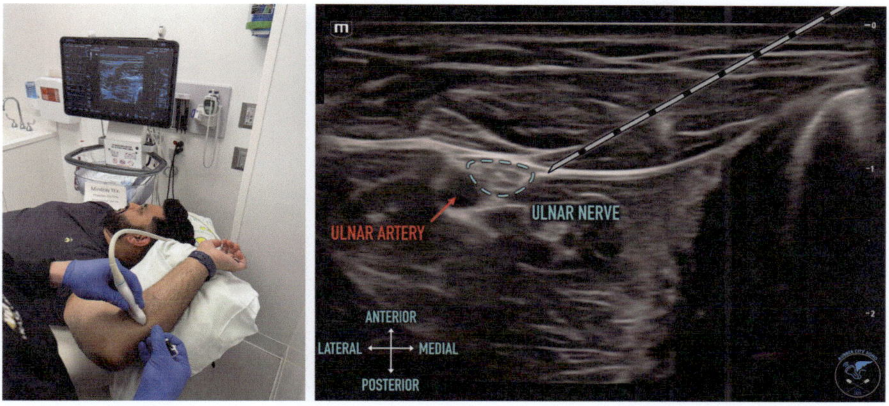

Fig. 22.5 Figure showing ulnar nerve block. Left, image showing setup and ergonomics for ulnar nerve block. Right, image showing ulnar nerve in proximal forearm just proximal to where the ulnar artery separates, with needle trajectory (arrow) aiming for adjacent fascial plane. (Created by Dr. Brian Makowski (with permission to share))

called the "donut sign" or circumferential spread (although this is debated by some) [23].

- Median Nerve Block
  - Indications:
    - Palmar/Hand lacerations and soft tissue injuries [27].
    - Adjunct to distal radius fractures [28].
    - Carpal tunnel syndrome [29].
  - Anesthetic Volume:
    - 5–10 mL
  - Procedure [30]:
    - Position affected arm supine, ideally planted on bed or table for stability.
    - Place probe in a transverse orientation and identify median nerve tracking along the most anterior aspect of forearm.
      - May identify entering carpal tunnel, but must ensure not confusing for tendons running adjacent to such (differentiated best by sweeping up arm and tendons form musculotendinous bodies then muscle whereas the nerve will remain appearing like a nerve).
      - Alternatively, may identify nerve running with artery in antecubital fossa.
    - Sweep probe to middle/proximal forearm where the nerve is isolated and has a clear approach (Fig. 22.6).
    - Blocking nerve in the distal forearm risks missing the palmar branches, depending on indication.
    - Insert needle in-plane toward adjacent fascial plane, with trajectory free of any nerves/vessels/tendons (Video 22.7).

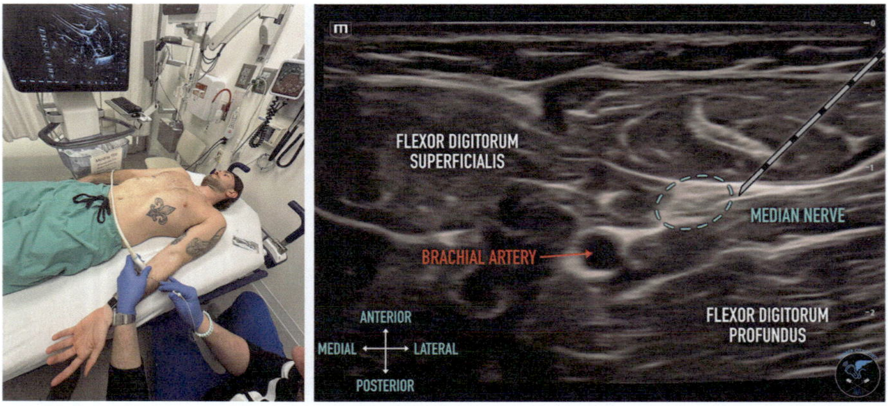

Fig. 22.6 Figure showing median nerve block. Left, photo showing setup and ergonomics for median nerve block. Right, image showing median nerve in mid forearm with needle trajectory (arrow) targeting adjacent fascial plane. (Created by Dr. Brian Makowski (with permission to share))

  - Surround nerve with anesthetic. If trying for a very dense block, consider placing needle on both sides of fascial plane while injecting to have the nerve completely surrounded in anesthetic, which is often called the "donut sign" or circumferential spread (although this is debated by some) [23].
- Alternative Approach, Above-the-Elbow [31].
  - At or slightly proximal to the crease of the elbow, the median nerve is located just medial to the brachial artery, making it a reliable site for identification and blockade.
  - Procedure:
    - Position the patient's arm abducted with palm facing up.
    - Place probe in a transverse orientation to the humerus along the medial aspect of the arm, just above the medial condyle.
    - Sweep back and forth distally/proximally to identify the median nerve and brachial artery.
      - If not immediately seen, position transducer slightly more medially or use Color Doppler to aid in locating.
    - Median nerve should be located along the medial side of the brachial artery (Fig. 22.7).
    - Insert needle, in-plane, medially to laterally, targeting the fascial plane adjacent to the median nerve.
    - Consider hydrodissection with 2–3 mL of saline to "peel away" the median nerve from the fascial plane and off the brachial artery (Video 22.8).
    - After negative aspiration, inject 5–10 mL of local anesthetic.

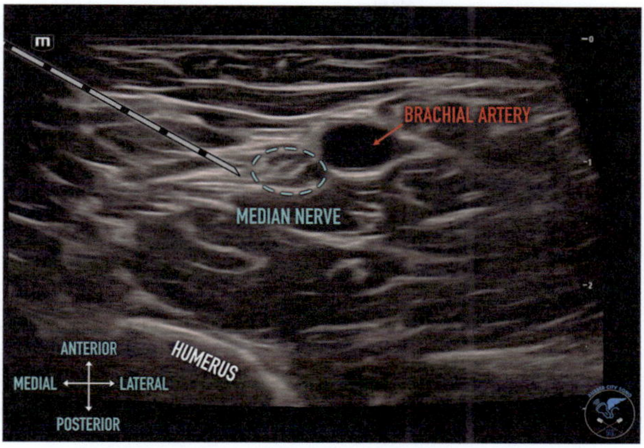

Fig. 22.7 Figure showing above the elbow median nerve block. Needle trajectory shown away from vessel. (Created by Dr. Brian Makowski (with permission to share))

References

1. Küpeli İ, Yazici KM. Anesthesia or analgesia? New block for shoulder surgery: pericapsular nerve group block. Braz J Anesthesiol. 2022;72(5):669–72. https://doi.org/10.1016/j.bjane.2021.05.009. Epub 2021 Jun 9. PMID: 34118263; PMCID: PMC9515664.
2. Ramadurai R, Bhoi D, Nagarajappa A, Amar P. Pericapsular nerve group block (PENG) at neutral position for shoulder manipulation: a feasible approach for a new indication. J Clin Anesth. 2021;75:110541. https://doi.org/10.1016/j.jclinane.2021.110541. Epub 2021 Oct 12.
3. Metri S, Gonzalez-Cobos C, Rose G. Treatment of shoulder pain with ultrasound-guided interfascial plane block. Am J Emerg Med. 2024;86:189.e1–3. https://doi.org/10.1016/j.ajem.2024.10.022. Epub 2024 Oct 13.
4. Xiao SJ, Fan CL. Pericapsular nerve group (PENG) block for shoulder manipulation: it may not be a real pericapsular block. J Clin Anesth. 2023;88:111123. https://doi.org/10.1016/j.jclinane.2023.111123. Epub 2023 Apr 12.
5. Yamak Altinpulluk E, Teles AS, Galluccio F, Simón DG, Olea MS, Salazar C, Fajardo PM. Pericapsular nerve group block for postoperative shoulder pain: a cadaveric radiological evaluation. J Clin Anesth. 2020;67:110058. https://doi.org/10.1016/j.jclinane.2020.110058. Epub 2020 Sep 26.
6. González-Arnay E, Galluccio F, Pérez-Santos I, Merlano-Castellanos S, Bañón-Boulet E, Jiménez-Sánchez L, Rivier-Julien C, Barrueco-Fernández M, Olea MS, Yamak-Altinpulluk E, Teles AS, Fajardo-Pérez M. Permeable spaces between glenohumeral ligaments as potential gateways for rapid regional anesthesia of the shoulder. Ann Anat. 2022;239:151814. https://doi.org/10.1016/j.aanat.2021.151814. Epub 2021 Sep 16.
7. Galluccio F, Fajardo Perez M, Yamak Altinpulluk E, Hou JD, Lin JA. Evaluation of interfascial plane and pericapsular nerve blocks to the shoulder joint: a preliminary analysis of shoulder anterior capsular block. Pain Ther. 2021;10(2):1741–54. https://doi.org/10.1007/s40122-021-00326-0. Epub 2021 Oct 20. PMID: 34669181; PMCID: PMC8586108.
8. Caliskan B, Ataoglu C, Ok M, Yamak AE. Comparison of shoulder anterior capsular block and interscalene brachial plexus block for shoulder arthroscopy: a preliminary analysis. Minerva Anestesiol. 2024;90(1–2):22–30. https://doi.org/10.23736/S0375-9393.23.17536-5. Epub 2023 Nov 23.
9. Kriwanek KL, Wan J, Beaty JH, Pershad J. Axillary block for analgesia during manipulation of forearm fractures in the pediatric emergency department a prospective randomized comparative trial. J Pediatr Orthop. 2006;26(6):737–40. https://doi.org/10.1097/01.bpo.0000229976.24307.30.

10. Mackay CA, Bowden DF. Axillary brachial plexus block–an underused technique in the accident and emergency department. J Accid Emerg Med. 1997;14(4):226–9. https://doi.org/10.1136/emj.14.4.226. PMID: 9248910; PMCID: PMC1342946.
11. https://pain.ucsf.edu/peripheral-nerve-blocks/axillary-brachial-plexus-block.
12. https://www.nysora.com/techniques/upper-extremity/axillary/ultrasound-guided-axillary-brachial-plexus-block/#toc_GENERAL-CONSIDERATIONS.
13. https://resources.wfsahq.org/atotw/ultrasound-guided-axillary-brachial-plexus-block/.
14. Chan VW, Perlas A, McCartney CJ, Brull R, Xu D, Abbas S. Ultrasound guidance improves success rate of axillary brachial plexus block. Can J Anaesth. 2007;54(3):176–82. https://doi.org/10.1007/BF03022637. Erratum in: Can J Anaesth. 2007 Jul;54(7):594.
15. He LD, Vlassakov KV, Bader AM, Chen Y-YK. Adverse event reporting in ultrasound-guided brachial plexus blocks: a scoping review. JCA Adv. 2025;2(1):100085. ISSN 2950-5534. https://doi.org/10.1016/j.jcadva.2024.100085.
16. Li S, Sviggum H, Hilliard P. Axillary blockade. ASRA Pain Med. 2019;7. https://asra.com/news-publications/asra-updates/blog-landing/legacy-b-blog-posts/2019/08/07/axillary-blockade.
17. Bigeleisen PE. Nerve puncture and apparent intraneural injection during ultrasound-guided axillary block does not invariably result in neurologic injury. Anesthesiology. 2006;105(4):779–83. https://doi.org/10.1097/00000542-200610000-00024.
18. Ecoffey C, Oger E, Marchand-Maillet F, Cimino Y, Rannou JJ, Beloeil H, SOS French Regional Anaesthesia Hotline. Complications associated with 27031 ultrasound-guided axillary brachial plexus blocks: a web-based survey of 36 French centres. Eur J Anaesthesiol. 2014;31(11):606–10. https://doi.org/10.1097/EJA.0000000000000063.
19. Hanouz JL, Grandin W, Lesage A, Oriot G, Bonnieux D, Gérard JL. Multiple injection axillary brachial plexus block: influence of obesity on failure rate and incidence of acute complications. Anesth Analg. 2010;111(1):230–3. https://doi.org/10.1213/ANE.0b013e3181dde023. Epub 2010 Apr 24.
20. Frenkel O, Herring AA, Fischer J, Carnell J, Nagdev A. Supracondylar radial nerve block for treatment of distal radius fractures in the emergency department. J Emerg Med. 2011;41(4):386–8. https://doi.org/10.1016/j.jemermed.2010.11.043. Epub 2011 Feb 5.
21. Mohanty CR, Radhakrishnan RV, Gupta A, Bellapukonda S. Ultrasound-guided superficial radial nerve block in the emergency Department for Pain Management following centipede bite. Wilderness Environ Med. 2023;34(4):528–31. https://doi.org/10.1016/j.wem.2023.05.010. Epub 2023 Jul 13.
22. Capek A, Dolan J. Ultrasound-guided peripheral nerve blocks of the upper limb. BJA Educ. 2015;15(3):160–5. https://doi.org/10.1093/bjaceaccp/mku048.
23. Dieguez-Garcia P, Lopez-Alvarez S, Juncal J, Lopez AM, Sala-Blanch X. Comparison of the effectiveness of circumferential versus non-circumferential spread in median and ulnar nerve blocks. A double-blind randomized clinical trial. Reg Anesth Pain Med. 2020;45(5):362–6. https://doi.org/10.1136/rapm-2019-101157. Epub 2020 Mar 11.
24. Mori T, Nomura O, Ihara T. Ultrasound-guided peripheral forearm nerve block for digit fractures in a pediatric emergency department. Am J Emerg Med. 2019;37(3):489–93. https://doi.org/10.1016/j.ajem.2018.11.033. Epub 2018 Nov 24.
25. Bowling JM, Zoumberakis E. Ultrasound-guided nerve blocks for flexor tenosynovitis. POCUS J. 2024;9(2):12–4. https://doi.org/10.24908/pocus.v9i2.17395. PMID: 39634685; PMCID: PMC11616797.
26. https://www.nysora.com/topics/anatomy/functional-regional-anesthesia-anatomy/.
27. Bhoi S, Gopinath B, Khandelwal U, Nayaka R, Bhaskararayuni J, Gupta D, Srivastava A, Anshu A, Katyal A, Sinha TP. Assessing the clinical impact of emergency physician-performed ultrasound-guided peripheral nerve blocks in a level 1 trauma center: a retrospective analysis. J Emerg Trauma Shock. 2024;17(4):193–200. https://doi.org/10.4103/jets.jets_8_24. Epub 2024 Dec 24. PMID: 39911459; PMCID: PMC11792750.

28. Abbasi S, Garjani N, Mahshidfar B, Farsi D, Mofidi M, Hafezimoghadam P, Rezai M, Javan A. Comparative study of radial and median nerve blocks with hematoma block under ultrasound guide in distal radius fracture reduction: a randomized clinical trial. Med J Islam Repub Iran. 2023;23(37):113. https://doi.org/10.47176/mjiri.37.113. PMID: 38145179; PMCID: PMC10744119.
29. Puebla DL, Luchitsky I, Montes De Oca R, Shalaby M, Farrow RA 2nd. Ultrasound-guided, mid-forearm median nerve block for relief of carpal tunnel syndrome pain in the emergency department: a case report. Clin Pract Cases Emerg Med. 2024;8(1):68–71. https://doi.org/10.5811/cpcem.1265. PMID: 38546317; PMCID: PMC10966504.
30. Wroe P, Nagdev A. How to perform ultrasound-guided forearm nerve blocks to provide non-drug pain relief for acute injuries. ACEP Now. 2016;13:2.
31. Lin J-A, Bendtsen TF, Lopez AM, Jalil H. Ultrasound-guided blocks at the elbow. NYSORA. https://www.nysora.com/topics/regional-anesthesia-for-specific-surgical-procedures/upper-extremity-regional-anesthesia-for-specific-surgical-procedures/anesthesia-and-analgesia-for-hand-procedures/ultrasound-guided-blocks-elbow/.

Ultrasound-Guided Regional Anesthesia: Trunk

23

Robert Stenberg, Brian Makowski, and Jordan Tozer

Ultrasound-guided nerve blocks of the trunk have revolutionized regional anesthesia by providing targeted, effective analgesia for thoracic and abdominal maladies. These blocks—ranging from superficial techniques like the transversus abdominis plane (TAP) block to deeper approaches such as the erector spinae plane (ESP) block—offer opioid-sparing pain control with improved safety profiles. Ultrasound guidance allows for precise needle placement and real-time visualization of anatomical structures, reducing the risk of complications. This chapter explores the key principles, sonoanatomy, techniques, and clinical applications of trunk nerve blocks.

Truncal Nerve Blocks

- Clavipectoral Fascial Plane Block (CPB)
  - Indications:
    - Clavicle fracture/pain [1].
  - Anesthetic Volume:
    - 5–15 mL [2]

Supplementary Information The online version contains supplementary material available at https://doi.org/10.1007/978-3-032-27643-8_23.

R. Stenberg (✉) · B. Makowski
Department of Emergency Medicine, Cleveland Clinic, Akron, OH, USA
e-mail: stenber@ccf.org; makowsb2@ccf.org

J. Tozer
Department of Emergency Medicine, Virginia Commonwealth University Health, Richmond, VA, USA
e-mail: jordan.tozer@vcuhealth.org

A. Lindsay et al. (eds.), *Clinical Ultrasound*,
https://doi.org/10.1007/978-3-032-27643-8_23

    - Often anesthesia will block each side of the fracture site (up to 15 mL per side), but some may argue this is unnecessary in the emergency department setting; with goals of achieving analgesia, and not anesthesia.
  - Procedure [3]:
    - Place transducer in a sagittal fashion adjacent to the fracture site along the clavicle (slightly caudally), until both the clavicle and pectoralis muscle are well seen. Slide probe until the clavicle is seen off-centered toward the edge of the screen (Fig. 23.1).
    - Insert needle in-plane, from caudal to cranial, aiming toward the superficial aspect of the clavicle (Video 23.1).
    - Adjust needle with hydrolocalization until fluid is seen lifting fascia off clavicle and surrounding clavicle; inject anesthetic. Consider spinning/rotating needle to get underneath clavipectoral fascia [4].
    - It can be challenging in low BMI patients to reach the superficial surface of clavicle. Consider bending the needle to sufficiently reach the surface, or using a regular needle in this scenario may help do such (which is overall safer for this block given the absence of neurovascular structures along the needle path). One can also consider a short axis out-of-plane approach to come down on top of clavicle and get spread; although it may be harder to get fascial spread with this method.
- Serratus Anterior/Serratus Anterior Fascial Plane Block (SAPB)
  - Indications [5]:
    - Chest wall abscess/hematoma/injury
    - Rib fractures
    - Adjunct for chest tube analgesia/anesthesia (does *not* provide pain relief for visceral pleura)
  - Anesthetic Volume:
    - 30–40 mL [6]

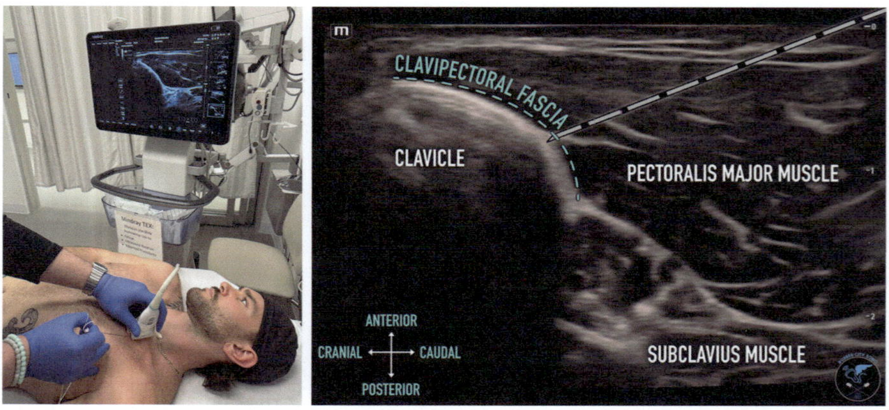

Fig. 23.1 Figure showing clavipectoral block. Left, photo showing set-up and ergonomics for the block. Right, image showing needle trajectory (arrow) inserting caudal to cranial along the inferior aspect of the clavicle, with the goal to see fluid spreading along the clavicle in between pectoralis and clavicle. (Created by Dr. Brian Makowski (with permission to share))

- Procedure:
  - Select level based on location of rib fractures and visualization of serratus muscle.
    - Traditionally, the level was designed to be injected at fifth rib, with spread from T2–T9 regions using 25–30 mL. Cadaveric studies have shown a spread of 15 cm superiorly to inferiorly with only 20 mL [7, 8].
    - The serratus muscle belly is inconsistent in thickness across different ribs. Targeting a rib adjacent to injury where there is a more robust muscle belly ensures an easier block.
    - If fractured ribs 10–12, targeting a more caudal rib site where there is still a clear target.
  - Position patient supine, semi-recumbent, or lateral decubitus (affected side up).
    - Depending on patient comfort/tolerance, it may be helpful to have the ipsilateral arm abducted to increase exposure and reduce soft tissue thickness.
  - Place the probe along the anterolateral chest wall at about the mid-axillary line.
    - There are multiple approaches to the axis/orientation of the probe; some perform with a transverse approach (Fig. 23.2).
    - The other consideration is placing the probe in an oblique orientation running along the long axis of the rib, which provides a consistent bony backboard to avoid inadvertent advancement of needle deep to such, and hopes to reduce pneumothorax (Fig. 23.3).

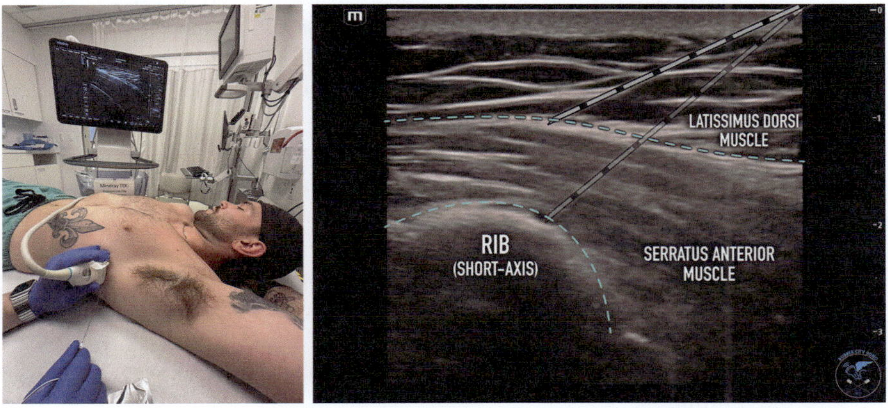

Fig. 23.2 Figure showing serratus anterior block. Left, photo showing room set-up and ergonomics for serratus anterior block. Right, image showing transducer orientation on the short axis of the rib, ensuring needle trajectory is toward rib to provide a safe back-stop. Needle trajectory (arrow) approaching both approaches: targeting either the fascia superficial to serratus or deep to serratus against bone. (Created by Dr. Brian Makowski (with permission to share))

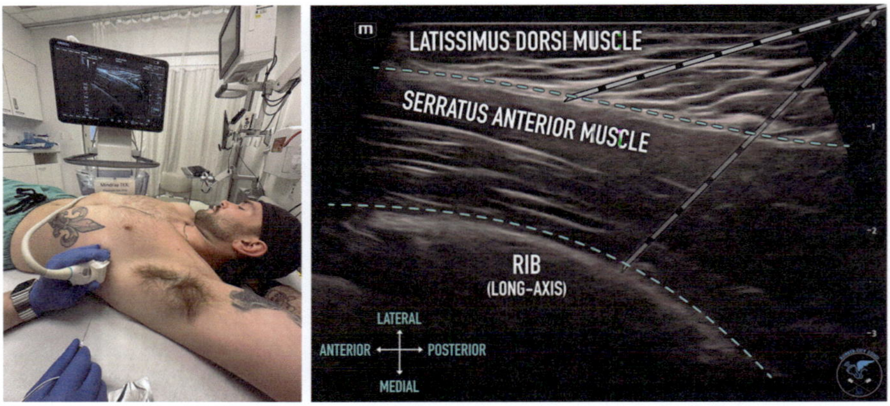

Fig. 23.3 Figure showing serratus anterior block. Left, photo showing room set-up and ergonomics. Right, image showing transducer orientation along rib providing a uniform back-stop, further protecting the lung from injury. (Created by Dr. Brian Makowski (with permission to share))

- Insert needle anteromedial to posterolateral toward the serratus anterior muscle belly.
  - Some sources highlight a posterolateral to anteromedial needle trajectory; ergonomics and safely reaching the correct fascial plane are of the utmost importance. This approach can also be helpful to get around a chest tube bandage. There should be increased caution to avoid the thoracodorsal artery, which runs more posteriorly [9].
- It can be effective to inject into either the superficial fascial layer of serratus, the fascial layer deep to serratus, or both [10, 11].
  - In elderly patients with less robust serratus muscle bellies, it can be challenging to identify the muscle and associated fascia; anecdotally, there may be increased ease to target the fascial layer deep to serratus between bone and serratus, given the challenge of the less demarcated fascial planes (Video 23.2).
  - There are some surgical studies comparing the superficial versus deep, with some favoring superficial approach. One theory is anesthetic placed deep to the serratus likely misses the long thoracic nerve, which may play a role into pain (Video 23.3) [5, 12, 13]. Some experts feel targeting the superficial fascial plane in a section where the serratus muscle belly is deep to latissimus dorsi is easier to identify correct fascial spread.
- After in desired fascial plane, inject anesthetic, aspirating every 5 mL during infiltration.

- Erector Spinae Plane (ESP) Block
  - Indications:

    - There is a marked potential to what this block can do, and the emergency indications have only expanded; largely, with appropriately targeting levels, it should be seen as a great means of visceral pain control.
    - Posterior rib fractures (target center of rib fracture pattern) [14]
    - Pneumonia (based on lung section) [15]
    - Cholecystitis (T7) [16]
    - Pancreatitis (T7/T8) [17]
    - Renal colic (T8) [18]
    - Small bowel obstruction
    - Appendicitis (T10/L1) [19]
    - Endometriosis [20]
    - Headaches (T4) [21]
  - Anesthetic Volume:
    - 30–40 mL (some institutions are using 60 + mL) [14]
  - Procedure:
    - Positioning
      - Prone, lateral decubitus with affected side up (especially for rib fractures and having affected side not being compressed against gurney), or sitting upright and leaning forward.
        - Anecdotally, laying prone can provide stability, and relaxing truncal musculature reduces discomfort associated with advancement of needle.
      - Probe selection
        - Consider either using linear probe or curvilinear probe based on patient's anatomy and habitus.
    - Traditional approach (thoracic vertebra) [22]:
      - Review anatomy/pathology and select desired level.
      - Place probe in a sagittal orientation along the midportion of the affected hemithorax. Identify the twelfth rib and slide probe cranially until desired rib/spinal level identified (may also start at first rib and count down to desired level) (Fig. 23.4) (Video 23.4).
      - After the desired rib/level is identified the probe is swept medially tracking the rib. As doing so, the rib will dive deep relative to probe (into far field), and the transverse process will appear as a bony prominence, slightly superficial to rib (prior to identifying the spinous process) (Video 23.5).
        - May also go to the, superficial spinous process at midline once the target level is identified, and sweep laterally until the transverse process is identified.
      - After identifying the transverse process, the needle is either inserted craniocaudally or caudocranially based on ergonomics, with an in-plane approach, until the corner/side of the transverse process is contacted. By aiming for corner aspect of the transverse process, it is felt generally easier to get underneath the erector spinae fascial plane [23].

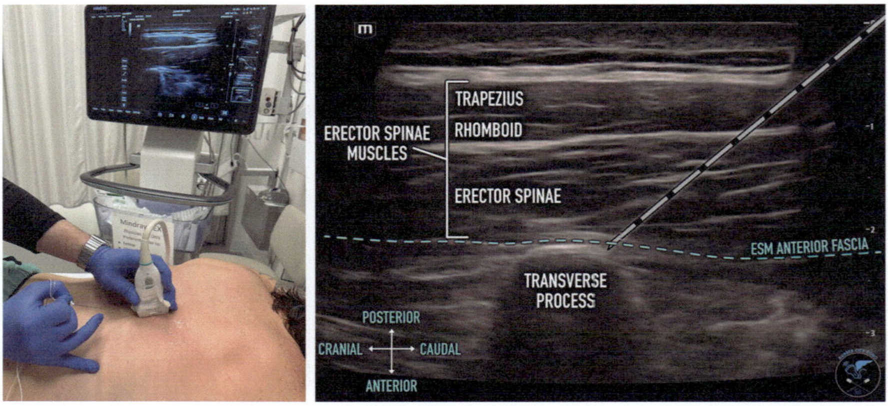

Fig. 23.4 Figure showing a thoracic erector spinae fascial plane block. Left, photo showing the conventional set-up and ergonomics for erector spinae fascial plane block. Right, image showing sagittal orientation of transverse process with needle trajectory (arrow) aiming toward the corner of the transverse process. (Created by Dr. Brian Makowski (with permission to share))

    - There is anesthesia literature that has evaluated targeting the erector spinae fascial plane in between transverse processes, but this does not provide a bony backstop to avoid puncture into the inter-transverse space [24, 25].
  - Inject fluid and adjust needle until fluid is seen underneath the bright hyperechoic erector spinae fascial plane (Video 23.6).
  - After needle is in the correct fascial plane, inject anesthetic, with intermittent aspiration (every ~5 mL) to ensure no vascular involvement; also consider color Doppler during the survey scan.
- Alternative approach (short axis/transverse orientation):
  - May be helpful when poorly visualizing TP, and more evidence in the pediatric population [26].
  - Place probe transversely in a paramedian region lateral to the spinous process (Fig. 23.5).
  - Identify transverse process lateral to spinous process in thoracic vertebra and lateral to the articular processes in the lumbar vertebra [27].
  - Insert needle in-plane (or out-of-plane until transverse process is contacted and fascial fluid seen spreading underneath erector spinae fascial plane (Video 23.7).
- Lumbar Vertebra (largely for back pain) [27, 28].
  - In a sagittal orientation, identify target by finding L1 as the first vertebra caudally without rib or find sacrum and count cranially.
  - Find the prominent spinous process midline. Sweep laterally, passing the first bony prominence (articular process), and identifying the transverse process as the second bony prominence. The transverse processes in the lumbar region tend to be longer and appear flatter (Fig. 23.6).

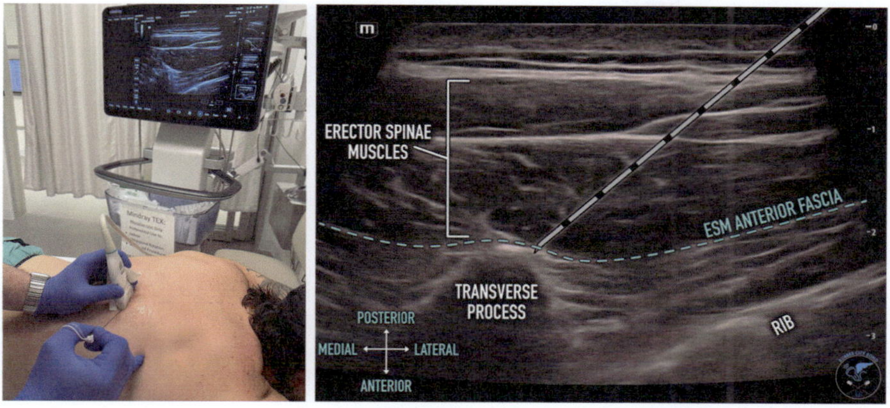

Fig. 23.5 Figure showing the alternate approach to the thoracic erector spinae fascial plane block. Left, photo showing the set-up and ergonomics for the block. Right, image showing a transverse orientation or short axis of the spine, with needle inserting in-plane to reach the transverse process. (Created by Dr. Brian Makowski (with permission to share))

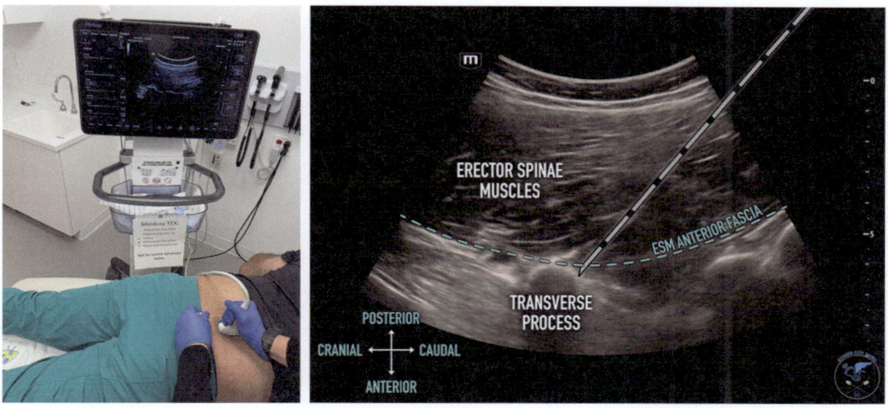

Fig. 23.6 Figure showing a lumbar erector spinae fascial plane block. Left, photo showing the room set-up and ergonomics for the block. Right, image showing sagittal orientation of lumbar transverse process with needle trajectory (arrow) aiming toward the corner of the transverse process. (Created by Dr. Brian Makowski (with permission to share))

- Insert needle in-plane until contacting transverse process. Adjust/inject until fluid is seen lifting erector spinae fascial plane off transverse process.
- Alternate approach for lumbar vertebra:
  - May also view the same anatomy in the short/transverse axis, and insert needle in-plane to reach transverse process (Fig. 23.7) (Video 23.8) [29].

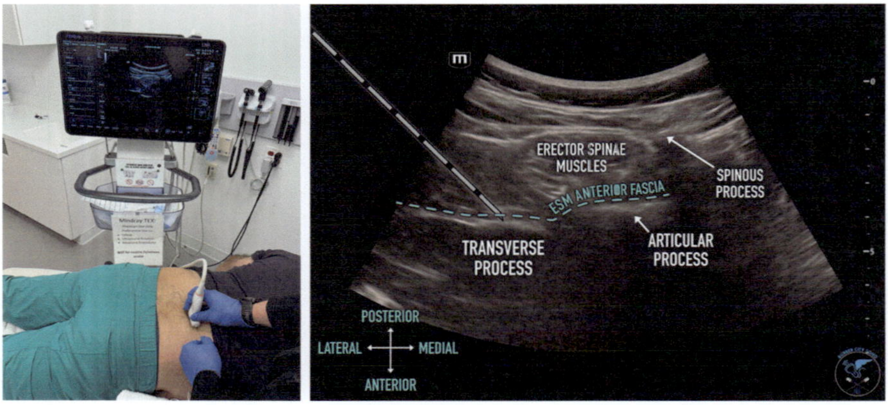

Fig. 23.7 Figure showing an alternate approach to lumbar erector spinae fascial plane block. Left, photo showing the room set-up and ergonomics for the block. Right, image showing transverse orientation or short axis of the lumbar spine, with needle inserting in-plane to reach the transverse process. (Created by Dr. Brian Makowski (with permission to share))

- Transversus Abdominis Plane (TAP) Block
  - Indications:
    - Somatic abdominal wall pain at level of umbilicus or below (area above umbilicus would require subcostal TAP block, which is not covered).
      - Rectus sheath hematoma [30]
      - Abdominal wall pain/strain
      - Abdominal wall abscess
    - Efforts to use as adjunct for analgesia with a component of parietal peritoneal irritation.
      - Appendicitis [31]/Abdominal wall hernia (again will not have any visceral pain coverage including with attempts at reduction)
  - Anesthetic Volume:
    - ~20 mL
  - Procedure [32]:
    - Place patient in lateral decubitus position with the affected side up.
    - Place transducer in transverse fashion along anterior/middle axillary line, in between the costal margin and iliac crest.
    - Identify the abdominal wall layers; usually easiest to identify structures deep first, with finding peritoneal stripe, then working externally: peritoneum, transversus abdominis, internal oblique, and external oblique.
    - There are two approaches with the TAP block, one being lateral, and one being posterior, varying based on where the anesthetic is injected along the superficial aspect of the transversus abdominis fascial plane. The more common practice, with literature showing better pain control, is performing the posterior TAP; this is done by sliding posteriorly until the transversus abdominis muscle is seen tapering into a triangular shape (Fig. 23.8) [33, 34].

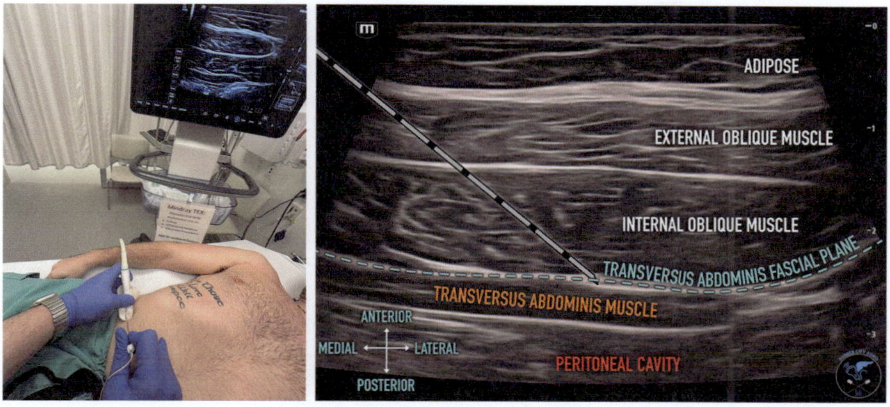

Fig. 23.8 Figure showing Transversus Abdominis Plane block (TAP) block. Left, photo showing set-up and ergonomics for posterior TAP block. Right, image showing needle trajectory (arrow) anterior to posterior, aiming toward the tapering portion of the transversus abdominis TA muscle (semi-oval) after piercing through the external (EO) and internal oblique (IO) muscles. (Created by Dr. Brian Makowski (with permission to share))

    - Needle is inserted in an in-plane approach anteromedially to posterolaterally until the fascial layer in between the transversus abdominis and internal oblique is reached (using hydro-localization) (Video 23.9) [35].
    - Once in the fascial plane, deposit anesthetic, aspirating every 5 mL.

- Dorsal Penile Nerve Block (DPNB)
  - Indications:
    - Penile trauma [36]
    - Penile fractures
    - Priapism [37]
    - Paraphimosis reduction [38]
  - Anesthetic Volume:
    - 5–10 mL
  - Procedure [39–41]:
    - Place probe transversely on the ventral (bottom) side of the penis near the base of penis. Can also consider stabilizing penis with the transducer hand to minimize movement [41].
    - Identify Buck's fascia dorsally, which is the fascial plane enveloping corpora cavernosa and dorsal artery, vein and nerve (Fig. 23.9).
    - With an in-plane approach insert needle dorsally (opposite side of transducer), along the superolateral aspect of penis around the 2 or 10 o'clock positions. Advance needle until underneath Buck's fascia but not violating the corpora cavernosa nor the neurovascular bundle.
    - Inject anesthetic once fascial spread seen underneath the fascial plane (Video 23.10).
    - An alternative approach from the dorsal side is feasible, but given the very superficial structures, it can make needle visualization difficult.

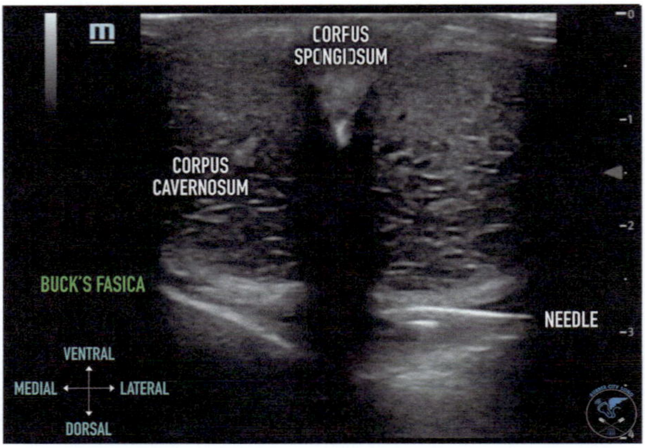

Fig. 23.9 Figure showing dorsal penile nerve block. Image showing transducer on ventral aspect of penis and needle inserting on dorsal side at ~2' O'Clock positioning with goal of getting underneath Buck's fascia. (Created by Dr. Brian Makowski (with permission to share))

References

1. Ashworth H, Martin D, Nagdev A, Lind K. Clavipectoral plane block performed in the emergency department for analgesia after clavicular fractures. Am J Emerg Med. 2023;74:197.e1–3. https://doi.org/10.1016/j.ajem.2023.09.056. Epub 2023 Oct 3.
2. Abu Sabaa MA, Elbadry AA, El Malla DA. Ultrasound-guided Clavipectoral block for postoperative analgesia of clavicular surgery: a prospective randomized trial. Anesth Pain Med. 2022;12(1):e121267. https://doi.org/10.5812/aapm.121267. PMID: 35433386; PMCID: PMC8995874.
3. Kukreja P, Davis CJ, MacBeth L, Feinstein J, Kalagara H. Ultrasound-guided Clavipectoral fascial plane block for surgery involving the clavicle: a case series. Cureus. 2020;12(7):e9072. https://doi.org/10.7759/cureus.9072. PMID: 32782888; PMCID: PMC7413568.
4. Rosales AL, Aypa NS. Clavipectoral plane block as a sole anesthetic technique for clavicle surgery - a case report. Anesth Pain Med (Seoul). 2022;17(1):93–7. https://doi.org/10.17085/apm.21085. Epub 2021 Dec 28. PMID: 34974646; PMCID: PMC8841259.
5. Serra S, Santonastaso DP, Romano G, Riccardi A, Nigra SG, Russo E, Angelini M, Agnoletti V, Guarino M, Cimmino CS, Spampinato MD, Francesconi R, Iaco F. Efficacy and safety of the serratus anterior plane block (SAP block) for pain management in patients with multiple rib fractures in the emergency department: a retrospective study. Eur J Trauma Emerg Surg. 2024;50(6):3177–88. https://doi.org/10.1007/s00068-024-02597-6. Epub 2024 Jul 17. PMID: 39020130; PMCID: PMC11666617.
6. https://www.asra.com/news-publications/asra-newsletter/newsletter-item/asra-news/2020/05/02/how-i-do-it-serratus-anterior-plane-block-for-rib-fractures.
7. Blanco R, Parras T, McDonnell JG, Prats-Galino A. Serratus plane block: a novel ultrasound-guided thoracic wall nerve block. Anaesthesia. 2013;68(11):1107–13. https://doi.org/10.1111/anae.12344. Epub 2013 Aug 7.
8. Allred C, et al. 209 Cadaveric study of serratus anterior block. Ann Emerg Med. 70(4):S84.
9. Nagdev A, Mantuani D, Durant E, Herring A. Ultrasound-guided serratus anterior plane block can help avoid opioid use for patients with rib fractures. ACEP NOW. 2017;5
10. Bhoi D, Selvam V, Yadav P, Talawar P. Comparison of two different techniques of serratus anterior plane block: a clinical experience. J Anaesthesiol Clin Pharmacol. 2018;34(2):251–3. https://doi.org/10.4103/joacp.JOACP_294_16. PMID: 30104841; PMCID: PMC6066876.
11. Lin J, Hoffman T, Badashova K, Motov S, Haines L. Serratus anterior plane block in the emergency department: a case series. Clin Pract Cases Emerg Med. 2020;4(1):21–5. https://doi.org/10.5811/cpcem.2019.11.44946. PMID: 32064417; PMCID: PMC7012558.

12. Tan KW, Sayed Masri SNN, Musthafa QA, Mohd Azidin A, Nik Mohamed Kamil A, Izaham A, Md NN. Analgesic efficacy of the superficial versus deep serratus plane blocks for mastectomy with axillary clearance: a randomized controlled trial. Medicine (Baltimore). 2022;101(35):e30515. https://doi.org/10.1097/MD.0000000000030515. PMID: 36107598; PMCID: PMC9439770.
13. Qiu L, Bu X, Shen J, Li M, Yang L, Xu Q, Chen Y, Yang J. Observation of the analgesic effect of superficial or deep anterior serratus plane block on patients undergoing thoracoscopic lobectomy. Medicine (Baltimore). 2021;100(3):e24352. https://doi.org/10.1097/MD.0000000000024352. PMID: 33546068; PMCID: PMC7837840.
14. Jiang M, Peri V, Ou Yang B, Chang J, Hacking D. Erector Spinae plane block as an analgesic intervention in acute rib fractures: a scoping review. Local Reg Anesth. 2023;12(16):81–90. https://doi.org/10.2147/LRA.S414056. PMID: 37334278; PMCID: PMC10275321.
15. Stenberg R, Goff L, Simon EL. Ultrasound-guided erector spinae nerve block for relief of chest pain from pneumonia in the emergency department. Am J Emerg Med. 2024;80:230.e1–2. https://doi.org/10.1016/j.ajem.2024.04.026. Epub 2024 Apr 21.
16. Bowling JM, Ray R, Stenberg R. Ultrasound-guided erector Spinae plane nerve block for relief of acute Cholecystitis pain. J Emerg Med. 2025;69:51–3. https://doi.org/10.1016/j.jemermed.2024.08.008. Epub 2024 Aug 21.
17. Mantuani D, Josh Luftig PA, Herring A, Mian M, Nagdev A. Successful emergency pain control for acute pancreatitis with ultrasound guided erector spinae plane blocks. Am J Emerg Med. 2020;38(6):1298.e5–7. https://doi.org/10.1016/j.ajem.2020.02.005. Epub 2020 Feb 5.
18. Candel BGJ, Visser LN, Ter Avest E, Ridderikhof ML, De Groot B, Jacobs R, Weltings S, Groenwold RHH, van Bodegom L, van den Hout WB, Kemper M, Hollmann MW. Efficacy of an erector spinae plane block for renal colic: a systematic review and meta-analysis. Emerg Med J. 2024. https://doi.org/10.1136/emermed-2024-214321. Epub ahead of print.
19. Brewer J, Conger H, Rash R. The erector spinae block: a novel approach to pain management in acute appendicitis. Ultrasound J. 2022;14(1):30. https://doi.org/10.1186/s13089-022-00281-7. PMID: 35881268; PMCID: PMC9325929.
20. Stenberg R, Septaric K, Simon EL. Ultrasound-guided erector spinae nerve block for relief of endometriosis pain in the emergency department. Am J Emerg Med. 2024;83:163.e1–3. https://doi.org/10.1016/j.ajem.2024.03.001. Epub 2024 Mar 15.
21. Hernandez N, Guvernator G, Ansoanuur G, Ge M, Tabansi P, Le TT, Obeidat SS, de Haan J. Relief of secondary headaches with high thoracic erector spinae plane block. Local Reg Anesth. 2020;13:49–55. https://doi.org/10.2147/LRA.S249250. PMID: 32606918; PMCID: PMC7319503.
22. https://www.asra.com/news-publications/asra-newsletter/newsletter-item/asra-news/2020/05/01/how-i-do-it-erector-spinae-block-for-rib-fractures-the-penn-state-health-experience.
23. Slama R, Lerner J, Kyle A. Ultrasound-guided erector spinae plane block: a case series demonstrating utility for acutely painful conditions in the emergency setting. Cureus. 2024;16(8):e67327. https://doi.org/10.7759/cureus.67327. PMID: 39301352; PMCID: PMC11412688.
24. Harbell MW, Langley NR, Seamans DP, Koyyalamudi V, Kraus MB, Carey FJ, Craner R. Evaluating two approaches to the erector spinae plane block: an anatomical study. Reg Anesth Pain Med. 2023;48(10):495–500. https://doi.org/10.1136/rapm-2022-104132. Epub 2023 Feb 16.
25. Yoshida T, Nakamoto T. Blockade of intercostobrachial nerve by an erector spinae plane block at T2 level: a case report. JA Clin Rep. 2023;9(1):49. https://doi.org/10.1186/s40981-023-00641-9. PMID: 37537322; PMCID: PMC10400509.
26. Lucente M, Ragonesi G, Sanguigni M, Sbaraglia F, Vergari A, Lamacchia R, Del Prete D, Rossi M. Erector spinae plane block in children: a narrative review. Korean J Anesthesiol. 2022;75(6):473–86. https://doi.org/10.4097/kja.22279. Epub 2022 Jul 5. PMID: 35790215; PMCID: PMC9726462.

27. Saadawi M, Layera S, Aliste J, Bravo D, Leurcharusmee P, Tran Q. Erector spinae plane block: a narrative review with systematic analysis of the evidence pertaining to clinical indications and alternative truncal blocks. J Clin Anesth. 2021;68:110063. https://doi.org/10.1016/j.jclinane.2020.110063. Epub 2020 Oct 5.
28. Silver D, Anderson K, Esener D, Rose G. Ultrasound guided lumbar erector spinae block: a case series on a novel technique for the treatment of acute low Back pain. Am J Emerg Med. 2023;72:223.e1–4. https://doi.org/10.1016/j.ajem.2023.07.047. Epub 2023 Jul 26.
29. Aksu C, Gürkan Y. Aksu approach for lumbar erector spinae plane block for pediatric surgeries. J Clin Anesth. 2019;54:74–5. https://doi.org/10.1016/j.jclinane.2018.10.043. Epub 2018 Nov 6.
30. Stenberg RT, Wahi-Singh B, Wahi-Singh P, Hill A, Simon EL. Transversus abdominis plane (TAP) block for pain management of rectus sheath hematoma in the emergency department (ED). Am J Emerg Med. 2023;63:183.e1–3. https://doi.org/10.1016/j.ajem.2022.10.036. Epub 2022 Nov 9.
31. Mahmoud S, Miraflor E, Martin D, Mantuani D, Luftig J, Nagdev AD. Ultrasound-guided transverse abdominis plane block for ED appendicitis pain control. Am J Emerg Med. 2019;37(4):740–3. https://doi.org/10.1016/j.ajem.2019.01.024. Epub 2019 Jan 26.
32. Tran DQ, Bravo D, Leurcharusmee P, Neal JM. Transversus abdominis plane block: a narrative review. Anesthesiology. 2019;131(5):1166–90. https://doi.org/10.1097/ALN.0000000000002842.
33. Yoshiyama S, Ueshima H, Sakai R, Otake H. A posterior TAP block provides more effective analgesia than a lateral TAP block in patients undergoing laparoscopic gynecologic surgery: a retrospective study. Anesthesiol Res Pract. 2016;2016:4598583. https://doi.org/10.1155/2016/4598583. Epub 2016 Jan 28. Retraction in: Anesthesiol Res Pract. 2022 Aug 20;2022:9768905. https://doi.org/10.1155/2022/9768905. PMID: 26941794; PMCID: PMC4749791.
34. Abdallah FW, Laffey JG, Halpern SH, Brull R. Duration of analgesic effectiveness after the posterior and lateral transversus abdominis plane block techniques for transverse lower abdominal incisions: a meta-analysis. Br J Anaesth. 2013;111(5):721–35. https://doi.org/10.1093/bja/aet214. Epub 2013 Jun 27.
35. Modi R. How I do it: TAP block. ASRA Pain Medicine Update. Aug 7, 2019, 14:00PM. https://www.asra.com/news-publications/asra-updates/blog-landing/legacy-b-blog-posts/2019/08/07/how-i-do-it-tap-block.
36. Rose G, Costa V, Drake A, Siadecki SD, Saul T. Ultrasound-guided dorsal penile nerve block performed in a case of zipper entrapment injury. J Clin Ultrasound. 2017;45(9):589–91. https://doi.org/10.1002/jcu.22459. Epub 2017 Feb 10.
37. Stenberg R, Sun J, Makowski B, Krizo J. Ultrasound guidance for real-time management of acute ischemic priapism. Am J Emerg Med. 2024;79:230.e3–5. https://doi.org/10.1016/j.ajem.2024.03.024. Epub 2024 Mar 25.
38. Flores S, Herring AA. Ultrasound-guided dorsal penile nerve block for ED paraphimosis reduction. Am J Emerg Med. 2015;33(6):863.e3–5. https://doi.org/10.1016/j.ajem.2014.12.041. Epub 2014 Dec 26.
39. McPhee AS, McKay AC. Dorsal penile nerve block. 2023. In: StatPearls [Internet]. Treasure Island: StatPearls Publishing; 2025.
40. Fujiwara T, Kagawa T. Ultrasound-guided dorsal penile nerve block in children: in-plane technique. Paediatr Anaesth. 2023;33(6):499. https://doi.org/10.1111/pan.14660. Epub 2023 Mar 16.
41. Zadrazil M, Feigl G, Opfermann P, Marhofer P, Marhofer D, Schmid W. Ultrasound-guided dorsal penile nerve block in children: an anatomical-based observational study of a new anesthesia technique. Children (Basel). 2023;11(1):50. https://doi.org/10.3390/children11010050. PMID: 38255363; PMCID: PMC10813842.

Ultrasound-Guided Regional Anesthesia: Lower Extremity

24

Robert Stenberg, Brian Makowski, and Jordan Tozer

Ultrasound-guided nerve blocks of the lower extremity offer precise, effective regional anesthesia and analgesia for procedures involving the hip, thigh, knee, leg, and foot. By visualizing neural structures in real time, ultrasound guidance improves the accuracy of needle placement and local anesthetic spread while reducing the risk of complications. Commonly performed blocks include the femoral, popliteal sciatic, and posterior tibial; each tailored to specific surgical and pain management needs. This chapter reviews the relevant anatomy, indications, and techniques for lower extremity blocks, emphasizing practical considerations for safe and successful application in diverse clinical settings.

Lower Extremity Nerve Blocks

- Hip PEricapsular Nerve Group (PENG) Block
  - Indications:
    - Hip fractures at level of intertrochanteric level or proximal to such (capsular nerve group block, therefore, will only cover bony portion in joint capsule) [1]

Supplementary Information The online version contains supplementary material available at https://doi.org/10.1007/978-3-032-27643-8_24.

R. Stenberg (✉) · B. Makowski
Department of Emergency Medicine, Cleveland Clinic, Akron, OH, USA
e-mail: stenber@ccf.org; makowsb2@ccf.org

J. Tozer
Department of Emergency Medicine, Virginia Commonwealth University Health, Richmond, VA, USA
e-mail: jordan.tozer@vcuhealth.org

A. Lindsay et al. (eds.), *Clinical Ultrasound*,
https://doi.org/10.1007/978-3-032-27643-8_24

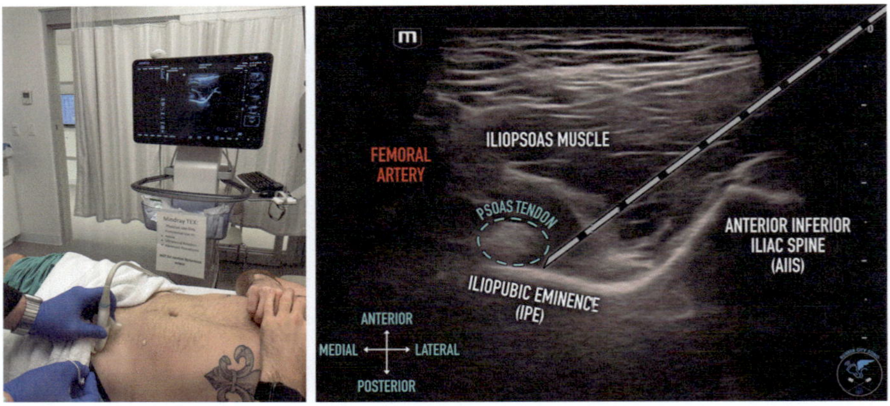

Fig. 24.1 Figure showing hip PENG block. Left, photo showing set-up and ergonomics for block. Right, image showing needle trajectory (arrow) for hip PENG, with goal to bring needle underneath psoas tendon (circle) along the valley of pubic bone between the pubic eminence medially and anterior inferior iliac spine laterally. (Created by Dr. Brian Makowski (with permission to share))

    - Acetabular fracture [2]
    - Pelvic fracture/pubic rami fractures [3]
    - Hip dislocation [4]
    - Hip pain with need to have motor-sparing block
  - Anesthetic Volume:
    - 20–30 mL
      - There is evidence in cadaveric models that going over 20 mL of anesthetic may cause further spread, which could result in some motor involvement and quadricep weakness; which may be relevant, depending on the goal of the block and mobilization [5].
  - Procedure [6]:
    - Place probe obliquely along the axis of the inguinal ligament near location where one would do a fascia iliaca or femoral central line.
    - Adjust depth until the proximal femur is seen and centered. Sweep proximally along this axis as the femur disappears into the pelvis, and the iliopubic eminence, anterior inferior iliac spine, and psoas tendon in the iliacus muscle are seen creating a bony valley (Fig. 24.1). Insert needle laterally to medially with an in-plane approach and advance until needle contact along pelvic bone deep to psoas tendon. Inserting the needle lateral away from ultrasound transducer can permit a better needle angle for this deeper block. Adjust with hydrolocalization until fascial fluid seen lifting off the bone and displacing the psoas tendon up off the bone (Fig. 24.1) (Video 24.1).
      - Consider spinning/rotating the needle to facilitate getting underneath the fascia if initially not getting good spread [7].
    - Administer anesthetic, aspirating every ~5 mL.

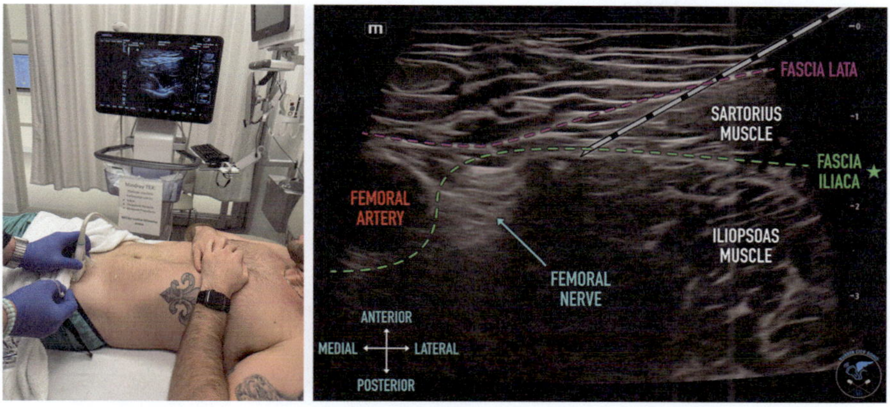

Fig. 24.2 Figure showing Fascia Iliaca Compartment Block (FICB). Left, photo showing set-up and ergonomics for fascia iliaca block. Right, image showing femoral artery and fascia iliaca tracking underneath and lateral to artery. Needle trajectory (arrow) showing target fascial plane. (Created by Dr. Brian Makowski (with permission to share))

- Infrainguinal Fascia Iliaca Compartment Block (FICB)
  - Indications
    - Hip fracture (femoral head, femoral neck, intertrochanteric and subtrochanteric regions) [8, 9]
    - Hip dislocation [10, 11]
    - Femur fracture [12]
    - Anterior thigh lacerations/abscesses/pain [13]
  - Anesthetic Volume
    - 30–40 mL
  - Procedure [14, 15]
    - Place probe in transverse orientation and consider rotating probe obliquely, matching the inguinal ligament to help accentuate fascial planes.
      - There is an alternate approach called the SupraInguinal Fascia Iliaca (SIFI) Block, which is not covered here.
    - Identify femoral artery and assure transducer is proximal to the femoral artery bifurcation (only see one artery). Identify fascia lata superficial to neurovascular bundle; identify fascia iliaca directly underneath the femoral artery, surrounding the iliacus muscle belly and running deep to sartorius laterally (Fig. 24.2).
    - Insert needle with an in-plane approach lateral to medial with hydrolocalization until needle reaches the fascia iliaca. Traditionally, this should be felt as the second "pop" through fascial layers, first being fascia lata and second fascia iliaca (Fig. 24.2).
    - Use hydro-localization, adjusting the needle until the fluid is seen spreading across the fascial plane (Video 24.2).
    - Inject total of anesthetic, aspirating every 5 mL.

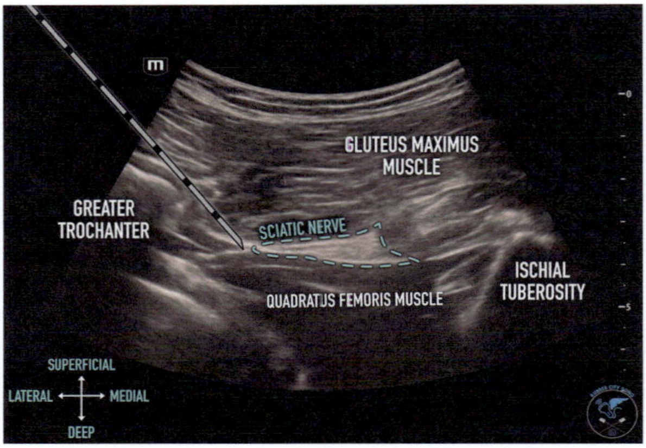

Fig. 24.3 Figure showing transgluteal sciatic nerve block. Image showing sciatic nerve in the transgluteal region. Needle trajectory (arrow) should target the fascial plane between the gluteus maximus (GM) and quadratus lumborum (QL) muscles. (Created by Dr. Brian Makowski (with permission to share))

- Transgluteal Sciatic Nerve Block (TGSN)
  - Indications:
    - Sciatica [16]
    - Burns, lacerations, abscesses, or injuries to the posterior thigh
  - Anesthetic/Medication Volume:
    - 10–20 mL
    - There is some consideration to use Dextrose 5% in Water (D5W) instead of anesthetic to specifically treat sciatica, by mitigating difficulties with ambulation (using anesthetic may cause motor blockade with hamstring weakness and/or foot drop) [17–19].
      - Further, there is thought dextrose has the potential to improve outcomes in the setting of compressive neuropathy not only by releasing it with fluid in general, but also reducing neural glycopenia and downregulating pain receptors [20, 21].
  - Procedure [22]:
    - Position the patient in lateral decubitus, affected side up, with hip and knee flexed to approximately 90 degrees.
    - Typically need a curvilinear transducer given the depth of the transgluteal sciatic nerve, which also provides a large field of view to identify bony landmarks; may consider linear on low BMI patients; extend the field of view if machine capable of doing such.
    - Place transducer in a transverse orientation on the gluteal region, between greater trochanter and ischial tuberosity. Identify sciatic nerve deep to gluteus muscle (Fig. 24.3). Consider color Doppler
    - Insert needle with an in-plane approach, and advance using hydrolocalization until there is fluid seen spreading in the fascial plane deep to gluteus Maximus muscle in which the nerve resides (Video 24.3).
    - Inject, aspirating every ~5 mL.

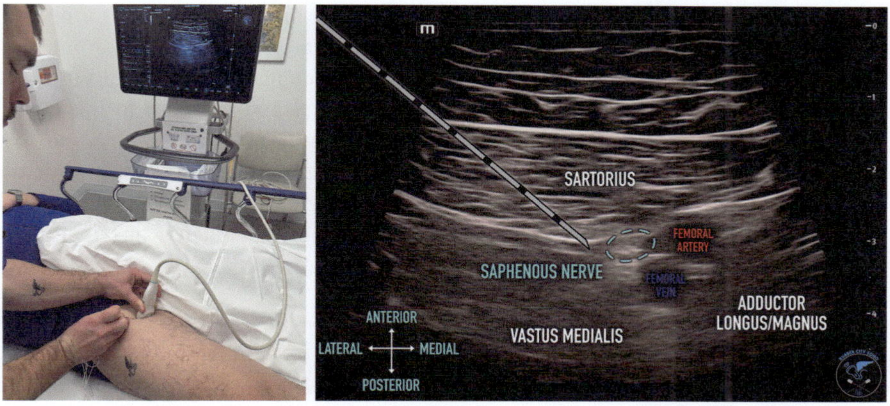

Fig. 24.4 Figure showing adductor canal block. Left, photo showing room set-up and ergonomics for block. Right, image showing saphenous nerve (sensory branch of femoral nerve) lateral to vessels in the proximal adductor canal. Needle trajectory (arrow) should target the fascial plane deep to sartorius. (Created by Dr. Brian Makowski (with permission to share))

- Adductor Canal/Saphenous Nerve Block (sensory branch of femoral nerve)
  - Indications:
    - Knee pain/injury [23]
    - Soft tissue injury along saphenous nerve distribution (medial lower leg) [24, 25]
    - Adjunct to popliteal sciatic nerve for ankle injuries for more comprehensive analgesia (adding medial malleolus coverage) [26]
  - Anesthetic Volume:
    - 10–20 mL
  - Procedure [27]:
    - Position patient supine, with leg in "frog-legged" position (slight external rotation and knee flexion), if possible.
    - Place probe transversely on the anteromedial mid-thigh (proximal third to middle third of thigh), near region where one would evaluate for DVT of the femoral vein. Can also start approximately 10 cm proximal to the medial femoral condyle. Alternatively, a simplified approach is placing the transducer at the halfway point between the the inguinal crease and the superior aspect of the patella.
    - Identify the area where the femoral artery is sitting centrally, deep to sartorius muscle, with the adductor longus muscle seen medially (Fig. 24.4).
    - In the proximal adductor canal, the saphenous nerve tends to run lateral to femoral vessels, then distally, traverses over the vessels, and runs medially as they dive deep toward the popliteal fossa [28].

    - Insert needle with an in-plane or out-of-plane approach, aiming for needle tip to be located deep to the sartorius fascial plane, while avoiding the femoral vessels. Position and adjust needle using hydrolocalization until fluid is seen spreading around femoral vessel and adjacent to the nerve (Video 24.4). If fluid is not seen tracking around and or displacing the femoral vessels, there is a chance of a failed block due to the vasoadductor membrane.
      - If unable to visualize nerve well, can consider placing anesthetic on both sides of artery [29].
    - Deposit anesthetic, aspirating every 5 mL.
- Genicular Nerve Block
  - Indications:
    - Acute, chronic, and acute-on-chronic knee pain, including intra-articular processes [30–33]
    - Acute knee injuries [32]
    - Tibial plateau fracture (caution due to risk of compartment syndrome; consider discussing with orthopedics prior to block) [34]
  - Anesthetic Volume:
    - 3–5 mL per site
  - Procedure [35, 36]:
    - There are up to 5 nerves documented that innervate knee.
      - The nerve to vastus intermedius is often excluded for time.
        - Some argue the extra time to bring the needle down to bone over one more site is minimal (all superior sites can be cleaned together), and may provide superior benefits.
      - The inferior lateral genicular nerve is often avoided due to its close proximity to the common peroneal nerve.
        - Nerve blockade could result in temporary foot drop, limiting mobility (especially if trying to discharge the patient home).
        - Nerve blockade could also result in affected distal neurovascular exam.
      - Due to their small size, genicular nerves (GN) are not typically visualized on ultrasound; however, they do have reliable/consistent anatomic relationships to bony landmarks (Fig. 24.5).
        - Additionally, Color/Power Doppler may be used to identify the genicular arteries as a landmark, as they run in the same path as the nerves.
      - Due to using a smaller block volume per site, consider using saline and only administering anesthetic once spreading fascia off bone.
    - Superolateral GN (SLGN):
      - Place transducer in a sagittal orientation superolateral to the knee, until the curved metaphyseal portion of the femur is noted, deep to the quadriceps, and with a sloping contour of the bone (lateral femoral epicondyle) (Fig. 24.6).

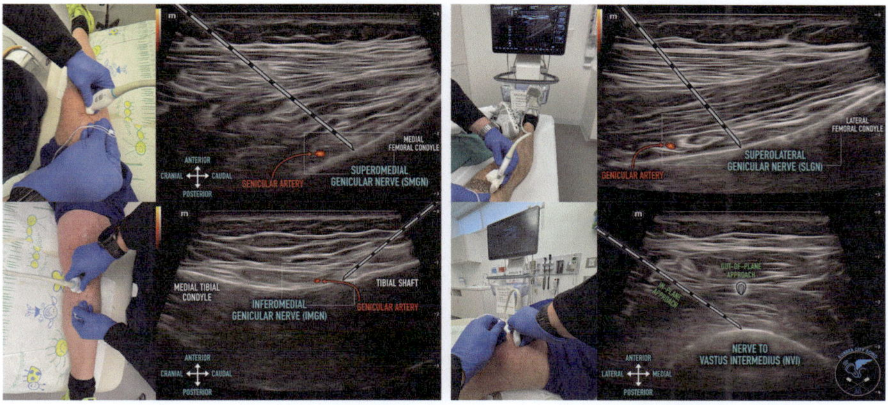

Fig. 24.5 Figure showing collage of genicular nerve blocks. Images highlight focusing on a landmark needle-to-bone technique over trying to find a small, very challenging to identify genicular nerve. Also Doppler is shown, highlighting nearby vessel which is a landmark demonstrating a good location, as the genicular nerve will often run with vessel. Needle trajectory is seen away from, but adjacent to vessel. (Created by Dr. Brian Makowski (with permission to share))

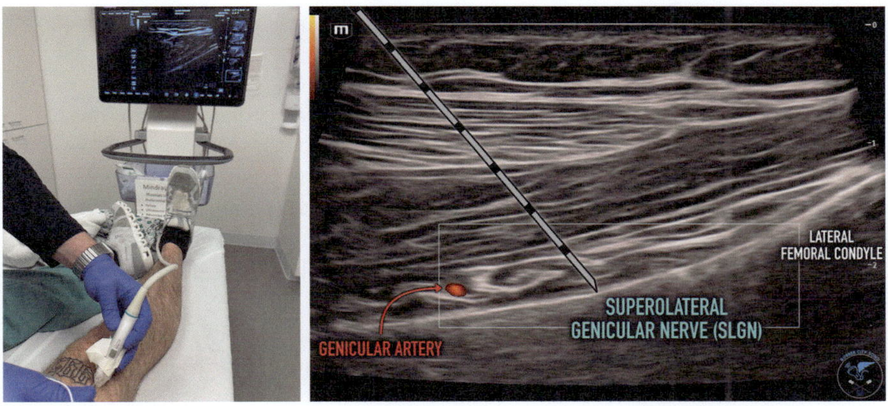

Fig. 24.6 Figure showing the superolateral portion of the genicular nerve block. Left, shows setup and ergonomics, including noting the transducer being near 10 O'clock positioning on the femur. Right, shows arrow with goal needle trajectory (arrow) and target which is down to bone and lifting muscle fascia off bone with anesthetic. (Created by Dr. Brian Makowski (with permission to share))

  - Insert needle in-plane, cranial to caudal, advancing until needle tip contacts bone, and fascial fluid is seen lifting fascia off bone. Deposit anesthetic (Video 24.5).
- Superomedial GN (SMGN):
  - Place transducer in a sagittal fashion superomedial to knee until the curved metaphyseal portion of the femur is noted deep to the quadriceps with the sloping contour of bone (Fig. 24.7).

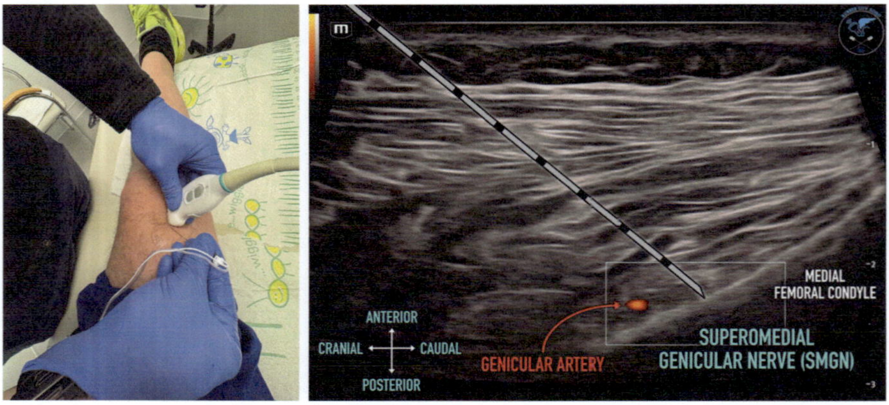

Fig. 24.7 Figure showing the superomedial portion of the genicular nerve block. Left, shows set-up and ergonomics, including noting the transducer being near 2 O'clock positioning on the femur. Right, shows arrow with goal needle trajectory (arrow) and target which is down to bone and lifting muscle fascia off bone with anesthetic. (Created by Dr. Brian Makowski (with permission to share))

  - Insert needle cranial to caudal with an in-plane approach advancing until needle contacts bone and fascial fluid is seen lifting fascia off bone. Deposit anesthetic.
- Inferomedial GN (IMGN):
  - Place transducer in a sagittal fashion inferomedial to knee, medial to tibial tuberosity where the contour of the tibia is seen sloping toward the knee joint. May see nerve and vessel in this region.
  - Insert needle in-plane caudal to cranial, advancing until down to bone adjacent to neurovascular bundle without violation of such. Needle positioned using hydro-localization until fluid is seen lifting fascia off bone. Deposit anesthetic (Fig. 24.8).
- Nerve to Vastus Intermedius (NVI), optional as described above:
  - Probe placed transversely on leg, ~3–5 cm superior to the patella, with femur visualized in short-axis. Insert needle, out-of-plane, cranial-to-caudally, through rectus femoris and vastus intermedius muscles, until boney contact is made with the needle tip. Local anesthetic spread should note elevation of the vastus intermedius muscle off the bone. Deposit anesthetic (Fig. 24.9).
- These can also be performed with a way-out-of-plane (WOOP) approach instead of an in-plane needle approach. This allows the needle trajectory to moreso match the path of the ultrasound waves where the desired target is seen [37].
- Rotating/spinning the needle while maintaining boney contact can help facilitate getting into the correct fascial plane if not seeing ideal spread.

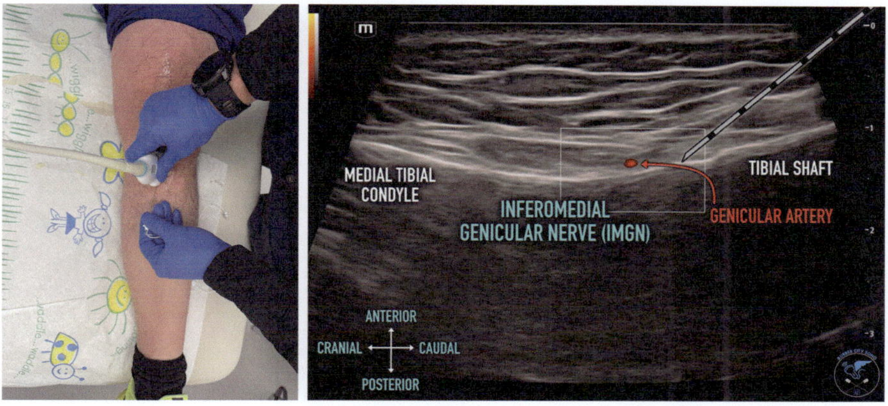

Fig. 24.8 Figure showing the inferomedial portion of the genicular nerve block. Left, shows set-up and ergonomics, including transducer near tibial intraosseous insertion site. Right, shows ideal needle trajectory, including needle coming adjacent to but not directly toward artery. (Created by Dr. Brian Makowski (with permission to share))

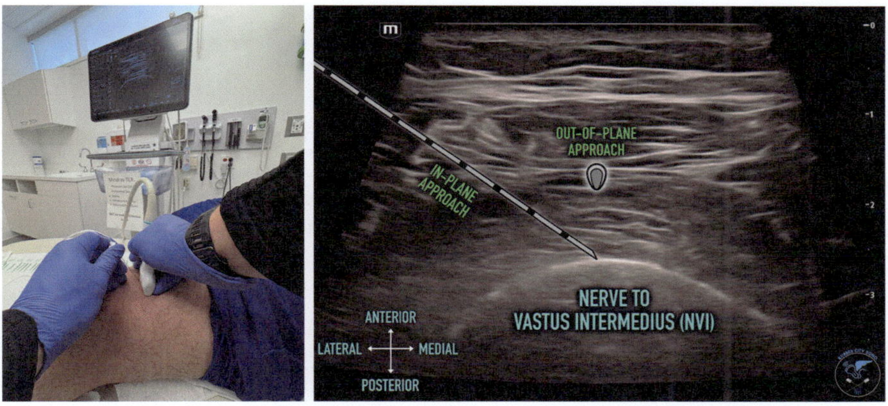

Fig. 24.9 Figure showing the genicular nerve portion associated with vastus intermedius. Left, shows set-up and ergonomics, including the transducer being 3–5 cm proximal to the patella. Right, shows arrow with goal needle trajectory (arrow) and target which is down to bone and lifting muscle fascia off bone with anesthetic. (Created by Dr. Brian Makowski (with permission to share))

- Popliteal Sciatic Nerve Block
  - Indications
    - Soft tissue injury to anterolateral lower leg (no coverage for the medial strip, which is provided by saphenous nerve) [38, 39].
    - Ankle fracture/dislocation [40]
      - Consider addition of Saphenous Nerve/Adductor Canal Block for complete analgesic coverage of the ankle.

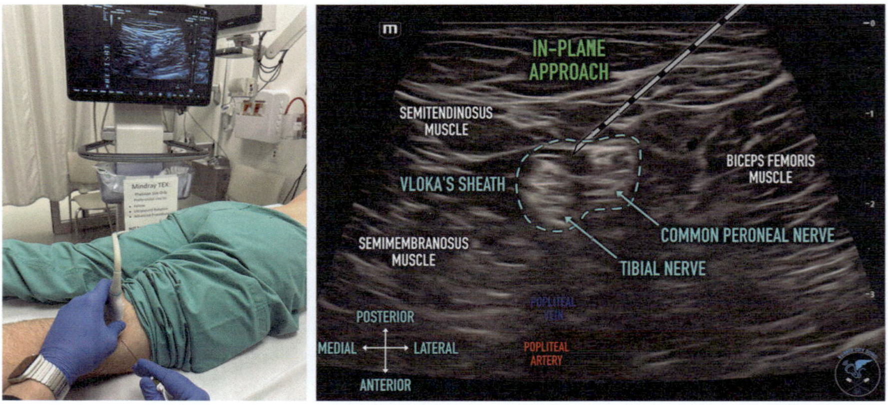

Fig. 24.10 Figure for popliteal sciatic nerve block. Left, picture showing set-up and ergonomics for posterior approach to popliteal sciatic nerve block. Right, image showing popliteal portion of sciatic nerve superficial to the vessels, at the point of bifurcation where one can see both the peroneal and tibial portions (arrows) branching away from each other. (Created by Dr. Brian Makowski (with permission to share))

- Anesthetic Volume
  - 10–20 mL [41]
- Procedure
  - There is some evidence that there is a more effective and faster onset nerve block if the nerve is blocked just distal to the sciatic nerve bifurcation into the tibial and common peroneal nerves, where the nerves still maintain a common epineural sheath (Vloka's sheath) [42, 43].
    - It is also important to ensure the visualized portion of the sciatic nerve contains the common peroneal nerve, as it is easy to scan too far distal; missing this nerve will result in an incomplete block. In order to not miss the common peroneal nerve, scan cranially and caudally superior to the popliteal fossa, while watching for the common peroneal nerve to dive from the lateral direction toward the popliteal vessels. Alternatively, one can also find peroneal nerve posteriorly near fibular head, then track proximally to popliteal sciatic nerve.
  - Posterior Approach (traditional) [44]:
    - Position patient prone or decubitus, with affected side up.
    - Place transducer in transverse orientation in the popliteal fossa (similar region for DVT study), and identify sciatic nerve (Fig. 24.10).
    - Insert needle in-plane, lateral to medially, in the clearest path trajectory.
    - Advance needle until tip reaches the epineural sheath. Aiming the needle between the two nerves, apply gradual pressure to the epineural sheath until tip is able to be advanced through it (sheath will often indent a lot, followed by a large give once underneath, thus it is critical to aim away from either nerve) (Video 24.6).
    - Inject anesthetic, aspirating every ~5 mL.

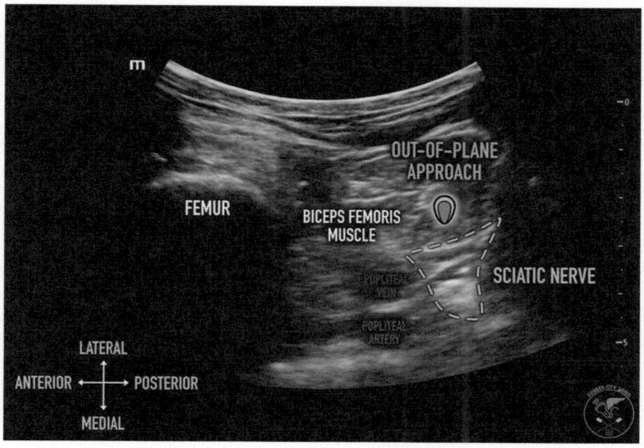

Fig. 24.11 Figure for alternate approach to popliteal sciatic nerve block, the CAPS block which allows for supine positioning. Left, picture showing set-up and ergonomics for block. Right, image showing an out-of-plane approach to reach the sciatic nerve. (Created by Dr. Brian Makowski (with permission to share))

    - Crosswise Approach to Popliteal Sciatic (CAPS) Block Crosswise approach [45]:
      - Positioning here does not require prone or decubitus positioning, which is favorable for those with unstable fractures.
      - Transducer (linear or curvilinear depending on habitus) is place along lateral aspect of leg and nerve identified running with vessels (Fig. 24.11).
      - With an out-of-plane approach, the needle is advanced carefully using hydro-localization until it is adjacent to nerve, and fluid is seen spreading in the fascial plane surrounding the nerve
      - Deposit anesthetic, aspirating every ~5 mL.
    - Lateral Approach [46]
      - While patient supine place transducer (linear or curvilinear depending on habitus) in popliteal fossa and identify popliteal sciatic nerve.
      - Insert needle in-plane, along the lateral aspect of the leg aiming toward needle.
- Posterior Tibial Nerve Block
  - Indications
    - Soft tissue injury to plantar surface [47]
    - Foreign body removal from plantar foot [48]
    - Calcaneus fracture [49, 50]; consider orthopedics consultation prior to block if higher risk for compartment syndrome
  - Anesthetic Volume
    - 5–10 mL [51]
  - Procedure [52, 53]
    - Place probe in transverse orientation posterior to the medial malleolus and identify neurovascular bundle including the posterior tibial nerve (Fig. 24.6).

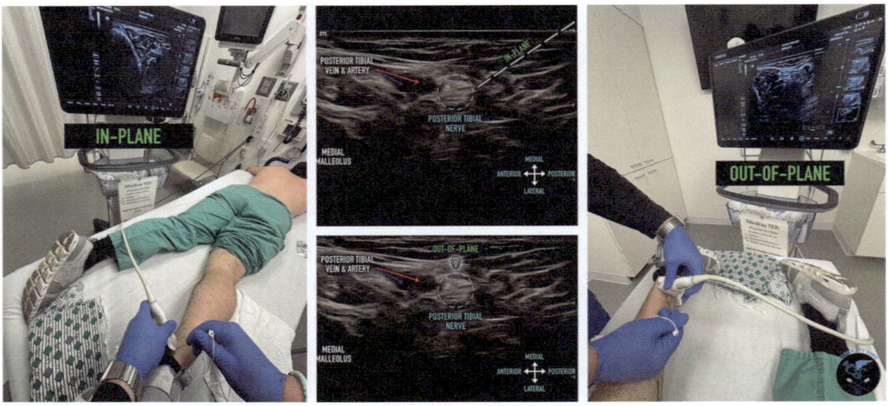

Fig. 24.12 Figure showing the approaches to the posterior tibial nerve block. Left/Right, photos showing room set-up and ergonomics. Center, images showing in-plane versus out-of-plane approaches to posterior tibial nerve. (Created by Dr. Brian Makowski (with permission to share))

- Standard Approach (Retromalleolar):
  - Sweep proximal and distal until the optimal window identified in terms of safe and feasible needle approach and to also confirm which structure is the nerve as several adjacent tendons have a very similar appearance at the ankle.
- Alternate Approach (supramalleolar) [54]:
  - Has advantage of theory catching more branches and often splitting off vessels, but is often deeper.
  - After identifying posterior tibial nerve in the retromalleolar region as part of the neurovascular bundle, sweep proximally past medial malleolus as far proximal as possible where the nerve is still well visualized and there remains a clear needle trajectory.
  - Some approaches recommend up to 10 cm above medial malleolus [55].
- Insert needle in-plane or out-of-plane approach and advance until adjacent to nerve, and hydro-localization shows fascial spread surrounding the nerve (Video 24.7).
- Inject anesthetic (Fig 24.12)

References

1. Rocha-Romero A, Arias-Mejia K, Salas-Ruiz A, Peng PWH. Pericapsular nerve group (PENG) block for hip fracture in the emergency department: a case series. Anaesth Rep. 2021;9(1):97–100. https://doi.org/10.1002/anr3.12118. PMID: 34027410; PMCID: PMC8131169.
2. Fahey A, Cripps E, Ng A, Sweeny A, Snelling PJ. Pericapsular nerve group block for hip fracture is feasible, safe and effective in the emergency department: a prospective observational comparative cohort study. Emerg Med Australas. 2022;34(6):884–91. https://doi.org/10.1111/1742-6723.14013. Epub 2022 Jun 14. PMID: 35701386; PMCID: PMC9796647.

3. Luftig J, Dreyfuss A, Mantuani D, Howell K, White A, Nagdev A. A new frontier in pelvic fracture pain control in the ED: successful use of the pericapsular nerve group (PENG) block. Am J Emerg Med. 2020;38(12):2761.e5–9. https://doi.org/10.1016/j.ajem.2020.05.085. Epub 2020 May 28.
4. Thomas R, Carr M, Fry J, Hoffman T. Pericapsular nerve group block for prosthetic hip reduction in the emergency department: case report. Clin Pract Cases Emerg Med. 2025;9(1):14–6. https://doi.org/10.5811/cpcem.21137.
5. Kim JY, Kim J, Kim DH, Han DW, Kim SH, Kim D, Chung S, Yu S, Lee UY, Park HJ. Anatomical and radiological assessments of Injectate spread stratified by the volume of the pericapsular nerve group block. Anesth Analg. 2023;136(3):597–604. https://doi.org/10.1213/ANE.0000000000006364. Epub 2023 Feb 17.
6. Del Buono R, Padua E, Pascarella G, Costa F, Tognù A, Terranova G, Greco F, Fajardo Perez M, Barbara E. Pericapsular nerve group block: an overview. Minerva Anestesiol. 2021;87(4):458–66. https://doi.org/10.23736/S0375-9393.20.14798-9. Epub 2021 Jan 12.
7. https://www.asra.com/news-publications/asra-newsletter/newsletter-item/asra-news/2023/08/01/how-i-do-it-pericapsular-nerve-group-(peng)-block.
8. Kolodychuk N, Krebs JC, Stenberg R, Talmage L, Meehan A, DiNicola N. Fascia Iliaca blocks performed in the emergency department decrease opioid consumption and length of stay in patients with hip fracture. J Orthop Trauma. 2022;36(3):142–6. https://doi.org/10.1097/BOT.0000000000002220.
9. Makkar JK, Singh NP, Bhatia N, Samra T, Singh PM. Fascia iliaca block for hip fractures in the emergency department: meta-analysis with trial sequential analysis. Am J Emerg Med. 2021;50:654–60. https://doi.org/10.1016/j.ajem.2021.09.038. Epub 2021 Sep 25.
10. Eyi YE, Arziman I, Kaldirim U, Tuncer SK. Fascia iliaca compartment block in the reduction of dislocation of total hip arthroplasty. Am J Emerg Med. 2014;32(9):1139. https://doi.org/10.1016/j.ajem.2014.06.007. Epub 2014 Jun 12.
11. Kaldirim Ü, Yolcu Ü. Fascia iliaca compartment block for hip dislocation. Eur J Emerg Med. 2015;22(2):145–6. https://doi.org/10.1097/MEJ.0000000000000190.
12. Shakya BM, Shrestha N. Continuous fascia Iliaca compartment block for post operative analgesia in fracture femur. J Nepal Health Res Counc. 2018;16(2):248–50.
13. Barton DJ, Marino RT, Pizon AF. Multimodal analgesia in crotalid snakebite envenomation: a novel use of femoral nerve block. Am J Emerg Med. 2018;36(12):2340.e1–2. https://doi.org/10.1016/j.ajem.2018.09.020. Epub 2018 Sep 14.
14. LaJeunesse M, Cronin A, Takahashi M, Knudsen J, Nagdev A. Control hip fracture pain without opioids using ultrasound-guided fascia Iliaca compartment block. ACEP Now. 2018;37(1). https://www.acepnow.com/article/control-hip-fracture-pain-without-opioids-using-ultrasound-guided-fascia-iliaca-compartment-block/.
15. O'Reilly N, Desmet M, Kearns R. Fascia iliaca compartment block. BJA Educ. 2019;19(6):191–7. https://doi.org/10.1016/j.bjae.2019.03.001. Epub 2019 Apr 24. PMID: 33456890; PMCID: PMC7808109.
16. Goldsmith AJ, Liteplo A, Hayes BD, Duggan N, Huang C, Shokoohi H. Ultrasound-guided transgluteal sciatic nerve analgesia for refractory back pain in the ED. Am J Emerg Med. 2020;38(9):1792–5. https://doi.org/10.1016/j.ajem.2020.06.001. Epub 2020 Jun 6.
17. Silver D, Esener D, Rose G. Ultrasound guided transgluteal sciatic nerve hydrodissection for the treatment of acute sciatica in the emergency department. Am J Emerg Med. 2023;69:219.e3–6. https://doi.org/10.1016/j.ajem.2023.02.026. Epub 2023 Feb 28.
18. Goldsmith A, Brown J, Herrala J, Nagdev A. How to relieve sciatica pain with new TransGluteal nerve block treatment. ACEP Now. 2022;41(6). https://www.acepnow.com/article/transgluteal-sciatic-nerve-block/.
19. Macias R, Diaz D, Prats MI. Motor blockade from transgluteal sciatic nerve block in the emergency department. Am J Emerg Med. 2022;60:193–4. https://doi.org/10.1016/j.ajem.2022.06.029. Epub 2022 Jun 21.
20. Lam KHS, Hung CY, Chiang YP, Onishi K, Su DCJ, Clark TB, Reeves KD. Ultrasound-guided nerve hydrodissection for pain management: rationale, methods, current literature, and

theoretical mechanisms. J Pain Res. 2020;13:1957–68. https://doi.org/10.2147/JPR.S247208. PMID: 32801851; PMCID: PMC7414936.

21. Buntragulpoontawee M, Chang KV, Vitoonpong T, Pornjaksawan S, Kitisak K, Saokaew S, Kanchanasurakit S. The effectiveness and safety of commonly used Injectates for ultrasound-guided hydrodissection treatment of peripheral nerve entrapment syndromes: a systematic review. Front Pharmacol. 2021;5(11):621150. https://doi.org/10.3389/fphar.2020.621150. PMID: 33746745; PMCID: PMC7973278.
22. Selame LA, McFadden K, Duggan NM, Goldsmith AJ, Shokoohi H. Ultrasound-guided Transgluteal sciatic nerve block for gluteal procedural analgesia. J Emerg Med. 2021;60(4):512–6. https://doi.org/10.1016/j.jemermed.2020.10.047. Epub 2020 Dec 15.
23. Hasabo EA, Assar A, Mahmoud MM, Abdalrahman HA, Ibrahim EA, Hasanin MA, Emam AK, AbdelQadir YH, AbdelAzim AA, Ali AS. Adductor canal block versus femoral nerve block for pain control after total knee arthroplasty: a systematic review and meta-analysis. Medicine (Baltimore). 2022;101(34):e30110. https://doi.org/10.1097/MD.0000000000030110. PMID: 36042669; PMCID: PMC9410636.
24. Allen KW, Moake MM. Ultrasound-guided paravenous saphenous nerve block for lower extremity abscess incision and drainage in a male adolescent. Pediatr Emerg Care. 2023;39(4):279–82. https://doi.org/10.1097/PEC.0000000000002768. Epub 2022 May 26.
25. Ransford G, Feyzeau K, Noble M, Jones M, Byars D. Saphenous and sciatic nerve block to treat acute lower limb ischemic pain in the emergency department. J Ultrasound. 2022;25(4):979–81. https://doi.org/10.1007/s40477-021-00629-0. Epub 2022 Apr 23. PMID: 35460505; PMCID: PMC9705610.
26. Park YU, Joe HB, Lee JW, Seo YW. Analgesic effectiveness of continuous versus single-injection adductor canal block in addition to continuous popliteal sciatic nerve block for bimalleolar and trimalleolar ankle fracture surgery: prospective randomized controlled trial. J Orthop Sci. 2025;30(1):159–63. https://doi.org/10.1016/j.jos.2024.01.002. Epub 2024 Feb 5.
27. Croft PE, Mackenzie D. How to perform an Adductor Canal nerve block. ACEP Now. 2020. https://www.acepnow.com/article/how-to-perform-an-adductor-canal-nerve-block/.
28. https://www.asra.com/news-publications/asra-newsletter/newsletter-item/asra-news/2020/05/02/how-i-do-it-saphenous-nerve-block2.
29. Vora MU, Nicholas TA, Kassel CA, Grant SA. Adductor canal block for knee surgical procedures: review article. J Clin Anesth. 2016;35:295–303. https://doi.org/10.1016/j.jclinane.2016.08.021. Epub 2016 Oct 11.
30. Kong C, Bubic IJ, Tran AA, Tan G, Medak AJ, Oswald J. Genicular nerve block for emergency department patient: a successful management of subacute osteoarthritic knee ain. Pain Manag. 2023;13(7):373–8. https://doi.org/10.2217/pmt-2022-0104. Epub 2023 Jul 17.
31. Kim DH, Choi SS, Yoon SH, Lee SH, Seo DK, Lee IG, Choi WJ, Shin JW. Ultrasound-guided genicular nerve block for knee osteoarthritis: a double-blind, randomized controlled trial of local anesthetic alone or in combination with corticosteroid. Pain Physician. 2018;21(1):41–52.
32. Bhattaram S, Shinde VS. Novel use of motor-sparing genicular nerve blocks for knee injuries in the emergency department. Am J Emerg Med. 2024;75:196.e1–4. https://doi.org/10.1016/j.ajem.2023.10.038. Epub 2023 Oct 28.
33. Radwan A, Ohrndorf S, Aly H, Hamed M, Khalifa A, Elsaman AM. Genicular nerve block in juvenile idiopathic arthritis: a randomized clinical trial. Clin Rheumatol. 2023;42(3):879–88. https://doi.org/10.1007/s10067-022-06389-4. Epub 2022 Oct 5. PMID: 36197647; PMCID: PMC9935707.
34. Sobel J, Oswald J. Novel use of 3-point genicular nerve block for acute knee pain in the emergency department. J Emerg Med. 2021;61(4):416–9. https://doi.org/10.1016/j.jemermed.2021.04.012. Epub 2021 Jun 25.
35. Eberle M, et al. The genicular nerve block for knee pain in the emergency department. ACEP EUS. 2023. https://www.acep.org/emultrasound/newsroom/oct2023/the-genicular-nerve-block-for-knee-pain-in-the-emergency-department.

36. Tan YL, Neo EJR, Wee TC. Ultrasound-guided genicular nerve blockade with pharmacological agents for chronic knee osteoarthritis: a systematic review. Pain Physician. 2022;25(4):E489–502.
37. https://www.asra.com/news-publications/asra-newsletter/newsletter-item/asra-news/2022/05/01/how-i-do-it-genicular-nerve-blocks-for-acute-pain.
38. Miguel Ruano G, Leal Quiñones F, Arribas Sánchez C, Álvarez Avello JM. Ultrasound-guided sciatic popliteal block performed at the emergency department in a patient with a scorpion bite and severe pain. Rev Esp Anestesiol Reanim (Engl Ed). 2023;70(6):358–61. https://doi.org/10.1016/j.redare.2022.06.007. Epub 2023 Jun 3.
39. Mori T, Hagiwara Y. Ultrasound-guided popliteal sciatic nerve block for an ankle laceration in a pediatric emergency department. Pediatr Emerg Care. 2017;33(12):803–5. https://doi.org/10.1097/PEC.0000000000001334.
40. Herring AA, Stone MB, Fischer J, Frenkel O, Chiles K, Teismann N, Nagdev A. Ultrasound-guided distal popliteal sciatic nerve block for ED anesthesia. Am J Emerg Med. 2011;29(6):697.e3–5. https://doi.org/10.1016/j.ajem.2010.06.015. Epub 2010 Aug 3.
41. Piacherski V, Marochkov A. The blockade of the sciatic nerve with different doses and volumes of lidocaine using ultrasound guidance: 8AP3-6. Eur J Anaesthesiol. 2013;30:123.
42. Buys MJ, Arndt CD, Vagh F, Hoard A, Gerstein N. Ultrasound-guided sciatic nerve block in the popliteal fossa using a lateral approach: onset time comparing separate tibial and common peroneal nerve injections versus injecting proximal to the bifurcation. Anesth Analg. 2010;110(2):635–7. https://doi.org/10.1213/ANE.0b013e3181c88f27. Epub 2009 Dec 8.
43. Soberón JR, McInnis C, Bland KS, Egger AL, Patterson ME, Elliott CE, Treuting RJ, Osteen K. Ultrasound-guided popliteal sciatic nerve blockade in the severely and morbidly obese: a prospective and randomized study. J Anesth. 2016;30(3):397–404. https://doi.org/10.1007/s00540-016-2143-z. Epub 2016 Feb 9.
44. https://www.asra.com/news-publications/asra-newsletter/newsletter-item/asra-ews/2022/02/07/how-i-do-it-ultrasound-guided-sciatic-nerve-block-at-the-popliteal-fossa.
45. Mistry T, Sonawane K, Keshri V, Balavenkatasubramanian J, Sekar C. Ultrasound-guided CAPS (crosswise approach to popliteal sciatic) block: a novel technique for supine popliteal fossa block. Cureus. 2022;14(1):e20894. https://doi.org/10.7759/cureus.20894. PMID: 35145799; PMCID: PMC8809205.
46. Hadzic A, Lopez A, Vandepitte C, Sala-Blanch X. Ultrasound-guided popliteal sciatic nerve block. NYSORA. https://www.nysora.com/topics/regional-anesthesia-for-specific-surgical-procedures/lower-extremity-regional-anesthesia-for-specific-surgical-procedures/foot-and-anckle/ultrasound-guided-popliteal-sciatic-block/.
47. Shalaby M, Sanoja A, Rosselli M. Posterior Tibial nerve block for the treatment of plantar fasciitis in the emergency department. J Emerg Med. 2023;65(5):e441–3. https://doi.org/10.1016/j.jemermed.2023.05.025. Epub 2023 Jun 18.
48. Moake MM, Presley BC, Barnes RM. Ultrasound-guided posterior Tibial nerve block for plantar foot foreign body removal. Pediatr Emerg Care. 2020;36(5):262–5. https://doi.org/10.1097/PEC.0000000000001897.
49. Clattenburg E, Herring A, Hahn C, Johnson B, Nagdev A. ED ultrasound-guided posterior tibial nerve blocks for calcaneal fracture analagesia. Am J Emerg Med. 2016;34(6):1183.e1–3. https://doi.org/10.1016/j.ajem.2015.11.002. Epub 2015 Nov 9.
50. Farbood A, Asadi S, Amini A, Hamze Moghaddam B, Asmarian N, Naderi Boldaji V, Vosoughi AR. The effect of posterior tibial and sural nerve blocks on postoperative pain of patients following open reduction and internal fixation of calcaneal fractures. Foot Ankle Surg. 2022;28(7):858–62. https://doi.org/10.1016/j.fas.2021.11.009. Epub 2021 Nov 24.
51. Burl T, Latshaw P, Dreyfuss A. Ultrasound-guided posterior Tibial nerve block for frostbite of the plantar surfaces: a case series. Clin Pract Cases Emerg Med. 2022;6(4):272–5. https://doi.org/10.5811/cpcem.2022.7.56727. PMID: 36427030; PMCID: PMC9697877.
52. Herring AA, Miss J, Nagdev AD. Ultrasound-guided posterior Tibial nerve block. ACEP Now; 2012. https://www.acepnow.com/article/ultrasound-guided-posterior-tibial-nerve-block/2/.

53. Shah A, Morris S, Alexander B, McKissack H, Jones JR, Tedder C, Jha AJ, Desai R. Landmark technique vs ultrasound-guided approach for posterior Tibial nerve block in cadaver models. Indian J Orthop. 2020;54(1):38–42. https://doi.org/10.1007/s43465-019-00012-6. PMID: 32211127; PMCID: PMC7065735.
54. Benimeli-Fenollar M, Montiel-Company JM, Almerich-Silla JM, Cibrián R, Macián-Romero C. Tibial nerve block: supramalleolar or retromalleolar approach? A randomized trial in 110 participants. Int J Environ Res Public Health. 2020;17(11):3860. https://doi.org/10.3390/ijerph17113860. PMID: 32485917; PMCID: PMC7312777.
55. Garcia Tomas V, DeLeon AM, Johnson PA, Vargas K, MacLyman S, Chung B. Proximal ultrasound-guided posterior Tibial nerve block for the removal of calcaneal hardware. Cureus. 2023;15(6):e41047. https://doi.org/10.7759/cureus.41047. PMID: 37383303; PMCID: PMC10299757.

Ultrasound-Guided Procedures

25

Taylor Brittan, Michael J. Vitto, and Lindsay Taylor

Introduction

This chapter focuses on ultrasound-guided procedures, including ultrasound-guided peripheral intravenous access, central venous access, paracentesis, and lumbar puncture. Indications, procedure preparation, landmarks, and techniques are described.

Ultrasound-Guided Peripheral Intravenous Access

(a) Procedure Indications
   - Difficult intravenous (IV) access:
     - Risk factors for difficult IV access include:
       Diabetic patient
       Morbidly Obese
       Vascular Disease
       End Stage Renal Disease or Dialysis
       Sickle cell patient Chemotherapy patient IV drug abuse

Supplementary Information The online version contains supplementary material available at https://doi.org/10.1007/978-3-032-27643-8_25.

T. Brittan (✉)
Department of Emergency Medicine, University of Florida College of Medicine, UF Jacksonville, Jacksonville, FL, USA
e-mail: taylor.brittan@jax.ufl.edu

M. J. Vitto · L. Taylor
Department of Emergency Medicine, Virginia Commonwealth University Health, Richmond, VA, USA
e-mail: michael.vitto@vcuhealth.org; Lindsay.Taylor@vcuhealth.org

A. Lindsay et al. (eds.), *Clinical Ultrasound*,
https://doi.org/10.1007/978-3-032-27643-8_25

History of difficult access
Dehydration
Edema

- Multiple (>2) previous attempts without successful IV placement

(b) Contraindications
- Infection near or at the site of interest
- Lymphedema
- Burned Extremities
- Previous intravenous infiltrations
- Excessive Scar tissue
- AV Fistula (for dialysis patients)
- Sclerosed vein
- Phlebitis

(c) Procedure Complications
- Infection, phlebitis, hematoma
- Extraluminal placement
- Dislodgement and infiltration

(d) Transducer Selection
- Linear array
- optimize depth and gain

(e) Equipment
- IV needle with angiocatheter:
  - Long (>1.25 inches) vs short IV catheters.
  - Length of catheter in vein directly related to long-term function.
  - Echogenic needle.
- Ultrasound gel:
  - Sterile surgical lubricant.
  - Not multi-use containers.
- Probe cover or adhesive barrier.
- Antiseptic swab
- Tourniquet
- Luer lock adapter
- Saline flush
- Adhesive dressing
- Gloves

(f) Patient Position and Anatomical Landmarks
- Optimize patient positioning.
  - i.e. for brachial vein position supine with arm extended and externally rotated:
  - Figure 25.1—Patient position for PIV placement
- Optimize ultrasound machine position so that you can see the patient and the ultrasound machine screen.
- Blood vessels appear anechoic:
  - Veins are thin-walled and compressible.
  - Arteries have thicker walls, typically pulsate, and are not compressible.
  - Figure 25.2—Ultrasound of the artery and vein.

- Vein selection: in order of preference
  1. Lower arm cephalic
  2. Lower arm median vein
  3. Antecubital fossa
     (a) Often large and superficial veins, but don't last as long when patients bend their arm frequently.
     (b) Better for short term or urgent use.
  4. Upper arm cephalic vein
  5. Basilic vein
     (a) Can be found in the lower arm, but difficult to position the patient.
     (b) Often the largest vein in the upper arm, not accompanied by arteries, but can be deep.
  6. Brachial Veins
     (a) Technically challenging because they are accompanied by arteries and nerves.
  7. External jugular vein
- Figure 25.3—Cephalic, basilic, and brachial vein positions.

(g) Preparation
- Universal precautions should be utilized at all times.
  – At least gloves, probe cover, and sterile gel.
- Apply a tourniquet.
- Identify the vessel with ultrasound: IMPORTANT
  – Find vein direction and depth.
  – Increased success associated with veins <1.5 cm [1].
  – *Map out vein course and trajectory.*
    - Identifying turns/tortuous course, valves, clots, or other obstructions.

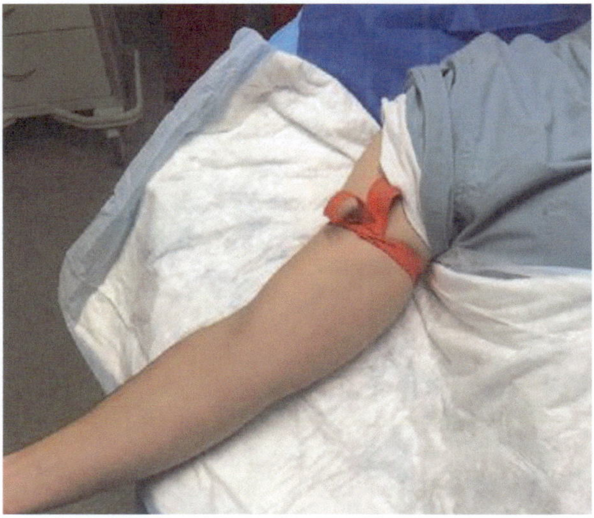

Fig. 25.1 Patient position for PIV placement. Extend and externally rotate the patient's arm when preparing for ultrasound-guided peripheral intravenous catheter placement

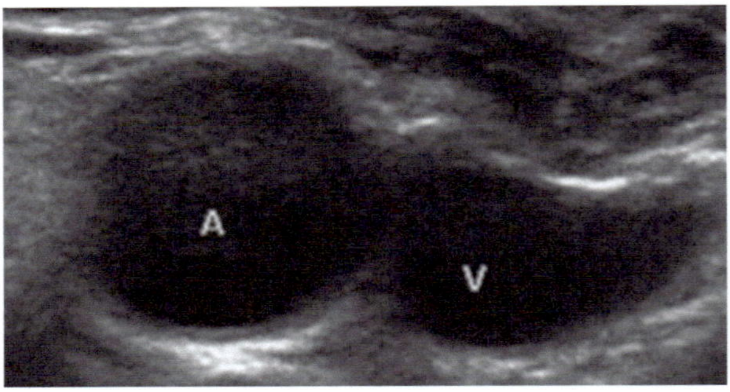

Fig. 25.2 Ultrasound of the artery and vein. Arteries are circular with thick walls and pulsate when pressure is applied. Veins have thinner walls and will compress with pressure

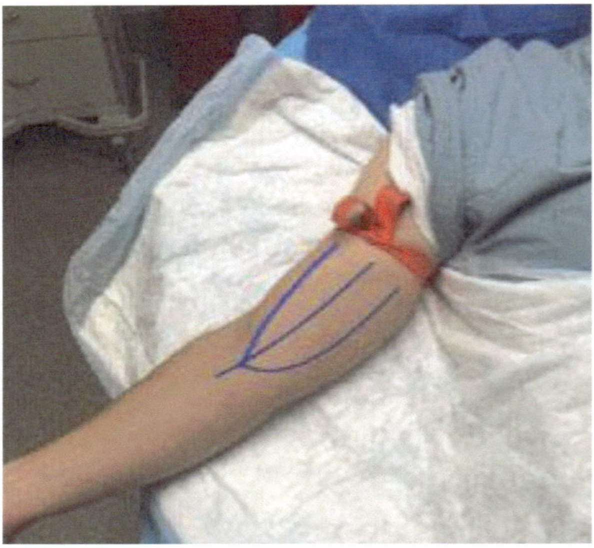

Fig. 25.3 Cephalic, brachial, and basilic vein positions. Approximate location

- Anchor hand holding transducer:
  - Be careful not to apply pressure with the transducer as this will displace the vessel deeper within the arm and compress the vein.
  - Figure 25.4 Transducer placement.
- Optimize Image:
  - Adjust depth so that the vessel is in the center of the screen.
  - Increase gain so that needle will show up bright on the screen.

(h) Figure 25.5—Ideal image for ultrasound-guided peripheral IV placement. Technique
- After practice, determine which hand holds the needle vs. probed. Some prefer dominant hand to hold a needle.
- Two approaches (in-plane or out-of-plane):
  - Figure 25.6a—In-plane
  - Figure 25.6b—Out-of-plane

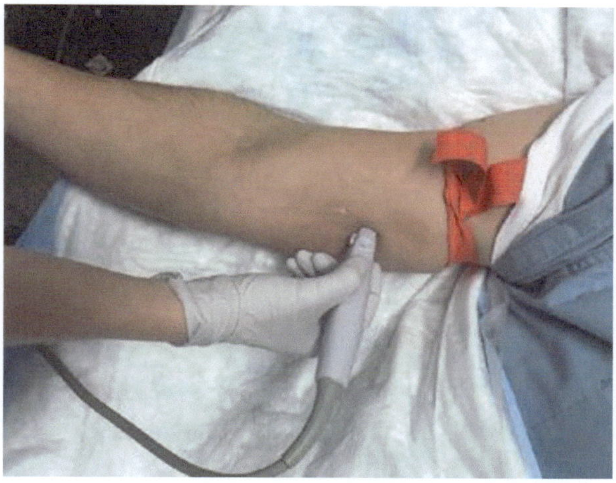

Fig. 25.4 Transducer placement over the area of the basilic vein

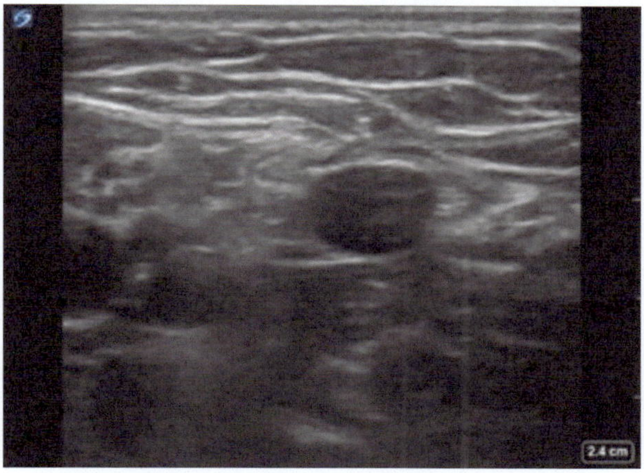

Fig. 25.5 Ideal image for ultrasound-guided peripheral IV placement. Success rate increases when the target vessel is within 1–1.5 cm depth and in the center of the screen

- Out-of-plane:
  - The vein will be imaged using a transverse or cross-sectional view.
  - The transducer marker should point in the same direction on the patient as on the ultrasound monitor.
  - Identify the vein in cross-section.
  - Insert the needle just distal to the transducer and enter the skin. Ideally at angle 15–30 degrees to maximize needle visualization.
    - More shallow angle for superficial vessels (<0.5 cm)
    - Steeper angle for deeper vessels (>1 cm)
      Figure 25.7—Needle position relative to transducer

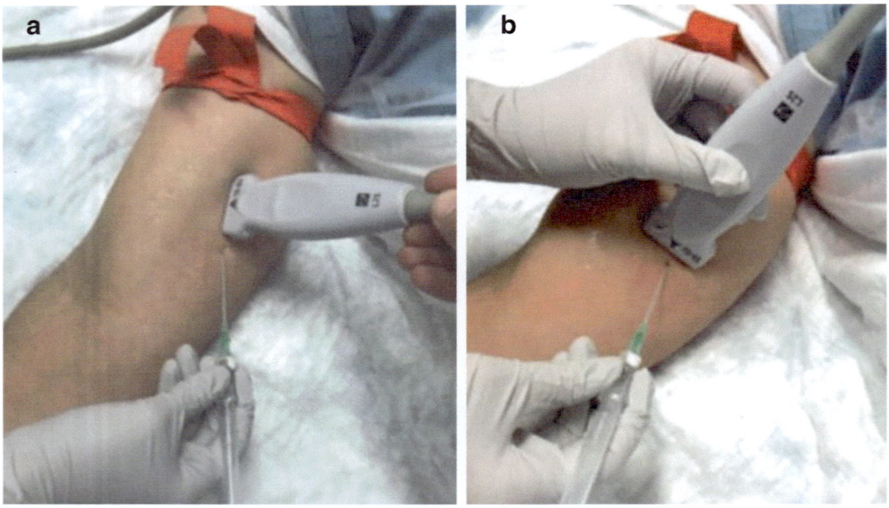

Fig. 25.6 In-plane vs. out-of-plane. (**a**) Is an in-plane approach and (**b**) is an out-of-plane approach

Fig. 25.7 Transducer with needle entering into the skin. Place the transducer centrally over the vessel of choice with the nondominant hand. The dominant hand holds the needle with catheter at the center of the transducer ready to enter the skin at a 15–30° angle

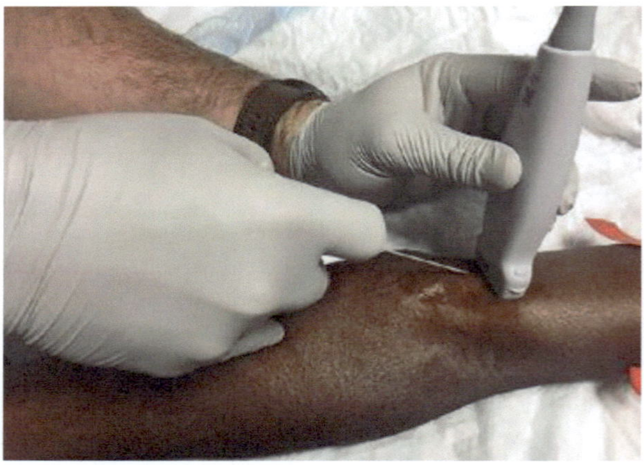

- After entering skin, find the needle tip on the US before advancing the needle any further.
  - Needle tip will be visualized in the subcutaneous tissue as a small bright white dot:
    Figure 25.8—Needle tip
  - Advance your needle 1 mm to 2 mm at a time, and always follow the needle tip as it enters the vein.
  - Once the needle tip enters the vessel, drop the angle of the needle, and advance in the same 1 mm to 2 mm step-wise movements to ensure the needle and the catheter are within the vessel lumen.

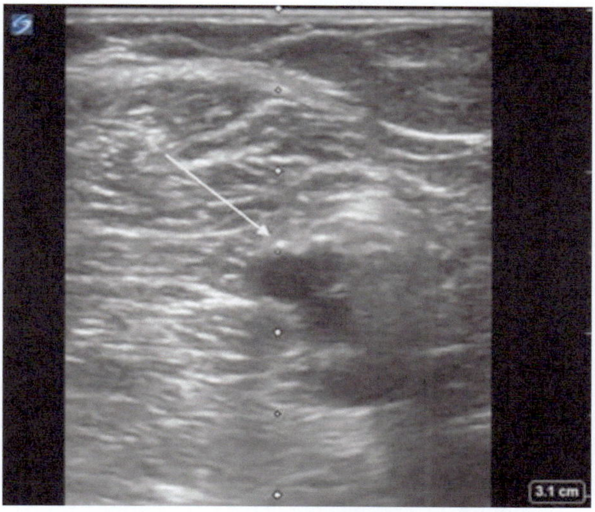

Fig. 25.8 Needle tip above the vessel. The needle tip is hyperechoic and seen just anterior to the vessel. Follow the needle tip through the layers of the skin and into the vein

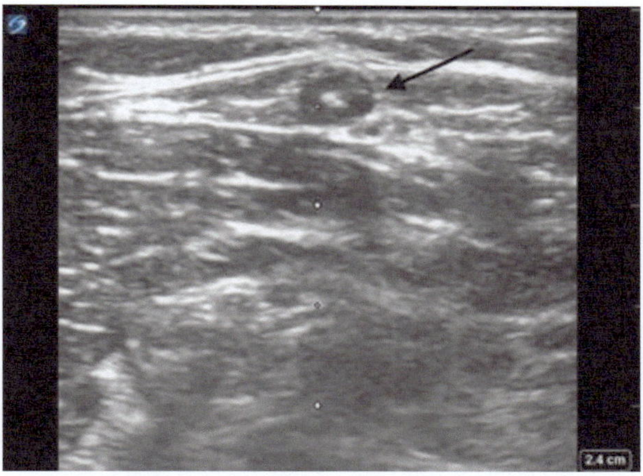

Fig. 25.9 Needle in the vessel, out-of-plane. The hyperechoic needle tip is seen within the center of the vein

- Figure 25.9—Needle in the vessel.
- Remember: Do not rely solely on flash. Catheter tip sits back slightly from needle bevel so at the initial flash, it may not be far enough into the vessel to advance the catheter.
- Stabilize the needle and slowly advance the catheter until it is completely within the vessel lumen.
- Advancing the catheter to the hub will increase the success rate.
- Video 25.1—Out-of-plane peripheral IV placement.

- In-plane:
  - The vein will be imaged using a longitudinal view of the vessel.
  - Place the transducer over the vessel with the marker pointed toward the needle: This can also be done with the marker pointed away from the needle.
  - In this view, the vein will appear as an anechoic tube.
  - Insert the needle just distal to the leading edge of the transducer and enter the skin at a 15–30° angle:
    Figure 25.10—Transducer and needle placement in long axis
  - If the needle is directly under the transducer beam, it will reflect the entire needle, and you can visualize it along its course into the vessel.
  - The benefit of this view is you do not have to proceed in a step-wise approach to localize needle tip. The drawback is it is easy to lose the entire needle and/or vein from view.
  - Figure 25.11—Long axis of needle toward the vein
  - Once the needle tip enters the vessel, drop the angle, and advance to ensure the needle and the catheter are within the vessel lumen:
  - Figure 25.12—Needle in the vessel, long axis. Stabilize the needle and slowly advance the catheter until it is completely within the vessel lumen.
  - Video 25.2—In-plane peripheral IV placement.
- Completing the procedure:
  - Gently place the US down, and cast off the catheter and retract the needle with free hand.
  - Once the catheter is in, you may ensure the blood flow is dark and nonpulsatile.
  - Then apply your gloved finger over the hub to decrease bleeding from IV.

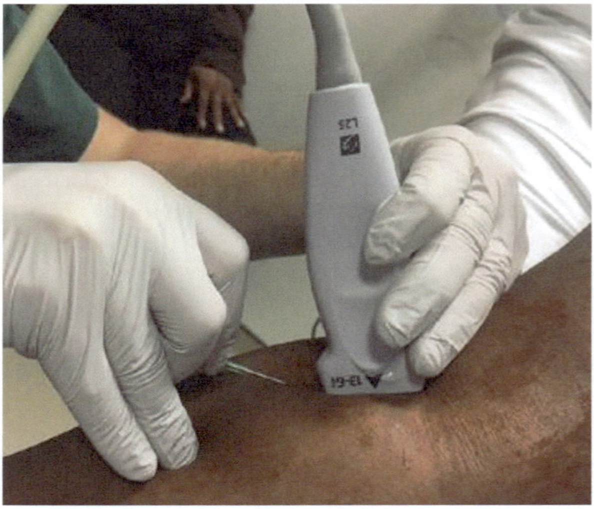

Fig. 25.10 Transducer and needle placement in the long axis. Place the transducer centrally over the vessel of choice with a catheter at the center of the transducer ready to enter the skin at a 15–30° angle

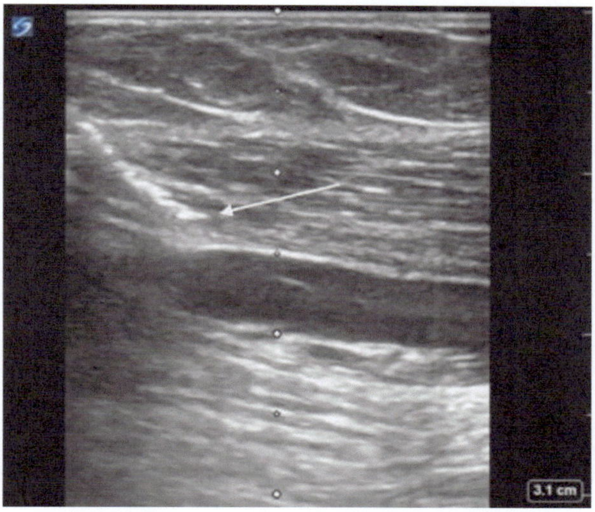

Fig. 25.11 Long axis of needle toward the vein. Advance the needle toward the vessel, ensuring to visualize the entire needle and vessel the entire time

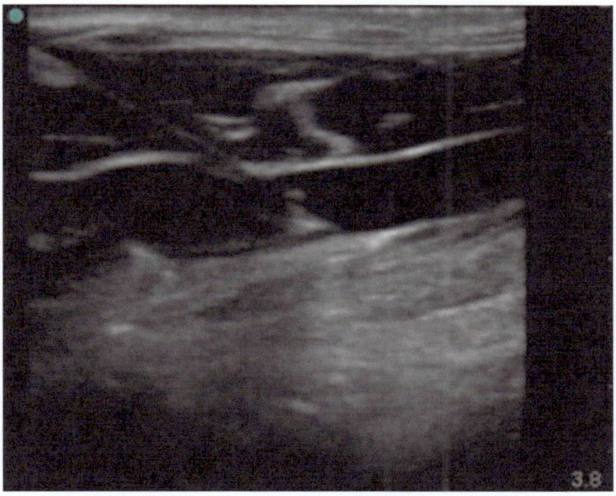

Fig. 25.12 Needle in the vessel, in-plane. The in-plane approach allows for visualization of the entire needle as it enters the vein

- Attach the catheter extension tubing, aspirate blood, then flush the line with saline
  - Saline should flow easily without resistance or pain.
  - If there is no good forward flow, the IV is likely extraluminal, or the vessel has been too diseased and damaged to be used.
- Release the tourniquet.
- Use the Tegaderm to secure.
  - Consider also wrapping in Coban to secure.

- Key Points
  - Preparation:
    - Selecting the ideal vessel based on depth, direction, and free of obstruction [2].
  - Technique:
    - Maintaining needle tip visualization and localization is the key to successful cannulation.
    - Probe angle in relation to needle to optimize needle visualization.
- Possible Complications of US-Guided PIV
  - Infiltration or extravasation
  - Thrombophlebitis
  - Nerve injury
  - Arterial Puncture

Central Venous Catheterization

1. Procedure Indications
   (a) Inability to obtain peripheral IV access
   (b) Emergent venous access
      - Keep in mind blood flow through a large-bore IV is faster than the standard triple-lumen central catheter.
   (c) Hemodynamic resuscitation
   (d) Transvenous pacer placement
   (e) Use of caustic or vasoactive medications such as parenteral nutrition or vasopressors.
   (f) Poor peripheral access
   (g) Dialysis (renal replacement therapy)
   (h) Plasma exchange
   (i) Frequent lab draws
2. Procedure Contraindications
   (a) Absolute:
      - Thrombosis/stenosis
        - Ultrasound provides the advantage of viewing the vessel to rule this out prior to the procedure.
        - Infection over the site of needle insertion
   (b) Relative:
      - Anticoagulation.
      - Bleeding dyscrasia.
      - The patient is unable to cooperate.
3. Procedure Complications
   (a) Arterial puncture
   (b) Bleeding or hematoma
   (c) Pneumothorax
   (d) Thrombosis
   (e) Infection
   (f) Nerve injury

4. Transducer Selection
   (a) Linear array
   (b) Vascular access or venous preset
5. Equipment
   (a) Trash bin
   (b) 3 claves
   (c) 3 flushes
   (d) Sterile ultrasound probe cover kit
   (e) Cap, mask, gloves
   (f) Sterile gown
   (g) ChloraPrep/chlorhexidine (If central line kit does not have)
   (h) Biopatch (If kit does not have)
   (i) Lidocaine (If kit does not have)
   (j) Sterile dressing/Tegaderm dressing (If kit does not have)
   (k) Central Line Kit (should contain the following):
      - Chlorhexidine
      - Sterile drape
      - 1% lidocaine without epinephrine
      - 5 mL syringe
      - 18-ga needle
      - Guidewire
      - Scalpel with 11-blade
      - Dilator
      - Triple-lumen catheter (or introducer catheter/Cordis)
      - Silk suture
      - Needle driver
      - Tegaderm dressing
6. Patient Position and Anatomical Landmarks
   (a) Patient Positioning:
      - Place patient and ultrasound machine in location allowing dual visualization during procedure.
   (b) Pre-scan to select target vein.
      - Similar to PIV you should map out veins.
   (c) Internal jugular (IJ) vein:
      - The patient should be supine with their head turned slightly to the opposite side of the insertion site.
        - In critically ill preferably left IJ to preserve right IJ for hemodialysis catheter.
      - If the patient is hypovolemic, position the patient in Trendelenburg, or have them Valsalva to assist visualizing the IJ lumen.
      - Figure 25.13—Internal jugular vein.
      - Video 25.3—Internal jugular vein.

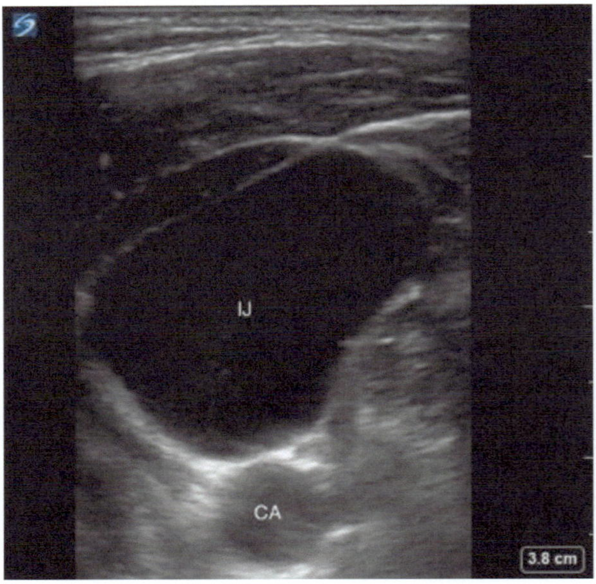

Fig. 25.13 Internal jugular vein on ultrasound. The internal jugular (IJ) vein is a larger vessel with thin walls that is compressible under pressure. The carotid artery (CA) is seen below the IJ vein

(d) Subclavian Vein:
- Compared to landmark, ultrasound guidance reduces the rates of arterial puncture, pneumothorax, brachial plexus injury, and hematoma formation.
- Supraclavicular Approach
  - Where the subclavian vein (SCV) meets the internal jugular vein to form the brachiocephalic vein.
  - This approach may be more difficult in patients with higher BMI or short necks since it's more difficult to probe and needle into the supraclavicular notch.
  - Always clearly visualize the needle tip with the in-plane technique and remember that the SCV is anterior to the subclavian artery (SCA).
  - Color Doppler can be used to discern between SCV and SCA.
- Infraclavicular Approach
  - Place the probe in the infraclavicular fossa
  - Identify the vasculature 2–3 cm distal to where the SCV courses below the clavicle.
  - Cannulation occurs near the junction of the axillary vein and SCV.
    - This is more lateral as compared to the landmark approach.
  - Obtain a long-axis view of the axillary vein and distal subclavian vein.
  - Use compressibility and/or pulse-wave Doppler to confirm visualization of the vein (as opposed to the artery).
  - Take note of the lung pleura beneath the vessels.
  - Alternative, can be done in short axis.

(e) Femoral Vein

- Place the transducer at the inguinal ligament, and slide distally until the thin-walled vein is visualized just medial to the femoral artery:
  - Alternatively, feel for a femoral pulse, and place the transducer over this site to locate the femoral vein.
- For patients who are hypovolemic, reverse Trendelenburg may assist to expand the vessel:
  - Use caution with collapsed veins as it is easier to penetrate the posterior wall.
- Figure 25.14—Femoral vein.
- Video 25.4—Femoral vein.

	Pros	Cons
Internal jugular vein	Easily seen with ultrasound	Difficult in morbidly obese patients Higher risk of arterial puncture
Subclavian vein	Lower risk of DVT Usually patent Usually in the same anatomical position	Higher risk of pneumothorax due to proximity to pleura Clavicle can obstruct view
Femoral vein	Fast	Higher risk of mechanical complications Higher risk of infection Higher risk of thrombosis

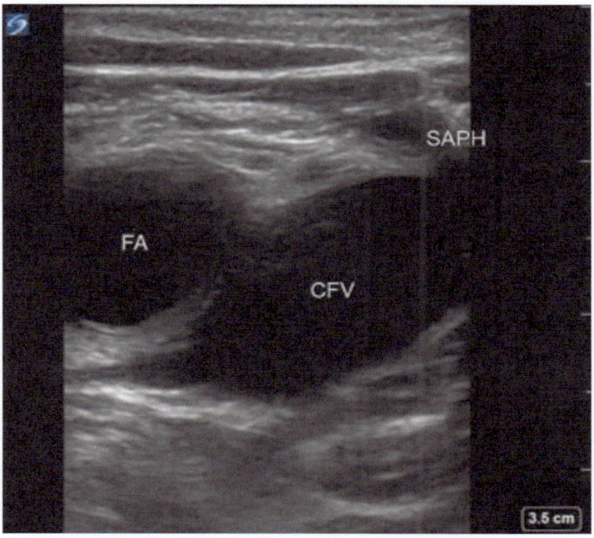

Fig. 25.14 Femoral vein on ultrasound. The common femoral vein on the left is compressible under pressure, and the femoral artery on the right with a thick muscular wall is pulsatile under pressure

7. Procedure Preparation
   (a) Gather equipment.
      - Central Line Kit
      - Sterile ultrasound probe cover with sterile gel
      - Caps
      - Sterile flushes
      - Biopatch
   (b) Hand hygiene before starting the procedure.
   (c) Identify target vessels with pre-procedural vein imaging using ultrasound.
   (d) Obtain personal protective equipment and maximal barrier precautions, which include:
      - Nonsterile cap
      - Nonsterile mask
      - Sterile gloves
      - Sterile gowns
      - Wide sterile field over the patient
      - Long sterile cover over the transducer.
   (e) Clean transducer.
   (f) Perform skin antisepsis with 2% chlorhexidine in 70% isopropyl alcohol in large area around target sit
   (g) Apply sterile field to the patient.
   (h) Apply sterile transducer cover:
      - Assistance will be required for this.
   (i) Flush all three ports of the CVC with normal saline to remove air bubbles.
8. Ultrasound Technique
   (a) TIP: Have the open side of the bevel aligned with the numbers on the syringe. This way, once the needle is in the vessel, you know where the bevel opening is pointing.
   (b) Ultrasound assistance for this procedure is similar to peripherally inserted catheters.
   (c) Hold transducer with nondominant hand:
      - Be careful not to apply pressure with the transducer as this will displace the vessel deeper within the arm and can compress the vein.
      - You can ask for assistance to adjust the depth so that the vessel is in the center of the screen and to adjust the gain.
   (d) Locate the vein entry site using ultrasound.
      - Use the depth of the vessel you just measured and track that same distance away from the center of the probe.
      - For example, if the vein is 2 cm deep, the best skin puncture site is 2 cm away from the probe.
   (e) Out-of-plane cannulation:
      - The vein will be imaged using a transverse or cross-sectional view. The transducer marker should point in the same direction on the patient as on the ultrasound monitor.

- Identify the vein in cross-section:
  - Make sure the vessel is compressible before attempting access.
- Insert the needle at an appropriate distance from the transducer and enter the skin at a 30–45° angle.
- Needle tip will be visualized in the subcutaneous tissue as a small bright white, hyperechoic dot.
- While advancing the needle, constant back pressure should be applied to the syringe plunger.
- The transducer should slide concomitantly with needle advancement to keep the needle tip visualized at all times ("Creep Method").
- Look for the anterior wall "tenting."
- Change the angle of the needle to 20–30°
- Once the needle tip enters the vessel, drop the angle further
- Advance needle a minimum of 2 mm to ensure the needle is within the vessel lumen.
- Under constant back pressure of the syringe plunger, blood will fill the syringe effortlessly once inside the lumen of the vessel.
- At this point, stabilize the needle to prevent movement out of the vessel.
- Videos 25.5 and 25.6—Out-of-plane central line placement.

(f) In-plane confirmation:
- Rotate the transducer 90° so that the marker is pointed toward the needle insertion site.
- Using an in-plane technique with the vessel in long axis, identify the needle tip within the vessel and compress the vessel to ensure line placement is within the vein and not the artery:
  - Video 25.7—In-plane central line needle
  - Video 25.8—In-plane wire confirmation

(g) Stabilize the needle, slowly advance the wire, and visualize it in the vessel lumen.
- The above steps should be performed before dilating the skin and placing the CVC.
- For complete CVC procedural details, please reference a procedural book or other resources as needed.

(h) Completing the procedure:
- Draw back and flush each line of the CVC to assess for adequate flow.
- Secure the CVC in place with a suture, and cover the area at the skin with a biodisc and sterile dressing.

(i) Confirmation of correct CVC placement:
- Traditional method:
  - Placement can be confirmed by ordering a STAT chest X-ray to evaluate the location of the catheter tip.
  - Chest X-ray can also identify a pneumothorax for a CVC that was placed in the IJ (or subclavian) vein.

- Ultrasound method: "Bubble Study"
  - Place a phased array transducer in the subxiphoid region, and obtain a subxiphoid view of the heart:
    See Chap. 3 for more detailed information.
  - Inject saline into the CVC, and watch for bubbles to reach the right atrium and ventricle; this is called rapid atrial swirl sign (RASS):
    Figure 25.15a—Before RASS
    Figure 25.15b—RASS
    Video 25.9—RASS
  - If the catheter is appropriately located, the rapid atrial swirl should be seen within 2 s after flushing the CVC from an IJ or less than 3 s after flushing from a femoral CVC.
- Check for pneumothorax
  - Evaluate the ipsilateral lung for sliding lung to make sure there is no pneumothorax:
    See Chap. 4 for more detailed information.

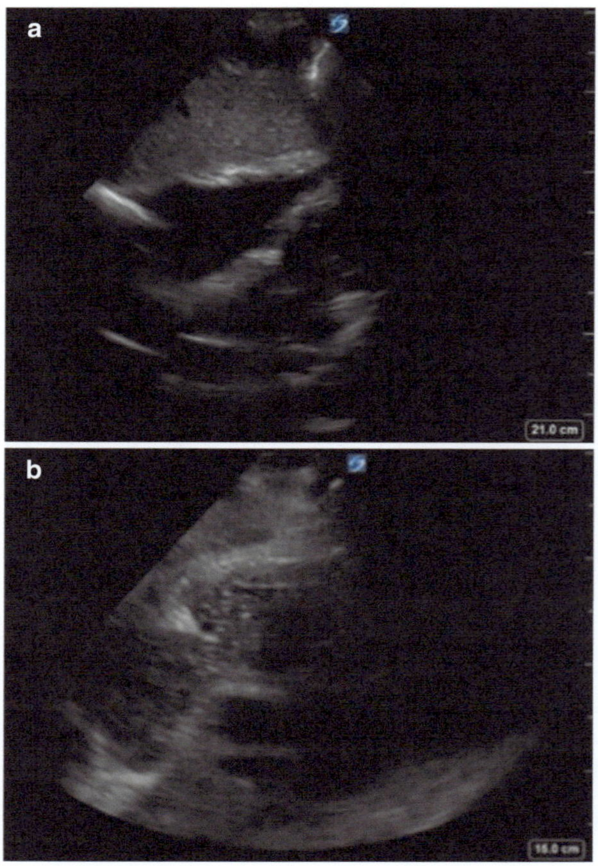

Fig. 25.15 Bubbles in RA/RV—RASS. (**a**) Is taken before injection of the saline flush, and (**b**) shortly after injection of saline into the CVC, bubbles will reach the right atrium and ventricle; this is called rapid atrial swirl sign (RASS)

9. Key Points
   (a) Anatomic variations occur among patients:
      - The internal jugular vein and femoral vein can be seen anterior to the artery. In this situation, use caution to not penetrate the posterior wall of the vein as this can cause perforation of the artery.
      - The internal jugular vein and femoral vein can also be seen posterior to the artery. In this situation, it is advised to look at the opposite side for a more optimal location.
   (b) Ultrasound improves success rate of central venous access and has become the standard of care. Map the vein.
   (c) Maintain needle tip visualization. ("Creep Method")
   (d) Confirm needle tip is in the center of the vessel.
   (e) Use agitated saline to confirm placement. ("Bubble study")

Paracentesis

- Procedure Indications
  - Diagnostic:
    - Evaluation of the fluid for blood, ascites, stool, gastric contents, urine, and malignancy
    - Diagnosis of infection, specifically spontaneous bacterial peritonitis (SBP)
  - Therapeutic:
    - Respiratory compromise secondary to ascites
    - Abdominal pain secondary to ascites
- Procedure Contraindications
  - Absolute:
    - Acute surgical abdomen
  - Relative:
    - Abdominal wall cellulitis
    - Dilated bowel
    - Distended bladder
    - Abdominal adhesions
    - Pregnancy
    - Intra-abdominal adhesions
    - Thrombocytopenia (platelet count <20 × 10 uL)
    - Coagulopathy (INR >2.0)
    - Disseminated intravascular coagulation
- Procedure Complications
  - Blood vessel puncture
  - Bleeding and/or hematoma
  - Bowel perforation
  - Inferior epigastric artery aneurysm
  - Vessel laceration (aorta, mesenteric artery, iliac artery)
  - Infection at site of insertion or into the peritoneum causing bacterial peritonitis
  - Persistent ascitic fluid leak

- Transducer Selection
  - Curvilinear
- Equipment
  - Paracentesis kit may contain many, if not all, items listed:
    - Skin disinfectant
    - Local anesthetic
    - Scalpel
    - 14- to 16-gauge paracentesis needle/catheter or straight needle such as 3.5″ spinal needle
    - Large syringe
    - Gauze
    - Bandage
  - Items usually not available in kits that will need to be obtained:
    - Vacuum bottles (or tubing to wall suction, if applicable)
    - Sterile gloves
    - Sterile towels/drape
    - Sterile transducer cover Sterile ultrasound gel
    - Antiseptic swab (chlorhexidine)
    - Sterile personal protective equipment
- Patient Position and Anatomical Landmarks
  - Place the patient in a lateral decubitus position rotated toward the side of insertion with the head raised to maximize a gravity-dependent fluid collection.
  - Alternatively, if unable to tolerate, the patient can be in a supine position.
- Preparation
  - Universal precautions.
  - Clean the transducer with antiseptic cloth and cover the transducer in a sterile sheath.
  - Hold the transducer with the nondominant hand.
  - Adjust depth so that the bowel is identified in the far field:
    Figure 25.16—Ascites with the bowel in far field
    Video 25.10—Ascites with the bowel in far field

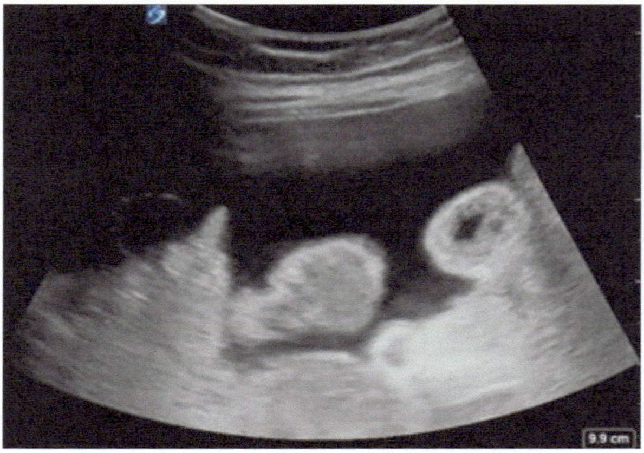

Fig. 25.16 Ascites with the bowel in far field. Ascites is anechoic, and the bowels are seen in the far field

- Technique
  - Pre-scan the abdomen to evaluate for pockets of fluid.
    - Should be >50 mL
  - Identify the location of the bowel, mesentery, and bladder.
    - Avoid upper quadrants due to liver and spleen
    - Avoid suprapubic due to bladder. Consider emptying.
  - Look in the low3er quadrants for adhesions, dilated loops of the bowel, or overlying arterial structures.
    - Avoid left lower quadrant due to cecum
  - Aspiration lateral to the rectus muscle avoids damaging the epigastric vessels.
  - Avoid surgical scars which may have adhesions to the bowel.
  - TIP: Measure the thickness of the skin to help pick the correct needle length: Figure 25.17—Skin measurement
    TIP: Identify the largest pocket of fluid.
  - Note the depth of the pocket of fluid and how deep the bowel is from the insertion point.
  - Choose a long enough needle that can penetrate through the thickness of the skin and penetrate the peritoneum.
  - Once the largest pocket is identified, make a mark on the skin to locate the site of needle insertion.
  - Using sterile precautions, use chlorhexidine to sterilize the skin, and drape the site of insertion with sterile towels or paper sheets.
  - Using a small-gauge needle, anesthetize the insertion site with lidocaine with or without epinephrine.
  - Use the "Z-track" technique by pulling superficial skin caudad approximately 2 cm relative to deep abdominal wall before perpendicular needle entry.
  - Using ultrasound guidance to allow direct visualization, insert the needle and advance into the peritoneum:
    Figure 25.18—Needle in the peritoneum and ascites
    Video 25.11—Needle in the peritoneum and ascites

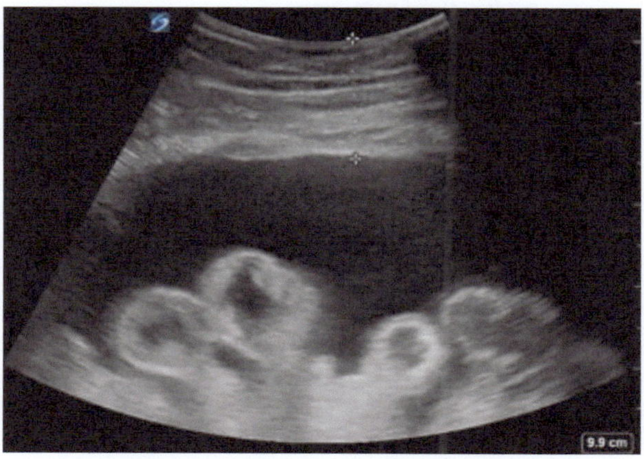

Fig. 25.17 Skin measurement. Measurement of the thickness of the skin. This will help determine how long the needle will need to be get into the peritoneum

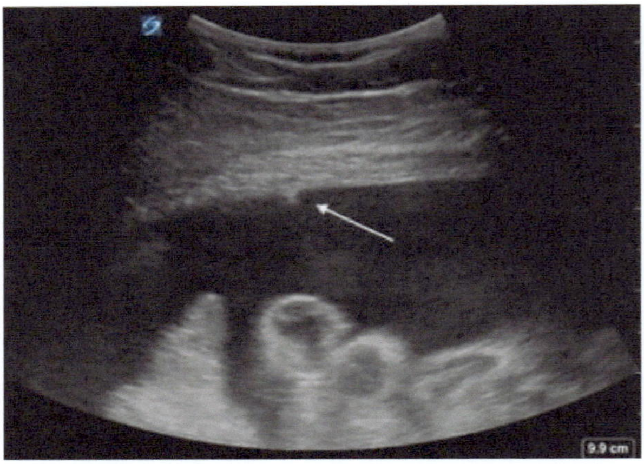

Fig. 25.18 Needle in the peritoneum and ascites. Direct visualization of the needle entering into the peritoneum. The needle will appear hyperechoic

- Once the needle is within the ascites, pull back on the plunger of the syringe and aspirate the fluid.
- Remove the needle, leaving the catheter in place.
- For diagnostic paracentesis aspirate ascitic fluid into the syringe (20–60 mL).
- Attach the catheter to the tubing and vacuum bottle if performing a therapeutic paracentesis.

- Completing the Procedure
  - Apply gauze with pressure to the insertion site as ascites and blood may continue to ooze from the puncture site.
  - Label all collection tubes with patient identification and order labs if considering spontaneous bacterial peritonitis.
  - Discard waste in the proper sanitary location.
  - Monitor vitals, such as blood pressure.
  - Consider infusion of intravenous albumin for large-volume paracentesis (>5 L of ascitic fluid) or if spontaneous bacterial peritonitis is confirmed.
    - Recommended administration of 6–8 g of albumin intravenous per liter of ascitic fluid removed.
  - Start empiric, broad-spectrum antibiotics if spontaneous bacterial peritonitis is suspected.
- Key Points
  - Thrombocytopenia and elevated international normalized ratio (INR) are not contraindications to paracentesis [3, 4].
  - The ultrasound-guided technique decreases the complication rate and improves first-time success rate [4].
  - Success rates are best when the patient is in left or right lateral decubitus forming a gravity-dependent fluid collection.
  - Ultrasound improves efficiency of paracentesis when compared to blind landmark attempts.
  - All emergency physicians should be proficient at US- guided paracentesis.

Lumbar Puncture

(a) Procedure Indications
- Evaluation of cerebral spinal fluid (CSF) to identify meningitis and subarachnoid hemorrhage.
- Improve success of lumbar puncture (LP) in patients who are obese and infants and after multiple failed attempts by traditional technique.

(b) Procedure Contraindications
- Cellulitis of the skin over the insertion site
- Increased intracranial pressure

(c) Procedure Complications
- Infection
- Bleeding and/or hematoma
- Post-LP headache
- Damage to nerves or surrounding structures

(d) Transducer Selection
- Linear array for thin and pediatric patients
- Curvilinear for obese patients

(e) Equipment
- Sterile personal protective equipment
- Lumbar puncture kit
- 22-gauge spinal needle:
- Longer needles for more obese patients 10 cc syringe
- 1% lidocaine
- Ultrasound gel:
  - Sterile surgical lubricant recommended
- Antiseptic swab:
  - Chlorhexidine recommended
- Sterile dressing surrounding the insertion site
- Face mask with eye protection
- Bouffant cap

(f) Patient Position and Anatomical Landmarks
- Lateral decubitus or sitting upright.
- In either position, the low back should be rounded and chest flexed anteriorly resembling a fetal position.

(g) Preparation
- Universal precautions.
- Clean transducer with antiseptic cloth.

(h) Technique
- Static approach:
  - The goal is to identify the interspinous space.

- Place the transducer over the pre-identified lumbar space using traditional landmarks with the marker pointed toward the patient's right:
  - Center the transducer over the spinous process:
    The bony spinous process will appear as a hyper- echoic crescent with posterior shadowing [5].
    Figure 25.19—Spinous process in transverse.
    Video 25.12—Spinous process in transverse.
  - Mark the skin above and below the transducer to illustrate the midline [6]:
  Figure 25.20—Midline LP marks
- Rotate the transducer into a sagittal plane with the marker pointed cephalad:
  - Center the interspinous space in the middle of the screen:
    Figure 25.21—Spinous process in sagittal
    Video 25.13—Spinous process in sagittal
    Mark the skin at the middle of the transducer
  - Mark the skin at the middle of the transducer [5, 6]. This will mark the site for needle insertion:

- Figure 25.22—Sagittal plane marks
- Figure 25.23—Needle insertion mark on the skin
  - Use ultrasound to assess the optimal angle to insert the needle and navigate between the spinous processes.
  - Assess the depth where the subarachnoid space is located to help choose the proper length of the spinal needle.
  - After the insertion site has been identified and marked, place the transducer down, and sterilize the insertion site as directed in the LP kit.
  - Once the area has been imaged and marked, the patient cannot be moved; any movement can change the underlying anatomy and trajectory.
  - Proceed with performing the lumbar puncture in typical fashion.

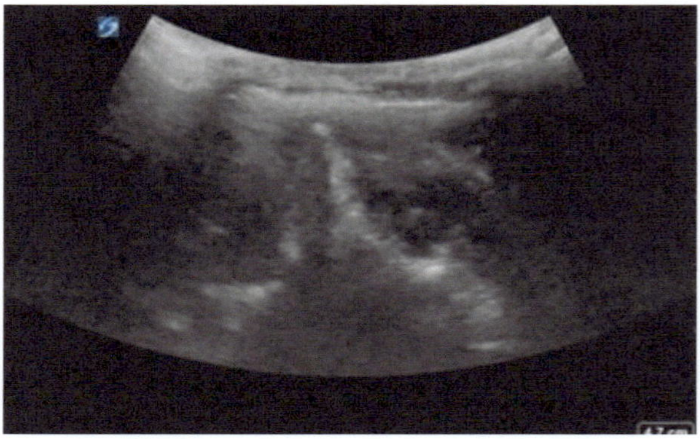

Fig. 25.19 Spinous process in transverse. The spinous process appears as a hyperechoic crescent with posterior shadowing

Fig. 25.20 Mid-line LP marks with transducer in transverse plane. Mark the skin above and below the transducer to help map out the midline of the spine

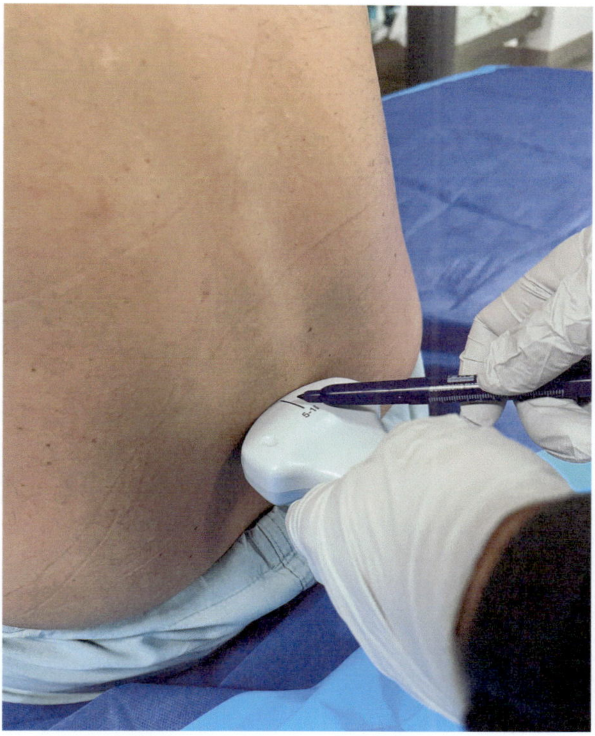

Fig. 25.21 Spinous process in sagittal view. The interspinous space is centered in the middle of the screen

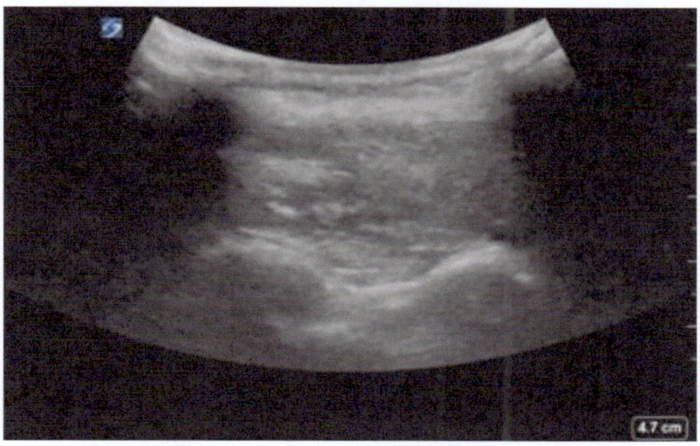

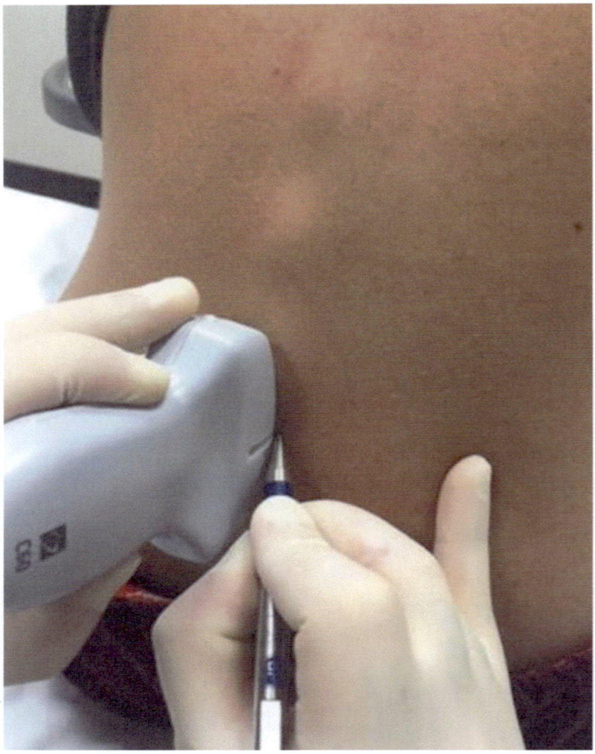

Fig. 25.22 Sagittal plane marks

(i) Completing the Procedure
- Remove the spinal needle and sterile dressing.
- Hold pressure.
- Place a bandage over the insertion site.

(j) Key Points
- Sterile transducer cover is not necessary because sterile technique is used after ultrasound localization.
- Keep the patient still after the area has been marked to avoid distortion of pre-identified landmarks.
- Using ultrasound decreases the rate of failed lumbar punctures, saves time, is easy to use, and decreases post-lumbar puncture complications [5].

Fig. 25.23 LP needle insertion site. Once the two planes have been mapped out from the sagittal and transverse views, the combined skin markings make a site for needle insertion. Note: this is a demonstration of how to use the landmarks, in reality the patient would have a sterile drape and the procedure is performed with universal precautions

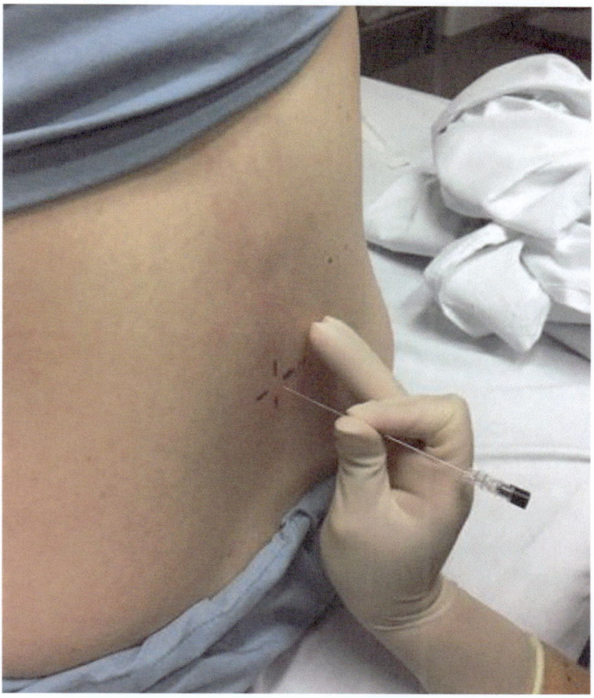

References

1. McNamee J, Jeong J, Patel N. 10 tips for ultrasound-guided peripheral venous access. ACEP Now website. http://www.acep- now.com/article/10-tips-ultrasound-guided-peripheral-venous- access/4/. December 17, 2014. Accessed 27 Apr 2017.
2. Rose JS, Bair AE, Parikh AK. Chapter 21: Vascular access. In: Ma OJ, Mateer JR, Reardon RF, Joing SA, editors. Emergency ultrasound. 3rd ed. Beijing: McGraw-Hill Education; 2014. p. 631–44.
3. AIUM practice parameter for the use of ultrasound to guide vascular access procedures. http://www.aium.org/resources/guidelines/usgva.pdf. Accessed 10 Apr 2024.
4. Runyon BA, Chopra S, Robson KM. Diagnostic and therapeutic abdominal paracentesis. UpToDate website. https://www.upto- date.com/contents/diagnostic-and-therapeutic-abdominal-para- centesis. Updated Sept 23, 2015. Accessed 27 Apr 2017.
5. Bramante RM. Lumbar puncture. https://www.acep.org/sonoguide/procedures/lumbar-puncture. Accessed 10 Apr 2024.
6. Dewitz A, Jones RA, Resnick JG, Stone MB. Chapter 22: Additional ultrasound-guided procedures. In: Ma OJ, Mateer JR, Reardon RF, Joing SA, editors. Emergency ultrasound. 3rd ed. Beijing: McGraw-Hill Education; 2014. p. 645–708.

Index

A. Lindsay et al. (eds.), *Clinical Ultrasound*,
https://doi.org/10.1007/978-3-032-27643-8

V

W

Y

Z

MIX
Papier aus verantwortungsvollen Quellen
Paper from responsible sources
FSC® C105338

If you have any concerns about our products,
you can contact us on
ProductSafety@springernature.com

In case Publisher is established outside the EU,
the EU authorized representative is:
Springer Nature Customer Service Center GmbH
Europaplatz 3, 69115 Heidelberg, Germany

Printed by Libri Plureos GmbH
in Hamburg, Germany